CLINICAL COM

TO ACCOMPANY

HEALTH ASSESSMENT & PHYSICAL EXAMINATION

THIRD EDITION

CLINICAL COMPANION
TO ACCOMPANY
HEALTH ASSESSMENT & PHYSICAL EXAMINATION
THIRD EDITION

Tamera D. Cauthorne-Burnette, RN, MSN, FNP, CS
Family Nurse Practitioner
James E. Jones, Jr., MD & Associates
Obstetrics & Gynecology
Richmond, Virginia
and
Family Nurse Practitioner
Montpelier Family Practice
Montpelier, Virginia
and
Graduate Clinical Faculty
Virginia Commonwealth University
School of Nursing
Richmond, Virginia

**Mary Ellen Zator Estes,
RN, MSN, FNP, APRN-BC, NP-C**
Family Nurse Practitioner
in Internal Medicine
Fairfax, Virginia
and
Clinical Faculty
Nurse Practitioner Track
School of Nursing
Ball State University
Muncie, Indiana

THOMSON
DELMAR LEARNING

Australia Canada Mexico Singapore Spain United Kingdom United States

THOMSON
DELMAR LEARNING

Clinical Companion to Accompany Health Assessment & Physical Examination, Third Edition
by Tamera D. Cauthorne-Burnette and Mary Ellen Zator Estes

Vice President, Health Care Business Unit:
William Brottmiller

Editorial Director:
Cathy L. Esperti

Executive Editor:
Matthew Kane

Editorial Assistant:
Tiffiny Adams

Marketing Director:
Jennifer McAvey

Marketing Coordinator:
Michele Gleason

Production Director:
Carolyn S. Miller

Art and Design Specialist:
Robert Plante

Production Coordinator:
Mary Ellen Cox

Senior Project Editor:
David Buddle

Printed in Canada
1 2 3 4 5 6 7 8 XXX 09 08 07 06 05

For more information, contact
Thomson Delmar Learning
5 Maxwell Drive
Clifton Park, NY 12065

Or find us on the World Wide Web at
http://www.delmarlearning.com

ISBN 1-4018-7207-7

Dedication

To Dr. Frank M. Sasser, Jr., who has faithfully provided medical service to the citizens of the Commonwealth of Virginia for over 50 years. You have been an example to us all in the art of compassionate care.

—TDCB

To Marcella, Joseph, Mary Brooke, and George.

—MEZE

Contents

Contributors

Mitzi Boilanger, MS, RNC
Clinical Nurse Specialist
Clarian Health Partners, Inc.
Indianapolis, Indiana

Tamera D. Cauthorne-Burnette, RN, MSN, FNP, CS
Family Nurse Practitioner
James E. Jones, Jr., MD & Associates
Obstetrics & Gynecology
Richmond, Virginia
and
Family Nurse Practitioner
Montpelier Family Practice
Montpelier, Virginia
and
Graduate Clinical Faculty
Medical College of Virginia
Virginia Commonwealth University
School of Nursing
Richmond, Virginia

Catherine Wilson Cox, RN, PhD, CCRN, CEN, CCNS
Assistant Professor
School of Nursing and Health Studies
Georgetown University
Washington, D.C.

Jane L. Echols, RN, PhD
Professor of Nursing
School of Health Professions
Marymount University
Arlington, Virginia

Barbara Springer Edwards, RN, BSN, MTS
Former Director
Cardiac Surgical Unit
Alexandria Hospital
Alexandria, Virginia

Joseph Haymore, MS, RN, CNRN, CCRN, ACNP
Nurse Practitioner
Clinical Consultants, LCC
Silver Springs, Maryland
and
Adjunct Clinical Faculty
School of Nursing and Health Studies
Georgetown University
Washington, D.C.

Randie R. McLaughlin, MS, CRNP
Certified Adult and Geriatric Nurse Practitioner
Urology Private Practice
Frederick, Maryland

Kathy Murphy, RN, MSN, CS
Clinical Nurse Specialist
Children's Healthcare of Atlanta
Sibley Heart Center
Atlanta, Georgia

Jo Anne Peach, RN, MSN, FNP
Family Nurse Practitioner
Forest Lakes Family Medicine
Charlottesville, Virginia

Susan Abbott Rogge, RN, NP
Department of Obstetrics and Gynecology
University of California, Davis
Sacramento, California
and
Private Practice
Sacramento, California

Bonnie R. Sakallaris, RN, MSN
Director of Cardiac Services
Washington Hospital Center
Washington, D.C.

Preface

Health assessment forms the foundation of all nursing care. Whether the patient is young or old, well or ill, assessment is an ongoing process of evaluating the whole person—the person as a physical, psychosocial, functional being. *Clinical Companion to Accompany Health Assessment & Physical Examination*, third edition, provides a fresh and innovative approach to the process of holistic assessment, including physical assessment skills, clinical examination techniques, and patient teaching guidelines.

Conceptual Approach

Clinical Companion to Accompany Health Assessment & Physical Examination, third edition, is developed from a parent text, *Health Assessment & Physical Examination*, third edition, by Mary Ellen Zator Estes, and is designed to be used in the clinical setting, both in conjunction with the parent text and as a stand-alone product. *Clinical Companion to Accompany Health Assessment & Physical Examination*, third edition, takes a user-friendly approach to delivering a wealth of information. The consistent, easy-to-follow format with recurring pedagogical features is based on two frameworks:

1. The IPPA method of examination (inspection, palpation, percussion, auscultation) is applied to body systems in describing complete, detailed physical assessments.
2. The ENAP format (examination, normal findings, abnormal findings, pathophysiology) follows every IPPA technique, providing a useful, valuable source of information. In acknowledgment of the fact that nurses' clinical decisions must be based on scientific rationale, pathophysiology is included for each abnormal finding.

Readers of *Clinical Companion to Accompany Health Assessment & Physical Examination*, third edition, must have an understanding of anatomy and physiology as well as familiarity with basic nursing skills and the nursing process.

Organization

Clinical Companion to Accompany Health Assessment & Physical Examination, third edition, comprises 25 chapters organized into five units. Unit 1 lays the foundation for the entire assessment process by guiding the reader through the nursing process, the patient interview, and the health history. Unit 2 highlights developmental, cultural, spiritual, and nutritional areas of assessment, emphasizing the holistic nature of the assessment process.

Unit 3 opens with a description of fundamental assessment techniques, including measuring vital signs, then details assessment procedures and findings for specific body systems. The format used for all applicable physical assessment chapters in this unit is as follows:

1. Anatomy and physiology overview
2. Modified health history
3. Physical assessment
    a. Inspection
    b. Palpation
    c. Percussion
    d. Auscultation

Because assessment techniques and findings for pregnant women and children may differ from those for nonpregnant women and adults, those populations are discussed in separate chapters in Unit 4. Unit 5 helps the reader assimilate and synthesize the wealth of information presented in the text in order to perform a thorough, accurate, and efficient health assessment.

Features

- Nursing Checklists offer an organizing framework for the assessment process or for approaching certain tasks.
- Nursing Tips help the reader apply basic knowledge to real-life situations and offer hints and shortcuts useful to new and experienced nurses alike.
- Nursing Alerts highlight serious or life-threatening signs or critical assessment findings that require immediate attention.
- The index facilitates access to material and includes specific entries for tables and illustrations.
- A list of abbreviations includes and defines abbreviations and symbols frequently used in charting.

New to This Edition

The content of the *Clinical Companion*, third edition, has been revised to reflect the changes made in *Health Assessment & Physical Examination*, third edition. These changes include:

- Updated photos and illustrations
- A section on HIPAA guidelines
- A new section on Domestic and Intimate Partner Violence
- References to holistic nursing
- The new USDA dietary guidelines
- Addition of Dietary Reference Intakes and MyPyramid
- Updated text on determining body mass index (BMI)
- Addition of transmission-based precautions
- Updated blood pressure tables
- A completely new section on pain assessment
- Coverage of ductal lavage
- Updated childhood immunization charts
- Assessment of voice sounds
- Risk factors for thyroid, colorectal, oral, and lung cancers
- Risk factors for hearing loss

Unit 1 Laying the Foundation

1

Critical Thinking and the Nursing Process

The nursing process comprises six phases: assessment, nursing diagnosis, outcomes identification, planning, implementation, and evaluation. It is a dynamic process that uses information in a meaningful way through problem-solving strategies to place the patient, family, or community in an optimal health state. The primary focus of this text is assessment.

Assessment

Assessment is the first step of the nursing process. It is the orderly collection of information concerning the patient's health status. The assessment process aims to identify the patient's current health status, actual and potential health problems, and areas for health promotion. The sources of information for the assessment include the health history, physical assessment, and diagnostic and laboratory data.

Health History

The health history interview is a means of gathering subjective data, usually from the patient. The data are considered subjective because you cannot verify all information. The subjective data can be obtained from the patient; the patient's relatives, neighbors, or friends; and medical records. Patient symptomatology is analyzed in this category. The health history is discussed in Chapter 3.

Physical Assessment Findings

Physical assessment findings constitute a second source of information in the assessment phase of the nursing process. These findings constitute the objective data, or information that is observable, measurable, and verifiable by more than one person. These data are also known as physical signs of illness or wellness.

The physical assessment data can be obtained via a body-system or head-to-toe approach. Table 1-1 lists the body systems that are assessed.

Diagnostic and Laboratory Data

The final source of information in the assessment phase of the nursing process is diagnostic and laboratory data. Results of serum, urine, or other body-fluid studies, cultures, radiographic studies, and diagnostic procedures constitute objective data about the patient's status.

The assessment phase of the nursing process is fluid and dynamic. You are continually compiling, validating, and interpreting the data. With this information, you are ready to progress to the second phase of the nursing process: the nursing diagnosis.

Nursing Diagnosis

The North American Nursing Diagnosis Association (NANDA) is the recognized

TABLE 1-1

Body System Assessment

1. General survey, vital signs, and pain
2. Skin, hair, and nails
3. Head and neck
4. Eyes
5. Ears, nose, mouth, and throat
6. Breasts and regional nodes
7. Thorax and lungs
8. Heart and peripheral vasculature
9. Abdomen
10. Musculoskeletal system
11. Mental status and neurological techniques
12. Female or male genitalia
13. Anus, rectum, and prostate

leader in the formulation, classification, and testing of nursing diagnoses. NANDA (2005) defines a nursing diagnosis as "a clinical judgment about individual, family, or community responses to actual or potential health problems/life processes." Nursing diagnoses provide the basis for selecting nursing interventions to achieve patient outcomes.

Outcomes Identification

Outcome identification represents the third step of the nursing process. After nursing diagnoses have been established, patient goals are established. The patient goal is directed toward removal of related factors or patient responses to an adverse condition. Goals are broad statements that are not measurable. For example, if the nursing diagnosis is *Anxiety related to a knowledge deficit of renal failure*, the patient goal might be, "The patient will experience a reduction in anxiety."

A patient outcome is a statement of the expected change in patient behavior denoting progress toward resolution of the altered human response over a specific period of time. Patient outcomes are reasonable and measurable and have a time frame. An example of a patient outcome would be, "The patient will lose 8 pounds over the next 2 months."

Planning

Planning is the fourth step in the nursing process. It involves prioritizing nursing diagnoses, formulating patient outcomes, and selecting nursing interventions.

The theoretical framework that can be employed to prioritize nursing diagnoses is Maslow's Hierarchy of Needs (Figure 1-1). According to Maslow, basic needs such as food and oxygen take priority over all other issues. For example, the patient experiencing a myocardial infarction must have his physical needs met before his safety needs are attended to.

Intervention Selection

Interventions are planned strategies, based on scientific rationale, that you devise to assist the patient in meeting the patient outcomes. When appropriate, include a frequency in each intervention, such as "turn patient every 2 hours." The interventions can be independent or collaborative nursing actions, or both. Independent nursing interventions are those that you are legally capable of implementing on the basis of education and experience. Collaborative interventions are prescribed by a physician or nurse practitioner and are implemented by a nurse.

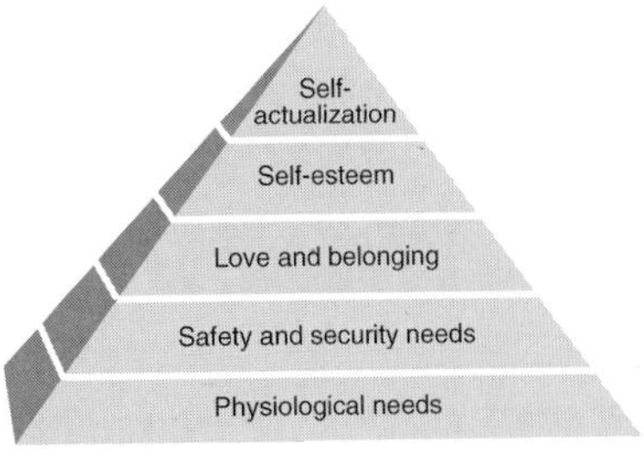

Figure 1-1 Maslow's Hierarchy of Needs

Evidence-Based Practice

There is a growing trend in health care toward evidence-based practice. This methodology uses the outcomes of well-designed and executed scientific studies to guide clinical decision making and clinical care rather than intuition or tradition.

Implementation

The fifth step in the nursing process is implementation. In this phase, you execute the interventions that were devised during the planning stage to help the patient meet predetermined outcomes. The time frame of the implementation phase varies depending on the patient and diagnosis.

Evaluation

Evaluation is the final phase of the nursing process. During evaluation, you determine the patient's progress in achieving the outcomes. Even before the time frame for assessing outcomes is reached, you are continually assessing the patient's progress toward the outcomes, making evaluation an ongoing and dynamic process. Note whether the outcome is met. If the outcome is not achieved, evaluate the factors that prevented achievement. After considering these factors, consult with the patient whether to revise the patient outcomes and nursing interventions or to eliminate them.

REFERENCE

North American Nursing Diagnosis Association. (2005). *Nursing diagnoses: Definitions and classification 2005–2006.* Philadelphia: Author.

2

The Patient Interview

The health assessment interview is initiated to collect specific information regarding the patient and the patient's health status. Other purposes include validating appropriate health and illness information presented by the patient or found in the patient's record and identifying the patient's knowledge of personal health and illness status.

The Patient Interview

The interview includes an assessment of physical, mental, emotional, social, cultural, and spiritual aspects of the patient. Data collected concern the patient's present and past states of health, including the patient's family status and relationships, cultural background, lifestyle preferences, and developmental level.

Roles of the Nurse and Patient

The nurse is often the first person from the health care team to interact with the patient. You will frequently assume the role of intermediary between the patient and the larger health care system. You can foster an atmosphere of safety and comfort by approaching each patient with an accepting, respectful, nonjudgmental attitude.

The patient is an active and equal participant in the interview process and should feel free to openly communicate thoughts, feelings, perceptions, and factual information.

Factors Influencing the Interview

Approach

Before approaching the patient:

1. Gather all available patient information.
2. Seek out an appropriate setting for the interview.
3. Set aside a block of time for the interview.
4. Assess yourself for possible problematic thoughts or feelings.
5. Begin the interview with a friendly introduction.
   a. Introduce yourself by name and title.
   b. Call the patient by formal name, for example, Mrs. Adams.
6. Provide the patient with an explanation of what is to follow and an approximate time frame for the interview. This information also helps to increase the patient's feeling of control.
7. Explain that you will be jotting down notes during the interview to facilitate discussion and ensure accuracy of information.

Environment

Whenever possible, the interview should be conducted in a private room with controlled lighting and temperature. When a private setting is impossible, control the environment to minimize distractions and interruptions and to increase the comfort level of the patient; use any physical barriers available in the room to provide as much privacy as possible.

Confidentiality

The patient's willingness to communicate private and personal information is predicated on the assumption that this information will be used with discretion and for the benefit of the patient. Your verbal assurance of confidentiality often eases the patient's concerns and fosters trust in the relationship.

HIPAA

Mandatory compliance with the Privacy Rule of the Health Insurance Portability and Accountability Act (HIPAA) began on April 14, 2003. This U.S. government regulation affects all health care providers as well as service organizations, information system vendors, and universities. The goal of HIPAA is to safeguard the confidentiality of all patient information, as well as to provide security for this information, whether it is in electronic or another form. In addition, HIPAA states that individuals have a right to access their medical records and to be informed of who else has been granted permission to view them. Inappropriate use and release of confidential patient information is now punishable by law. The extent to which HIPAA regulations have made an impact on the health care system varies greatly across the country.

Time, Length, Duration

When scheduling an interview, look at the patient's daily activities. Then select a block of time that does not conflict with the patient's mealtime, other planned activities, or sleep patterns.

Stages of the Interview Process

There are three stages to the interview process: the joining stage (or the introduction), the working stage, and the termination stage.

Stage I

The joining stage is the introduction or the first stage of the interview process, during which the nurse and patient establish trust and get to know one another.

Stage II

The working stage of the interview process is the time during which most of patient data is collected.

Stage III

The termination stage is the last stage of the interview process during which information is summarized and validated.

Factors Affecting Communication

Listening

Active listening, or the act of perceiving what is said both verbally and nonverbally, is a critical factor in conducting a successful health assessment interview. According to Bradley and Edinberg (1990), the primary goal of active listening is to decode patient messages in order to understand the situation or problem as the patient sees it.

Nonverbal Cues

Nonverbal communication is communicating a message without words. Nonverbal cues such as body position, nervous and repetitive movements of the hands or legs, rapid blinking, lack of eye contact, yawning, fidgeting, excessive smiling or frowning, and repetitive clearing of the throat may be indications of the patient's health or of feelings that the patient may not feel comfortable expressing verbally.

Distance

The amount of space a person considers appropriate for interaction is determined in part by cultural influences. In the United States, distances are generally categorized as follows:

Intimate distance is from the patient to approximately 1.5 feet.

Personal distance is approximately 1.5 to 4 feet.

Social distance is approximately 4 to 12 feet.

Public distance is approximately 12 feet or more.

Intimate and personal distance are the most intimate and often involve some touching or physical contact. Personal distance may provide for ease of communication in cases such as those involving hearing impairment. However, social distance is generally considered appropriate for the interview process because this distance allows for good eye contact, for ease in hearing, and for seeing the patient's nonverbal cues. Public distance is usually used in formal settings such as a classroom, where the teacher stands in front of the class.

Effective Interviewing Techniques

Effective interviewing techniques facilitate and support interaction between the nurse and the patient and foster continuation of interaction. These techniques encompass both verbal and nonverbal approaches.

Using Open-Ended Questions

Open-ended questions encourage the patient to provide general rather than specific information. Open-ended questions that begin with the words *how, what, where, when,* or *who* are usually effective in eliciting the maximum amount of information. A disadvantage of open-ended questions is that they can be time consuming. Furthermore, open-ended questions may not be appropriate in situations requiring rapid access to information and rapid response by health care providers.

Example of an open-ended question:

"How do you typically deal with an asthma attack?"

Using Closed Questions

Closed questions can frequently be answered with a yes or no. Closed questions can be used to focus the interview, pinpoint specific areas of concern, and elicit valuable information quickly and efficiently. However, closed questions can also serve to disrupt communication because they limit patient responses and interaction.

Example of an effective closed question:

"Has this type of allergic reaction ever happened to you before?"

Facilitating

There may be periods when the patient stops talking because of anxiety or uncertainty. You may nod or use the phrase "uh-huh" to prompt the patient to resume speaking.

Using Silence

Periods of silence can help structure and pace the interview, convey respect and acceptance and, in many cases, prompt additional patient data. The nurse must be sensitive to the possibility that silence on the part of the patient may indicate anxiety, confusion, embarrassment, a simple lack of understanding about the question asked, or an inability to speak English. As a nurse, you can handle silences by being quiet yourself and observing the patient's behavior for what is *not* being said verbally.

Grouping Communication Techniques

Communication techniques often seem mechanical and artificial to the beginning nurse; one way to make them less so is to group or cluster them according to their primary purposes. One simple way to group interview techniques is to divide them into two groups: listening responses and action responses.

Listening Responses

Listening responses are attempts to accurately receive and process and then respond to patient messages. They provide one way for you to communicate empathy, concern, and attentiveness.

Making Observations

Making observations involves verbalizing perceptions about the patient's behavior.

Example of making observations:

"Speaking about these symptoms seems to make you tense. I notice that you are clenching your fists and grimacing."

Restating

Restating involves repeating or rephrasing the main idea expressed by the patient and lets the patient know that you are paying attention.

Example of restating:

Patient: "I don't sleep well anymore. I find myself waking frequently at night."
Nurse: "You're having difficulty sleeping?"

Reflecting

Reflecting involves directing the patient's own questions, feelings, and ideas back to the patient and providing an opportunity for the patient to reconsider or expand on what was just said.

Example of reflecting:

Patient: "Do you think I should tell the doctor I stopped taking my medication?"
Nurse: "What do you think about that?"
Patient: "Well, yes, I think that I probably should. Not taking my medication could be one of the reasons I'm feeling so run down. But that medication just makes me so teary and agitated."
Nurse: "You sound a bit agitated now. It seems as if you've been thinking about this a lot."

Clarifying

Clarifying is a communication technique used to make clear something said by the patient or to pinpoint the message when the patient's words and nonverbal behavior do not agree.

Example of a clarifying response:

Patient: "During certain activities, I have the most awful pain in my back."
Nurse: "Tell me what you mean by awful."

Interpreting

When interpreting you have the opportunity to share your inferences or conclusions gathered from the patient's interview.

Example of interpreting:

Nurse: "Your headaches seem to occur every time you eat nuts."

Sequencing

To effectively assess the patient's needs, identify a time frame within which symptoms and problems developed or occurred. One way of obtaining this information involves asking the patient to place a symptom, problem, or event in its proper sequence.

Example of sequencing:

Nurse: "Did this sharp pain occur each time you had sexual intercourse or only when you didn't empty your bladder first?"

Encouraging Comparisons

Encouraging comparisons is a technique that enables both participants in the health assessment interview to become more aware of patterns, themes, or specific symptomatology in the patient's life.

Example of encouraging comparisons:

Nurse: "In what way was your reaction to this medication similar to or different from your reaction to other antibiotics you've taken before?"

Summarizing

Summarizing helps organize the patient's thoughts. A brief, concise review of the important points covered helps the patient identify anything that has been left out and provides you with an opportunity to make sure that what you understood the patient to say is actually what was said.

Example of summarizing:

"During this past hour, you've shared with me several health concerns of which the most vexing to you is your difficulty losing weight. Is that correct?"

Action Responses

Action responses stimulate the patient to make some change in thinking and behavior.

Focusing

Focusing allows you to concentrate on or "track" a specific point the patient has made.

Example of focusing:

"You've mentioned several times that your wife is concerned about your smoking. Let's go back to that."

Exploring

In exploring, you attempt to develop in greater detail a specific area of content or patient concern.

Example of exploring:

"Tell me more about how you feel when you do not take your medication."

Presenting Reality

The technique of presenting reality, although typically used with psychiatric or confused patients, is useful in the health assessment interview when you are confronted with a patient who exaggerates or makes large, grandiose statements.

Example of presenting reality:

Patient: "I can never get an appointment at this clinic."

Nurse: "But Mr. Jasper, I've seen you several times in the past 4 months."

Patient: "Well, yes, but I can never get an appointment at a time that is convenient for me."

Confronting

Confronting is a verbal response to some perceived discrepancy or incongruency in the patient's thoughts, feelings, or behaviors.

Example of confronting:

Patient: "I never know exactly which of my symptoms to pay attention to. I think I'm such a hypochondriac."

Nurse: "You say that you're not sure which symptoms are important, and yet it seems that you are very clear about which symptoms you thought serious enough for you to seek medical care and which ones you felt comfortable managing on your own."

Informing

Providing the patient with needed information, such as explaining the nature of and the reasons for any necessary tests or procedures, is called informing.

Example of informing:

Patient: "Dr. Jones told me that I need to have my gallbladder taken out."

Nurse: "Did you understand what Dr. Jones told you about your gallbladder surgery?"

Patient: "No, I didn't understand what she said about the new surgical technique. She said something about a tube."

Nurse: "There is a technique in which the surgeon inserts a tube in your abdomen to remove the gallbladder rather than making a cut, which is the usual procedure."

Patient: "Yes, that was it. Please tell me more about that."

Collaborating

In collaboration, you offer the patient a relationship wherein you and the patient work together, rather than one wherein you are in total control of the interaction.

Example of collaborating:

"Perhaps you and I can talk further about your asthma and discover what specifically is making you so anxious."

Limit Setting

During the interview with a seductive, hostile, or talkative patient, you may find it necessary to set specific limits on patient behavior. In such situations, patients may require some direction as to how to behave; provide guidance by calmly, clearly, and respectfully telling the patient your expectations regarding behavior. Limit only those behaviors that are problematic or detrimental to the interview.

Example of appropriate limit setting:

Nurse: "You know, it seems as if you are feeling pretty unsure of how to behave now."

Patient: "What do you mean?"

Nurse: "Well, you're asking me a lot of personal questions and generally making it difficult for me to find out what is bothering you. The reason you are here is because you have some health concerns. How can I help you more clearly tell me what brought you to the clinic?"

Normalizing

Normalizing is a technique to help decrease patient anxiety by helping the patient understand that his or her response to a situation may be quite common.

Example of normalizing:

"You seem shocked at finding a lump in your breast; most women have a similar reaction."

Interviewing the Patient with Special Needs

The Patient Who Is Hearing Impaired

1. Determine whether the patient wears a hearing aid. Ensure that it is in working order and turned on.
2. Make every effort to move the patient to a setting having minimal background noise.
3. Always face the patient.
4. Speak in a normal tone and at a normal pace.
5. Determine whether the patient uses sign language. If signing is used, enlist the assistance of an interpreter.
6. Pay particular attention to the patient's nonverbal cues and to your own nonverbal behavior.
7. Provide a pen and paper to facilitate communication, if possible.

The Patient Who Is Visually Impaired

1. Look directly at the patient when speaking.
2. Speak in a normal tone and at a normal volume.
3. Advise the patient as to when you are entering or leaving the room.
4. Orient the patient to the immediate environment; use clock hours to indicate the positions of items in relation to the patient.
5. Ask for permission before touching the patient.

The Patient Who Is Speech-Impaired or Aphasic

1. Assess the patient's usual method of communication and adapt the interview to the patient's abilities.
2. Allow plenty of time for the patient to respond to questions. Do not answer for the patient.
3. Use closed questions whenever possible.
4. Repeat or rephrase any question not understood or remembered by the patient.
5. Speak directly to the patient, rather than to an intermediary.
6. Use nonverbal behavior, including facial expressions, gestures, and voice tone, to supplement and reinforce your verbal messages.

The Patient Who Is Hostile

1. Before beginning the interview, review any available documentation that might alert you to potential problems. Be especially cautious of those patients with a history of violence or poor impulse control.
2. When interviewing patients with a potential for violence, do not position yourself in a corner from which you cannot easily exit if necessary. Arrange seating so that the patient is never between you and the door.

Do not turn your back on the patient, and do not allow the patient to walk behind you or to come between you and the exit.

3. Assess the risk for physical aggression. Be alert for signs of increasing tension (e.g., clenched fists; loud, angry tone of voice; narrowed eyes).
4. Remember that hostility tends to be contagious. Do not reciprocate anger and hostility.
5. Minimize the risk of aggression via nonthreatening interventions such as limit setting and refocusing.
6. If anxious, alert a colleague to your location and leave the door to the interview room open. These precautions will provide you with an added sense of security and will provide the patient with an added deterrent.
7. Respect the patient's feelings and right to have those feelings. However, do not encourage excessive venting of feelings.
8. Remove yourself from potentially threatening situations and call for assistance, if necessary.

The Patient Who Is Very Ill

1. Collect only immediately pertinent data from the patient; defer the remainder of the interview until later.
2. If a patient is very sick, it may be necessary to interview a family member or significant other.

REFERENCE

Bradley, J. C., & Edinberg, M. A. (1990). *Communication in the nursing context* (3rd ed.). East Norwalk, CT: Appleton & Lange.

3

The Complete Health History Including Documentation

The health history usually represents the first step of patient assessment. It is the collection of subjective information on the patient's health status from the well or ill patient and other sources. The health history can provide information on a patient's status, as well as social, emotional, physical, and spiritual identity. Patient strengths and areas of need can be identified. The health history is usually performed before the physical assessment. Analysis of the information obtained reveals areas needing attention in the physical assessment.

Types of Health History

There are four types of health history: complete, episodic, interval (or follow-up), and emergency. The complete health history, described in this text, is a comprehensive history of the patient's past and present health status and covers many facets of the patient's life. It is usually gathered during the patient's initial visit to a health care facility on a nonemergency basis and upon admission to the hospital. The episodic health history is shorter and is specific to the patient's current reason for seeking health care. For example, the patient who seeks care for a sore throat and fever would have an episodic health history taken. The interval, or follow-up, health history builds on a preceding visit to a health care facility. It documents the patient's recovery from illness, such as the sore throat and fever, or progress from a prior visit. Finally, the emergency health history is elicited from the patient and other sources in an emergency situation. Only information required immediately to treat the emergent need of the patient is gathered; after the life-threatening condition is no longer present, the nurse may elicit a more comprehensive history.

Preparing for the Health History

Taking a complete health history from a patient may require 30 to 60 minutes; before the interview starts, inform the patient of the amount of time that will be required. Refer to Chapter 2 for communication techniques and strategies for dealing with patients who have special needs. The health history may also be computerized, which is either patient or health care provider generated.

Identifying Information

Record the following biographical data:

Today's date
Patient's name
Address
Phone number
Date of birth
Birthplace
Social Security number
Occupation
Work address
Work phone number
Insurance
Usual source of health care
Source of referral
Emergency contact

The Complete Health History Assessment Tool

Source and Reliability of Information

The adult patient usually is the historian. However, in some instances, such as trauma, the historian may be someone other than the patient. Note the name of the historian as well as the relationship between the historian and the patient. In addition, assess the reliability of the historian. Consider the mental state of the historian because emotions and certain medical conditions can influence the retelling of events. For example, the information provided by a patient with severe Alzheimer's disease may be less than accurate. Note if an interpreter was used.

Patient Profile

The patient profile provides demographics that may be linked to health status. Record the patient's age, gender, race, and marital status.

Reason for Seeking Health Care and Chief Complaint

The reason for seeking health care is the reason for the patient's visit and is usually focused on health promotion. The chief complaint (CC) is the sign (objective finding) or symptom (subjective finding) that causes the patient to seek health care. A patient may present with multiple chief complaints in a single visit. The reason for seeking health care and CC should be recorded as direct quotes from the patient. The duration of the signs and symptoms should also be included in the CC.

"What concerns bring you here today?" or "What caused you to seek health care today?"

"How long has this condition been concerning you?"

Present Health and History of the Present Illness

If the patient is seeking health promotion, the present health states the patient's current health status.

The history of the present illness (HPI) is a chronological account of the patient's CC and the events surrounding it. Ten characteristics of each CC can be ascertained for a complete HPI:

1. Location
2. Radiation
3. Quality
4. Quantity
5. Associated manifestations
6. Aggravating factors
7. Alleviating factors
8. Setting
9. Timing
10. Meaning and impact

The CC may not have all 10 qualifiers; hoarseness, for example, may not be characterized by quantity.

Location

The location of the CC refers to the primary area where the symptom occurs or originates. Have the patient exactly state or point to where the symptom originates or occurs.

Radiation

The spreading of the CC or symptom from its original location to another part of the body is radiation.

Quality

The quality of the CC describes the way it feels to the patient. If the patient is having difficulty describing pain, suggest some quality terms such as *gnawing, burning, pounding, stabbing, pinching, aching, throbbing,* or *crushing.*

Quantity

The quantity is the severity, volume, number, or extent of the CC. The patient may refer to the CC using terms such as *minor, moderate,* or *severe,* or *small, medium,* or *large.* Another mechanism that can be used to assess the quantity of pain is a numerical scale known as the Visual Analog Scale, which rates pain from 0 (no pain) to 10 (worst pain imaginable). Ask the patient to rate the severity of pain at a particular point in time. Refer to Chapter 9 for additional information.

Associated Manifestations

The signs and symptoms that accompany the CC are termed associated manifestations. Rarely does a CC occur without affecting either other components of the involved body system or another body system. Positive findings are those associated manifestations that the patient has experienced along with the CC. Negative findings, also called pertinent negatives, are those manifestations expected in the patient having a suspected pathology but that are denied by the patient. If the patient does not mention specific signs or symptoms that might be present with a given pathology, ask whether they are present. Document both positive findings and pertinent negatives, because both give clues to the patient's condition. For example, a patient with chest pain may have nausea, diaphoresis, and anxiety as positive associated manifestations. Vomiting, fatigue, and restlessness are pertinent negatives because their presence might be expected in a patient with chest pain. Lack of these associated manifestations may lead to a different diagnosis.

Aggravating Factors

Events that worsen the severity of the CC are the aggravating factors.

Alleviating Factors

Alleviating factors are events that decrease the severity of the CC. This includes medications.

Setting

The setting can be the actual physical environment in which the patient is located, the mental state of the patient, or some activity in which the patient is involved.

Nursing Tip

PQRST Mnemonic

One way to remember the characteristics of a chief complaint is the PQRST mnemonic.

P is for what provokes the pain (aggravating factors) and for palliative measures (alleviating factors)
Q is for quality
R is for region (location) and radiation
S is for severity (quantity) and setting
T is for timing

The PQRST mnemonic does not include associated manifestations, so remember to ask about this characteristic of a chief complaint.

Timing

Timing, as used to describe a CC, encompasses three elements: onset, duration, and frequency. Onset refers to the time at which the CC began and is usually described as *gradual* or *sudden*. Duration refers to the amount of time that the CC is present. *Continuous* and *intermittent* are terms that can be used to describe the duration of a CC. Frequency refers to the number of times the CC occurs and how often it occurs (e.g., number of times per day, season of year).

Meaning and Impact

The last two pieces of information needed for the HPI are the meaning or significance of the CC to the patient and the impact that the CC has on the patient's lifestyle.

Past Health History

The past health history (PHH) or past medical history (PMH) provides information on the patient's health status from birth to the present. Sample questions for each element of the past health history are listed in the following discussion.

Medical History

The medical history comprises all medical problems that the patient has experienced during adulthood and their sequelae. Also included are chronic and serious episodic illnesses.

"Have you ever been diagnosed as having an illness? What was it?"

"When was the illness diagnosed?"

"Who diagnosed this problem?"

"What is the current treatment for this problem?"

"Have you ever been hospitalized for this illness? For what period of time? What was the treatment? What was your condition after the treatment?"

"Have you ever experienced any complications (sequelae) from this disease? What were they? How were they treated?"

Surgical History

Record a complete account of each surgical procedure, including year performed, hospital or office, practitioner, and sequelae.

"Have you ever had surgery? What type?"

"Who was your physician at the time?"

"When, where, and by whom was the surgery performed?"

"Were you hospitalized? For what period of time?"

"Were there any complications? How were they treated?"

"Are you currently receiving any treatment related to this surgery?"

"Have you ever had an adverse effect from anesthesia?"

Medications

Prescription Medication

"What prescription medications are you currently taking? Who prescribed them?"

"How long have you been taking this medication?"

"Have you ever experienced any side effects with this medication?"

"Have you ever had an allergic reaction to this medication? What happened?"

"Tell me the purpose of these medications."

Over-the-Counter Medication

"Do you currently take any over-the-counter medications? Which ones?"

"Why do you take this medication?"

"Do you take any home remedies? Which ones? For what purpose?"

"Are you taking herbs, supplements, minerals, or vitamins?"

Communicable Diseases

Communicable diseases can have a grave impact on the individual as well as on society. Some communicable diseases generate enough of a concern to a community that they are reportable to the public health department.

"Have you ever been told that you have had an infectious or communicable disease? Which one(s)?"

"What were your symptoms?"

"How were you treated?"

"Did you have any complications? What were they? Were there any permanent consequences?"

"Have you ever had gonorrhea, herpes, syphilis, chlamydia, or other sexually transmitted diseases?"

"Have you ever had measles, mumps, rubella, German measles, herpes, varicella (chickenpox), pertussis (whooping cough), tuberculosis (TB), scarlet fever, rheumatic fever, hepatitis, HIV, AIDS?" (If yes to any of the preceding, ask about symptoms, treatment, and complications.)

"Do you have any tattoos or body piercings?"

Allergies

Always note allergies in red ink.

"Are you allergic to any medications? Animals? Foods? Insect bites? Bee stings?"

"Are you allergic to anything in the environment?"

"What symptoms do you get when you are exposed to this substance?"

"What treatment do you use? Is it effective?"

"Have you experienced any complications from the allergies? Which?"

> **Nursing Tip**
>
> **Allergies versus Side Effects**
>
> Many patients report that they are allergic to specific medications. When questioned further on the specific reaction to a medication, patients frequently report symptoms such as nausea, headache, diarrhea, and vomiting. While not discounting the patient's experience with this medication, it is vital to keep in mind that these examples are not drug allergies. They are adverse reactions to the medication. True drug allergies usually manifest as urticaria, breathing difficulties, anaphylaxis, or a combination of these.

Injuries and Accidents

"Have you ever been involved in an accident or been injured?"

"Were there any long-term effects from this injury/accident?"

"Has this type of injury/accident occurred in the past?"

"Have you ever sustained an injury in a car accident?"

"Have you ever had a broken bone? Stitches? Burns?"

"Have you ever been assaulted? Raped? Shot? Stabbed?"

Special Needs

"Do you have any disability or special need? Describe the type of limitations."

Blood Transfusions

"Have you ever received a blood transfusion (whole blood or any of its components)? When? Why? What quantity?"

"Did you experience any reaction to this blood product? If yes, please describe."

Childhood Illnesses

"Have you ever had any of the following illnesses: varicella (chickenpox), diphtheria, measles, mumps, rubella, pertussis (whooping cough), polio, rheumatic fever, or scarlet fever?" (This question is eliminated if previously asked during the communicable disease section.)

"How old were you when the illness occurred?"

"Were there any complications? What were they?"

Immunizations

"As a child, did you receive the following immunizations: measles, mumps, rubella (MMR); polio; respiratory syncytial virus (RSV); varicella; diphtheria, pertussis, tetanus (DPT); hemophilus influenza type B (Hib); hepatitis B?"

"Have you received any immunizations as an adult, such as hepatitis A, hepatitis B, influenza, tetanus, pneumococcal, meningococcal, Lyme disease?"

"When was your last TB test, and what was the result?"

"Have you ever received any other immunizations such as for cholera, typhoid fever, or yellow fever?"

"Did you have any reaction to the immunizations?"

Family Health History

The family health history (FHH) records the health status of the patient as well as of the patient's immediate blood relatives. When feasible, obtain as complete a family history as possible. At a minimum, the history must contain the age and health status of the patient and of the patient's spouse, children, siblings, and parents. Ideally, the patient's grandparents, aunts, and uncles should be incorporated into the history as well. Documentation of this information is done in two parts: the genogram, or family tree, and a list of family diseases. Figure 3-1 demonstrates the appropriate method for constructing the genogram. The positive and pertinent negative findings are documented in the family genogram.

The second component of the FHH is the documentation of familial or genetic diseases.

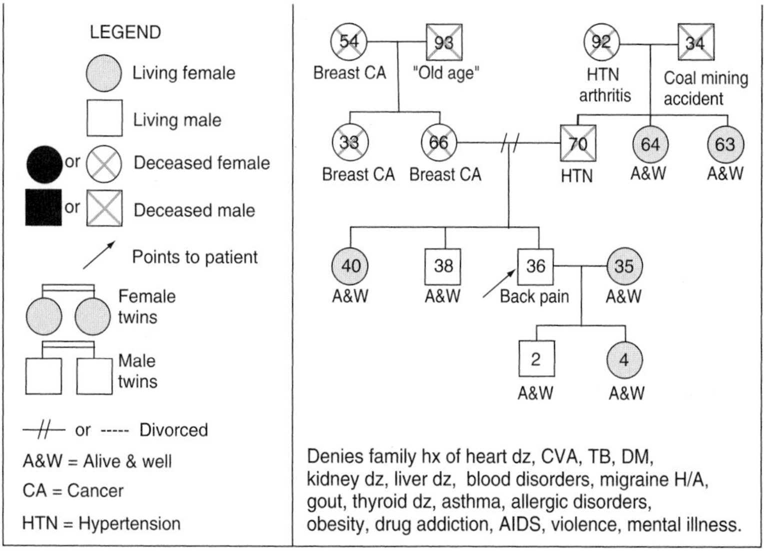

Figure 3-1 Family Health History and Genogram

Sample questions include:

"What are the current age and health status of each of the following members of your family: spouse, children, siblings, grandparents, aunts, and uncles?"

"Has anyone in your family ever had any of the following illnesses: heart disease, hypertension, stroke, TB, diabetes, cancer, kidney disease, blood disorders, sickle cell anemia, arthritis, epilepsy, migraine headaches, gout, thyroid disease, liver disease, asthma, allergic disorders, obesity, alcoholism, mental illness, mental retardation, drug addiction, AIDS or HIV? Who?"

"Has anyone in your immediate family died? Who? What was the cause of death?"

Patients who are adopted have varying degrees of information on their biologic parents. If the FHH of the biologic parents is unknown, document this fact in the chart.

Social History

The social history (SH) explores those elements of the patient's lifestyle that can affect health. Sample questions follow.

Alcohol Use

"How much alcohol do you drink a week? How often do you drink?"

"What type of alcohol do you drink (wine, beer, liquor spirits)?"

"How much do you consume at one time?"

"When did you first start drinking?"

"Have you ever lost consciousness or blacked out when drinking?"

"Do you ever drink and drive?"

"Do you binge drink?"

(For women) "Did you ever drink during pregnancy?"

"Do you have a drinking problem?"

Drug Use

The use of drugs in the SH section refers to the use of illegal substances, or abuse of prescribed medications.

"Do you or have you ever used street or recreational drugs?"

"At what age did you first use illegal substances?"

"What amount and form of drugs do you use? How often do you use drugs?"

"Do you sniff or inhale cleansers, paint, or other chemical products?"

"Do you share needles? Do you clean the needles between uses?"

"Have you experienced any health problems from drug use?"
"Have you ever overdosed? If yes, please describe."
"Have you ever been through a drug treatment program? What was the outcome?"
"Have you abused prescription medications?

Tobacco Use

"Do you or have you ever used tobacco products (cigarettes, pipe, cigars, chewing tobacco, snuff)?"
"At what age did you start using tobacco?"
"What is your daily consumption?"
"Have you ever tried to break this habit? What method did you use? What was the outcome?"
"Do you live or work with someone who smokes?"

Plot packs per day × number of years of use.

Sexual Practice

"What is your sexual orientation (heterosexual, homosexual, or bisexual)?"
"Does your current sexual orientation represent your past sexual practice? If not, how has it changed?"
"At what age was your first sexual experience?"
"With how many partners are you currently involved? Has this number changed? How many partners have you had during your lifetime?"
"What method of birth control do you use?"
"What measures do you use to prevent the spread of sexually transmitted diseases?"
"Do you engage in oral or anal sex?"
"Have you ever had a sexual partner who had a sexually transmitted disease?"
"Are you satisfied with your sexual performance?"
"Are there other activities that satisfy your sexual needs?"

Domestic and Intimate Partner Violence

It is estimated that up to 30% of injured women treated in emergency departments (ED) have suffered from domestic or intimate partner violence (IPV) (American College of Obstetricians & Gynecologists, 1995). Violence cuts across both sexes, as well as racial, cultural, geographic, and socioeconomic lines. It is vital to be familiar with your state's statutes regarding reporting actual and suspected violence and abuse.

Domestic and intimate partner violence involves more than physical abuse. It includes psychological, emotional, sexual, and financial abuse or coercion. Just as many health care providers advocate screening for tobacco and alcohol use for both men and women at each health care encounter, some providers recommend routine screening for domestic and intimate partner violence at every health care encounter for women. Though men can be the victims of domestic and intimate partner violence, the majority of victims are women.

Some clues that might alert you to the possibility of domestic and intimate partner violence are:

- Frequent injuries, accidents, or burns
- Previous injuries for which the individual did not seek health care
- Injury is inconsistent with the patient's report of how it occurred
- Refusal of the patient to discuss the injury
- Significant other accompanies the patient to the ED, answers questions for patient, and refuses to leave the patient's side
- Significant other has a history of previous violence or substance abuse

Using the communication technique of normalizing, the nurse can screen for potential domestic and intimate partner violence. Some appropriate introductory comments might be:

"Almost one-third of injured women who visit the ED have experienced some domestic and intimate partner violence. Is this what happened to you?"
"Domestic and intimate partner violence occur very frequently in our community. Keeping this in mind, I would like to ask you some questions."

A single broad question can also be used to screen for domestic and intimate partner violence:

"In the past year, have you been hit, kicked, punched, or hurt in other ways by someone close to you?"

If the patient answers yes to these questions, you need to inquire if the patient feels safe in his or her current environment or situation. Most EDs have resources available to assist the patient into a climate where he or she can receive help and feel safe.

It is imperative to document physical violence assessment findings concisely and accurately. Incorporate drawings of injury locations or use printed anatomical maps where injuries can be documented. Many EDs have cameras so that the staff can photograph injuries for the patient's records.

Travel History

"Where within the United States have you traveled? When? For how long?"

"Have you ever traveled outside of the United States? Where? When? For how long?"

"Did you receive any immunizations before you traveled to that area?"

"Were you ill while you were there?"

"What treatment did you receive? Were there any complications?"

"Since returning home, have you been ill?"

Work Environment

"Describe the work you do: is it physically, mentally, or emotionally demanding?"

"Do you spend the majority of your work day sitting, standing, walking, running, lifting, or biking?"

"Do you work with chemicals, toxins, radiation, fumes, or hazardous materials?"

"What safety measures do you practice at work?"

"What is the noise level at your place of employment?"

"Have you ever had a work-related accident or injury?"

"Is there any construction at your workplace/environment?"

Home Environment

Physical Environment

"In what type of structure do you live (e.g., house, trailer, apartment)?"

"How old is this structure?"

"Do you have heat, air conditioning, running water, electricity, smoke detectors for each floor, carbon monoxide detectors, running water, toilets, tub or shower, telephone, and fire extinguishers?"

"Do you have a pet? What kind? Does your pet live inside or outside? Describe your attachment to your pet."

"What type of transportation do you use?"

"Where do you store your medications, cleaning supplies, paint, gasoline, and other toxic or volatile substances?"

"Is there a firearm(s) in your home?"

Psychosocial Environment

"Do you feel safe in your neighborhood?"

"Does your neighborhood have a crime watch prevention program?"

Hobbies and Leisure Activities

"Do you engage in hobbies or other special activities? What are they?"

"Have you ever had an injury from your hobby?"

Stress

Distress is negative stress, while eustress is positive stress.

"What are the current stressors in your life? Which is the greatest stressor?"

"Have you ever progressed from the point of being stressed to being panicked? What were the circumstances? How did you handle it?"

"Are you able to recognize when you become stressed? What happens?"

Education

"What is the highest grade level you have completed?"

"Have you completed a GED certification program (if appropriate)?"

Economic Status

"What are the sources of your income?"
"How would you describe your economic status?"
"Are you able to meet food, medication, housing, clothing, and personal expenses for you and your family?"
"Are you able to save any money?"
"Do you hesitate seeking health care because of the cost? Do you have medical insurance?"

Military Service

"Are you now or have you ever been in the military? What branch?"
"How long have you been in the military? Are you on active or reserve duty?"
"To what regions have you been assigned? How long were you there? When?"
"Have you been in combat?"

Religion

"Are you affiliated with a specific religion?"
"Do you currently practice your faith?"
"Do you see your religious beliefs as affecting your health status? In what way?"
"Are there any religious practices that you may need assistance in practicing?"

Ethnic Background

"With what culture or ethnic group do you identify yourself?"

Roles and Relationships

"Who lives with you?"
"What type of relationship do you have with these individuals?"
"What is your role within your family (e.g., caregiver, breadwinner, child, student)?"
"What responsibilities go along with this role?"

Characteristic Patterns of Daily Living and Functional Health Assessment

"Describe a typical day for you, from the time you wake up to the time you go to bed."
"Do you need assistance with any activities of daily living? If yes, is assistance readily available?"
"Do you socialize, meet, or talk with people outside your home on a daily basis?"

The functional health assessment documents a person's ability to perform instrumental activities of daily living (IADLs).

Health Maintenance Activities

Health maintenance activities (HMAs) are those practices a person incorporates into his or her lifestyle that can promote healthy living. Sample questions related to HMAs follow.

Sleep

"What time do you usually go to bed?"
"What time do you usually awake?"
"How long does it take you to fall asleep?" "Do you snore?"
"Is this an adequate amount of sleep for you? How do feel when you awaken?"
"Do you ever have difficulty falling asleep? Have you ever been told that you have insomnia?"
"Do you ever have difficulty staying awake? Have you ever been told that you have sleep apnea or narcolepsy?"

Diet

Refer to Chapter 7 for a more thorough discussion of nutrition and diet history.

"Are you on any special therapeutic diet (e.g., low salt, low cholesterol, low fat, vegetarian)?"
"Do you follow any particular diet plan (e.g., vegetarian, liquid, commercially available diet food, rice diet, Atkins diet)?"
"How many meals a day do you eat? At what times do you eat? Do you snack? When?"

Exercise

An easy way to remember what questions to ask a patient regarding exercise is the use of the FIT acronym: *F* is for frequency, *I* is for intensity, *T* is for timing or duration.

"Do you participate in a formal or informal exercise program?"

"What type of exercise do you do? How many times per week and for how long?"

"Does your health pose any restrictions on your ability to exercise?"

Stress Management

"What activities do you do when you become stressed to help alleviate the stress? How are they helpful?"

Use of Safety Devices

"Do you wear a seat belt when riding in a motor vehicle?"

"Do you wear a helmet when riding a motorcycle?"

"Do your hobbies and leisure activities require the use of safety devices (such as a helmet for cycling)? Do you use them?"

"What precautions do you take when using pesticides or fertilizers?"

Health Check-ups

"When was the last time you had the following performed: pulse and blood pressure measurements, complete physical examination, chest X ray, TB test, EKG, urinalysis, complete blood count (CBC), blood chemistry, cholesterol or lipid panel? What were the results?"

"How often do you see a dentist? For what reason?"

"How often do you see an eye doctor? For what reason? Have you had a check for glaucoma?"

(For women) "How often do you have a gynecological check-up? Performed by whom? What was the date and result of your last Pap smear?"

(For women) "Do you know how to perform a breast self-examination? Who taught you? How often do you perform it? Do you have any questions about it?"

(For women) "What was the date and the result of your last mammogram?"

(For men) "Do you know how to perform a testicular self-examination? Who taught you? How often do you perform it? Do you have any questions about it?"

(For men) "How often do you have a prostate examination? What was the date and result of your last exam?"

"Do you have any other health care providers (e.g., psychiatrist, psychologist, occupational or physical therapist, podiatrist, chiropractor)? For what reason? How often do you see this person?"

Review of Systems

The review of systems (ROS) constitutes the patient's subjective response to a series of body system-related questions and serves as a double-check that vital information is not overlooked. Although the ROS covers a broad base of clinical states, it is by no means exhaustive. The ROS follows a head-to-toe, or cephalocaudal, approach and includes two types of questions: sign and symptom related and disease related. The sign, symptoms, and diseases are grouped according to physiological body parts and systems.

Both positive and pertinent negative findings are documented in the ROS. When a finding is positive, ask the patient to describe it as completely as possible. Refer to the 10 characteristics of a CC when gathering more information about positive findings. Table 3-1 lists the symptoms and diseases that can be ascertained during the ROS.

After completing the ROS, ask the patient whether there is any additional information to discuss. Inform the patient what the next step will be (e.g., physical assessment, diagnostic tests, or treatment) and when to expect it.

TABLE 3-1 Review of Systems

General
Patient's perception of general state of health at the present, difference from usual state, vitality and energy levels, body odors, fever, chills, night sweats

Skin
Rashes, itching, changes in skin pigmentation, ecchymoses, change in color or size of mole, sores, lumps, dry or moist skin, pruritus, change in skin texture, odors, excessive sweating, acne, warts, eczema, psoriasis, amount of time spent in the sun, use of sunscreen, skin cancer

Hair
Alopecia, excessive growth of hair or growth of hair in unusual locations (hirsutism), use of chemicals on hair, dandruff, pediculosis, scalp lesions

Nails
Change in nails, splitting, breaking, thickened, texture change, onychomycosis, use of chemicals, false nails

Eyes
Blurred vision, visual acuity, glasses, contacts, photophobia, excessive tearing, night blindness, diplopia, drainage, bloodshot eyes, pain, blind spots, flashing lights, halos around objects, floaters, glaucoma, cataracts, use of sunglasses, use of protective eyewear

Ears
Cleaning method, hearing deficits, hearing aid, pain, phonophobia, discharge, lightheadedness (vertigo), ringing in the ears (tinnitus), usual noise level, earaches, infection, piercings, use of ear protection, amount of cerumen

Nose and Sinuses
Number of colds per year, discharge, itching, hay fever, postnasal drip, stuffiness, sinus pain, sinusitis, polyps, obstruction, epistaxis, change in sense of smell, allergies, snoring

Mouth
Dental habits (brushing, flossing, mouth rinses), toothache, tooth abscess, dentures, bleeding or swollen gums, difficulty chewing, sore tongue, change in taste, lesions, change in salivation, bad breath, caries, teeth extractions, orthodontics

Throat and Neck
Hoarseness, change in voice, frequent sore throats, dysphagia, pain or stiffness, enlarged thyroid (goiter), lymphadenopathy, tonsillectomy, adenoidectomy

Breasts and Axilla
Pain, tenderness, discharge, lumps, change in size, dimpling, rash, benign breast disease, breast cancer, results of recent mammogram

Respiratory
Dyspnea on exertion, shortness of breath, sputum, cough, sneezing, wheezing, hemoptysis, frequent upper respiratory tract infections, pneumonia, emphysema, asthma, tuberculosis, tuberculosis exposure, result of last chest X ray or PPD

Cardiovascular and Peripheral Vasculature
Paroxysmal nocturnal dyspnea, chest pain, cyanosis, heart murmur, palpitations, syncope, orthopnea (state number of pillows used), edema, cold or discolored hands or feet, leg cramps, myocardial infarction, hypertension, valvular disease, intermittent claudication, varicose veins, thrombophlebitis, deep vein thrombosis, use of support hose, anemia, cyanosis, result of last EKG

continues

TABLE 3-1 Review of Systems *continued*

Gastrointestinal
Change in appetite, nausea, vomiting, diarrhea, constipation, usual bowel habits, melena, rectal bleeding, hematemesis, change in stool color, flatulence, belching, regurgitation, heartburn, dysphagia, abdominal pain, jaundice, ascites, hemorrhoids, hepatitis, gallstones, gastroesophageal reflux disease, appendicitis, ulcerative colitis, Crohn's disease, diverticulitis, hernia

Urinary
Change in urine color, voiding habits, dysuria, hesitancy, urgency, frequency, nocturia, polyuria, dribbling, loss in force of stream, bedwetting, change in urine volume, incontinence, urinary retention, suprapubic pain, flank pain, kidney stones, urinary tract infections

Musculoskeletal
Joint stiffness, muscle pain, cramps, back pain, limitation of movement, redness, swelling, weakness, bony deformity, broken bones, dislocations, sprains, crepitus, gout, arthritis, osteoporosis, herniated disc

Neurological
Headache, change in balance, incoordination, loss of movement, change in sensory perception or feeling in an extremity, change in speech, change in smell, syncope, loss of memory, tremors, involuntary movement, loss of consciousness, seizures, weakness, head injury, vertigo, tremor, tic, paralysis, stroke, spasm

Psychological
Irritability, nervousness, tension, increased stress, difficulty concentrating, mood changes, suicidal thoughts, depression, anxiety, sleep disturbances

Female Reproductive
Vaginal discharge, change in libido, infertility, sterility, pelvic pain, pain during intercourse, postcoital bleeding; menses: last menstrual period (LMP), menarche, regularity, duration, amount of bleeding, premenstrual symptoms, intermenstrual bleeding, dysmenorrhea, menorrhagia, fibroids; menopause: age of onset, duration, symptoms, bleeding; obstetrical: number of pregnancies, number of miscarriages or abortions, number of children, type of delivery, complications; type of birth control, hormone replacement therapy

Male Reproductive
Change in libido, infertility, sterility, impotence, pain during intercourse, age at onset of puberty, testicular or penile pain, penile discharge, erections, emissions, hernias, enlarged prostate, type of birth control

Nutrition
Present weight, usual weight, desired weight, food intolerances, food likes and dislikes, where meals are eaten, caffeine intake

Endocrine
Exophthalmos, fatigue, change in size of head, hands, or feet, weight change, heat and cold intolerances, excessive sweating, polydipsia, polyphagia, polyuria, increased hunger, change in body hair distribution, goiter, diabetes mellitus

Lymph Nodes
Enlargement, tenderness

Hematological
Easy bruising or bleeding, anemia, sickle cell anemia, blood type, exposure to radiation

REFERENCE

American College of Obstetricians & Gynecologists. (1995). Technical Bulletin on domestic violence (No. 209). Washington, DC: Author.

Unit 2 Special Assessments

4

Developmental Assessment

All individuals, from birth to death, pass through identifiable, cyclical stages of growth and development that determine who and what they are and can become. *Growth* refers to an increase in body size and function to the point of optimum maturity. *Development* refers to patterned and predictable increases in the physical, cognitive, socioemotional, and moral capacities of individuals that enable individuals to successfully adapt to their environments.

Developmental Theories

The theories most widely used for clinical assessment of patients are the "ages and stages" theories of Piaget (1952), Freud (1946), Erikson (1974), and Kohlberg (1981). The ages and stages developmental theories are based on the premise that individuals experience much the same sequential physical, cognitive, socioemotional, and moral changes during the same age periods, each of which is termed a developmental stage. During each developmental stage, specific physical and psychosocial skills, known as developmental tasks, must be achieved. An individual's readiness for each new developmental task is dependent on success in achieving prior developmental tasks and on the presence of environmental opportunities to develop the new skills. If prior developmental tasks have been insufficiently achieved or appropriate environments in which the tasks can be achieved are not available, mastery of subsequent developmental skills may not occur, may be delayed, or may occur in a defective way, thereby decreasing the individual's capacity to successfully adapt to the environment during his or her life span.

A second group of theories includes the life events or transitional theories of development. Life event or transitional developmental theories are based on the premise that development occurs in response to specific events, such as new roles (e.g., parenthood) and life transitions (e.g., career changes), each of which serves as an impetus for growth; excessive stress can disrupt an individual's equilibrium and lead to a variety of physical and psychological health problems (Wykle, Kahana, & Kowal, 1992; Grey, 1993; Aguilera, 1994). In identifying life events and stressors, the nurse can play a critical role in helping patients maintain health and control stress.

Ages and Stages Developmental Theories

The major tenets of Piaget, Freud, Erikson, and Kohlberg are discussed next; these are summarized in Table 4-1.

Piaget's Theory of Cognitive Development

Jean Piaget's (1952) theory of cognitive development depicts age-related, sequential stages through which all developing children must progress to learn to think, reason, and exercise judgment and to learn the cognitive life skills (e.g., language development, problem solving,

TABLE 4-1 Summary of Ages and Stages Developmental Theories

STAGE/AGE	PIAGET'S COGNITIVE STAGES	FREUD'S PSYCHOSEXUAL STAGES	ERIKSON'S PSYCHOSOCIAL STAGES	KOHLBERG'S MORAL JUDGMENT STAGES
1. **Infancy** Birth to 1 year	**Sensorimotor** (birth to 2 years): begins to acquire language Task: Object permanence	**Oral:** pleasure from exploration with mouth and through sucking Task: Weaning	**Trust vs. Mistrust** Task: Trust Socializing agent: Mothering person Central process: Mutuality Ego quality: Hope	
2. **Toddler** 1 to 3 years	**Sensorimotor** continues **Preoperational** (2 to 7 years) begins: use of representational thought Task: Use language and mental images to think and communicate	**Anal:** control of elimination Task: Toilet training	**Autonomy vs. Shame and Doubt** Task: Autonomy Socializing agent: Parents Central process: Imitation Ego quality: Self-control and willpower	**Preconventional Level:** **1. Morality Stage:** Avoid punishment by not breaking rules of authority figures
3. **Preschool** 3 to 6 years	**Preoperational** continues	**Phallic:** attracted to opposite-sex parent Task: Resolve Oedipus/Electra complex	**Initiative vs. Guilt** Task: Initiative and moral responsibility Socializing agents: Parents Central process: Identification Ego quality: Direction, purpose, and conscience	**2. Individualism, Instrumental Purpose, and Exchange Stage:** "Right" is relative, follow rules when in own interest

continues

TABLE 4-1 Summary of Ages and Stages Developmental Theories *continued*

STAGE/AGE	PIAGET'S COGNITIVE STAGES	FREUD'S PSYCHOSEXUAL STAGES	ERIKSON'S PSYCHOSOCIAL STAGES	KOHLBERG'S MORAL JUDGMENT STAGES
4. School Age 6 to 12 years	**Preoperational** continues **Concrete Operations** (7 to 12 years) begins: engage in inductive reasoning and concrete problem solving Task: Learn concepts of conservation and reversibility	**Latency:** identification with same-sex parent Task: Identify with same-sex parent and test and compare own capabilities with peer norms	**Industry vs. Inferiority** Task: Industry, self-assurance, self-esteem Socializing agents: Teachers and peers Central process: Education Ego quality: Competence	**Conventional Level:** **3. Mutual Expectations, Relationships, and Conformity to Moral Norms Stage:** Need to be "good" in own and others' eyes, believe in rules and regulations
5. Adolescence 12 to 18 years	**Formal Operations** (12 years to adulthood): engage in abstract reasoning and analytical problem solving Task: Develop a workable philosophy of life	**Genital:** develop sexual relationships Task: Establish meaningful relationship for lifelong pairing	**Identity vs. Role Confusion** Task: Self-identity and concept Socializing agents: Society of peers Central process: Role experimentation and peer pressure Ego quality: Fidelity and devotion to others, personal and sociocultural values	**4. Social System and Conscience Stage:** Uphold laws because they are fixed social duties
6. Young Adult 18 to 30 years	**Formal Operations** continues		**Intimacy vs. Isolation** Task: Intimacy Socializing agent: Close friends, partners, lovers, spouse Central process: Mutuality among peers Ego quality: Intimate affiliation and love	**Postconventional Level:** **5. Social Contract or Utility and Individual Rights Stage:** Uphold laws in the interest of the greatest good for the greatest number; uphold laws that protect universal rights

continues

STAGE/AGE	PIAGET'S COGNITIVE STAGES	FREUD'S PSYCHOSEXUAL STAGES	ERIKSON'S PSYCHOSOCIAL STAGES	KOHLBERG'S MORAL JUDGMENT STAGES
7. Early Middle Age 30 to 50 years			**Generativity vs. Stagnation** (30 to 65 years) Task: Generativity Socializing agent: Spouse, partner, children, sociocultural norms Central process: Creativity and person-environment fit Ego quality: Productivity, perseverence, charity, and consideration	
8. Late Middle Age 50 to 70 years			**Generativity vs. Stagnation** continues	**6. Universal Ethical Principles Stage:** Support universal moral principles regardless of the price for doing so
9. Late Adult 70 years to death			**Ego Integrity vs. Despair** (65 years to death) Task: Ego integrity Socializing agent: Significant others Central process: Introspection Ego quality: Wisdom	

decision making, critical thinking, and oral and written communication) needed to successfully adapt to their environment. Piaget divides cognitive development into four periods: the sensorimotor stage, the preoperational stage, the concrete operational stage, and the formal operational stage.

Freud's Psychoanalytic Theory of Personality Development

Sigmund Freud (1946) contended that human behavior is motivated by psychodynamic forces within an individual's unconscious mind. Driven to act by these internal forces, individuals repeatedly interact with their external environment. An individual's personality and psychosexual identity are developed through the accumulation of these interactional experiences.

Personality

Personality, according to Freud, consists of three components with distinctly separate functions: id, ego, and superego. The id, evident at birth, is inborn, unconscious, and driven by biologic instincts and urges to seek immediate gratification of needs such as hunger, thirst, and physical comfort. The ego is conscious and rational and emerges during the first year of life, as infants begin to test the limits of the world around them. The ego seeks realistic and acceptable ways to meet needs. The superego, appearing in early childhood, is the internalization of the moral values formed as children interact with their parents and significant others. The superego acts as a moral arbitrator by blocking unacceptable behavior that is generated by the id and that could threaten the social order, creating feelings of guilt when the internalized moral code is compromised and generating feelings of pride when the moral code is upheld.

Psychosexual Stages

Freud perceived the desire to satisfy biologic needs, primarily sexual needs, as the major drive governing human behavior. Each developmental stage is centered on a specific body region and the conflicts associated with that region; an individual experiences tension and seeks gratification via the associated body region. If an individual's needs are met and the conflicts are resolved during a given stage, development will proceed normally to the next stage, and the developing personality will be healthily integrated. If resolution of the conflict does not occur, however, the individual will become fixated at that given stage and the individual's personality and psychosexual identity will be arrested or impaired. Freud identified five psychosexual stages of development: oral, anal, phallic, latency, and genital.

Erikson's Epigenetic Theory of Personality

The most frequently used theory of personality development is Erikson's (1974) epigenetic theory, which is based on the biologic concept that all growing organisms have an inherent plan of growth for all parts of the entity. Each part of a growing entity has a designated time of ascendancy and forms the basis for growth of the next part until the functional whole is fully developed. Erikson's theory was built on Freud's theory of personality but goes beyond it by depicting personality development as a passage through eight sequential stages of ego development from infancy through old age.

According to Erikson, the developing individual must master and resolve, to some extent, a core conflict or crisis during each stage by integrating personal needs and skills with the social and cultural demands and expectations of the environment. Passage to each developmental stage is dependent on the resolution of the core conflict of the preceding stage. No core conflict is ever completely mastered, however. These stages include trust versus mistrust, autonomy versus shame and doubt, initiative versus guilt, industry versus inferiority, identity versus role confusion, intimacy versus isolation, generativity versus stagnation, ego integrity versus despair.

Kohlberg's Theory of Moral Development

The basic premise of Kohlberg's (1981) theory of moral development is that when a conflict occurs between any of several universal values (e.g., punishment, affection, authority, truth, law, life, liberty, justice), the moral choice that must be made and justified requires cognitive capabilities, including systematic problem solving, which constitutes moral reasoning. According to Kohlberg, moral development is contingent on children's ability to learn and internalize parental and societal rules and standards, develop the ability to empathize with others' responses, and form their own personal standards of conduct. Moral development progresses through three levels with two distinct stages per level for a total of six stages.

Developmental Stages, Tasks, and Life Events

The following section outlines the developmental tasks, life events, and transitions from each major theory of development in conjunction with fine motor, language, and sensory milestones that characterize each developmental stage from birth to adolescence.

Developmental Tasks of Infants (Birth to 1 Year)

Infancy is a period of dramatic and rapid physical, motor, cognitive, emotional, and social growth, which marks it as one of the most critical periods of growth and development. Key gross and fine motor, language, and sensory milestones associated with this period are listed in Table 4-2.

Developmental tasks that must be achieved during the infancy stage are to:

1. Develop a basic, relative sense of trust.
2. Develop a sense of self as dependent but separate from others, particularly the mother.
3. Develop and desire affection for and response from others, particularly the mother.
4. Develop a preverbal communication system, including emotional expression, to communicate needs and desires.
5. Begin to develop conceptual abilities and a language system.
6. Begin to learn purposeful fine and gross motor skills, particularly eye-hand coordination and balance.
7. Begin to explore and recognize the immediate environment.
8. Develop object permanence.

Developmental Tasks of Toddlers (1 to 3 years)

The toddler period is one of steadily increasing motor development and control, intense activity and discovery, rapid language development, increasingly independent behaviors, and marked personality development. Key gross and fine motor, language, and sensory milestones associated with the toddler period are listed in Table 4-3.

The principal developmental tasks that must be mastered during the toddler stage are to:

1. Interact less egocentrically with others.
2. Acquire socially acceptable behaviors.
3. Differentiate self from others.
4. Tolerate separation from key socializing agents (mother or parents).
5. Develop increased verbal communication skills.
6. Tolerate delayed gratification of wants and desires.
7. Control bodily functions (toilet training) and begin self-care (feed and dress self almost completely).

Developmental Tasks of Preschoolers (3 to 6 years)

During the preschooler period, children are focused on developing initiative and purpose. Play provides the means for physical, mental, and social development and becomes the "work" of children as they use it to understand, adjust to, and work out experiences with the environment.

TABLE 4-2 Growth and Development during Infancy

AGE	GROSS MOTOR	FINE MOTOR	LANGUAGE	SENSORY
Birth to 1 month	• Assumes tonic neck posture • When prone lifts and turns head	• Holds hands in fist • Draws arms and legs to body	• Cries	• Comforts with holding and touch • Looks at faces • Follows objects when in line of vision • Alert to high-pitched voices • Smiles
2 to 4 months	• Can raise head and shoulders when prone to 45°–90°; supports self on forearms • Rolls from back to side	• Hands mostly open • Looks at and plays with fingers • Grasps and tries to reach objects	• Vocalizes when talked to; coos, babbles • Laughs aloud • Squeals	• Smiles • Follows objects 180° • Turns head when hears voices or sounds
4 to 6 months	• Turns from stomach to back and then back to stomach • When pulled to sitting almost no head lag • By 6 months can sit on floor with hands forward for support	• Can hold feet and put in mouth • Can hold bottle • Can grasp rattle and other small objects • Puts objects in mouth	• Squeals	• Watches a falling object • Responds to sounds

continues

AGE	GROSS MOTOR	FINE MOTOR	LANGUAGE	SENSORY
6 to 8 months	• Puts full weight on legs when held in standing position • Can sit without support • Bounces when held in a standing position	• Transfers objects from one hand to the other • Can feed self a cookie • Can bang two objects together	• Babbles vowel-like sounds, "ooh" or "aah" • Imitation of speech sounds ("mama," "dada") beginning • Laughs aloud	• Responds by looking and smiling • Recognizes own name
8 to 10 months	• Crawls on all fours or uses arms to pull body along floor • Can pull self to sitting • Can pull self to standing	• Beginning to use thumb-finger grasp • Dominant hand use • Has good hand-mouth coordination	• Responds to verbal commands • May say one word in addition to "mama" and "dada"	• Recognizes sounds
10 to 12 months	• Can sit down from standing • Walks around room holding onto objects • Can stand alone	• Picks up and drops objects • Can put small objects into toys or containers through holes • Turns many pages in a book at one time • Picks up small objects	• Understands "no" and other simple commands • Learns one or two other words • Imitates speech sounds • Speaks gibberish	• Follows fast-moving objects • Indicates wants • Likes to play imitative games such as patty cake and peek-a-boo

TABLE 4-3 Growth and Development during Toddlerhood

AGE	GROSS MOTOR	FINE MOTOR	LANGUAGE	SENSORY
12 to 15 months	• Can walk alone well • Can crawl up stairs	• Can feed self with cup and spoon • Puts raisins into a bottle • May hold crayon or pencil and scribble • Builds a tower of two cubes	• Says four to six words	• Binocular vision is developed
18 months	• Runs, falling often • Can jump in place • Can walk up stairs holding on • Plays with push and pull toys	• Can build a tower of three to four cubes • Can use a spoon	• Says 10 or more words • Points to objects or body parts when asked	• Visual acuity 20/40
24 months	• Can walk up and down stairs • Can kick a ball • Can ride a tricycle	• Can draw a circle • Tries to dress self	• Talks a lot • Approximately 300-word vocabulary • Understands commands • Knows first name, refers to self • Verbalizes toilet needs	
30 months	• Throws a ball • Jumps with both feet • Can stand on one foot for a few minutes	• Can build a tower of eight blocks • Can use crayons • Learning to use scissors	• Knows first and last name • Knows the name of one color • Can sing • Expresses needs • Uses pronouns appropriately	

The preschooler stage of development is characterized by the refinement of many of the tasks that were achieved during the toddler stage and the development of the skills and abilities that prepare children for the significant lifestyle change of starting school. Readiness for school is demonstrated by the increased attention span and memory, ability to interact cooperatively, ability to tolerate prolonged periods of separation from family, and independence in performing basic self-care activities. Key gross and fine motor, language, and sensory milestones associated with the preschooler period are listed in Table 4-4.

Among the principal developmental tasks that must be mastered during the preschooler stage are to:

1. Develop a sense of separateness as an individual.
2. Develop a sense of initiative.
3. Use language for increasing social interaction.
4. Interact in socially acceptable ways with others.
5. Develop a conscience.
6. Identify sex role and function.
7. Develop readiness for school.

Developmental Tasks of School-Age Children (6 to 12 years)

With a well-developed sense of trust, autonomy, and initiative, the school-age child increasingly reduces dependency on the family as the primary socializing agents and moves to the broader world of neighborhood and school peers (primarily same-sex peers) as well as teachers and adult leaders of social, sports, and religious groups. Key gross and fine motor, language, and sensory milestones associated with this period are listed in Table 4-5.

The principal developmental tasks that must be mastered during the school-age stage are to:

1. Become a more active, cooperative, and responsible family member.
2. Learn the rules and norms of a widening social, religious, and cultural environment.
3. Increase psychomotor and cognitive skills needed for participation in games and working with others.
4. Master concepts of time, conservation, and reversibility as well as master oral and written communication skills.
5. Win approval from peers and adults.
6. Obtain a place in a peer group.
7. Build a sense of industry, accomplishment, self-assurance, and self-esteem.
8. Develop a positive self-concept.
9. Exchange affection with family and friends without seeking an immediate payback.
10. Adopt moral standards for behavior.

Developmental Tasks of Adolescents (12 to 18 Years)

The adolescent period is one of struggles and sometimes turmoil as the adolescent strives to develop a personal identity and achieve a successful transition from childhood to adulthood.

Adolescents who have the support and trust of their families as they tackle the developmental tasks of this period are likely to have smooth and successful transitions from the dependency of childhood to the independence of adulthood. If their parents have been too controlling, too permissive, or too confrontational during this period, adolescents will experience difficulty in judging the appropriateness of their behaviors and in forming their self-identity as competent, worthwhile individuals. Key gross and fine motor, language, and sensory milestones associated with this period are listed in Table 4-6.

The principal developmental tasks that must be mastered during the adolescent stage are to:

1. Develop self-identity and appreciate own achievements and worth.
2. Form close relationships with peers.
3. Gradually grow independent from parents.
4. Evolve own value system and integrate self-concept and values with those of peers and society.

TABLE 4-4 Growth and Development during Preschool Years

AGE	GROSS MOTOR	FINE MOTOR	LANGUAGE	SENSORY
3 to 6 years	• Can ride a bike with training wheels • Can throw a ball overhand • Skips and hops on one foot • Can climb well • Can jump rope	• Can draw a six-part person • Can use a scissors • Can draw circle, square, or cross • Likes art projects, likes to paste and string beads • Can button • Learns to tie and buckle shoes • Can brush teeth	• Language skills are well developed with the child able to understand and speak clearly • Vocabulary grows to over 2,000 words • Talks endlessly and asks questions	• Visual acuity well-developed • Focused on learning letters and numbers

TABLE 4-5 Growth and Development during School-Age Years

AGE	GROSS MOTOR	FINE MOTOR	LANGUAGE	SENSORY
6 to 12 years	• Can use in-line skates or ice skates • Able to ride two-wheeler • Plays baseball	• Can put models together • Likes crafts • Enjoys board games, plays cards	• Vocabulary increases • Language abilities continue to develop	• Reading • Able to concentrate on activities for longer periods

TABLE 4-6 Growth and Development during Adolescence

AGE	GROSS MOTOR	FINE MOTOR	LANGUAGE	SENSORY
12 to 19 years	• Muscles continue to develop • At times awkward, with some lack of coordination	• Well-developed skills	• Vocabulary is fully developed	• Development is complete

5. Develop academic and vocational skills and related social, work, and civic sensitivities.
6. Develop analytic thinking.
7. Adjust to rapid physical and sexual changes.
8. Develop a sexual identity and role.
9. Develop skill in relating to people from different backgrounds.
10. Consider and possibly choose a career.

Developmental Tasks of Young Adults (18 to 30 Years)

By young adulthood, motor, language, and sensory skills are fully developed; however, adults continue to work through developmental tasks for the remainder of their natural lives in order to progress through the four stages of adulthood.

Young adulthood is a time of separation and independence from the family and of new commitments, responsibilities, and accountabilities in social, work, and home relationships and roles. These major changes can often lead to conflict between parent and offspring. When parents and young adult offspring are able to resolve normal generational differences in philosophy and lifestyles, mastery of the young adult developmental tasks is greatly facilitated. Among the developmental tasks that the young adult must achieve are to:

1. Establish friendships and a social group.
2. Grow independent of parental care and home.
3. Set up and manage own household.
4. Form an intimate affiliation with another and choose a mate.
5. Learn to love, cooperate with, and commit to a life partner.
6. Develop a personal style of living (e.g., shared or single).
7. Choose and begin to establish a career or vocation.
8. Assume social, work, and civic responsibilities and roles in social, professional, political, religious, and civic organizations.
9. Learn to manage life stresses accompanying change.
10. Achieve a realistic outlook and acceptance of cultural, religious, social, and political diversity.
11. Form a meaningful philosophy of life and implement it in home, employment, and community settings.
12. Begin a parental role for own or life partner's children or for young people in a broader social parenting framework (e.g., teaching, health care, volunteer work).

Developmental Tasks of Early Middle Adulthood (30 to 50 years)

Middle age, spanning the ages of 30 to 70 years, is the longest stage of the life cycle and is often divided into early and late middle adulthood. During early middle adulthood, individuals experience relatively good physical and mental health; settle into their chosen careers, socioeconomic lifestyles, patterns of relationships (married, parental, partnered, single), and political, civic, social, professional, and religious affiliations and activities; and achieve maximum productivity in work and in influence over themselves and their environment. Among the developmental tasks that must be achieved during early middle adulthood are to:

1. Achieve desired level of achievement and status in career.
2. Review, evaluate, refine, and redirect career goals consistent with personal value system.
3. Continue to learn and refine competencies in areas of personal and career interests.
4. Manage life stress accompanying change.
5. Continue developing mature relationships with life partner and significant others.
6. Participate in social, professional, political, religious, and civic activities.
7. Cope with an empty nest and possibly a refilled nest.
8. Adjust to aging parents and help plan for when they will need assistance.
9. Develop currently enjoyable hobbies and leisure activities and begin to develop ones for post retirement.
10. Begin to plan for personal, financial, and social aspects of retirement.

Developmental Tasks of Late Middle Adulthood (50 to 70 years)

During late middle adulthood, many individuals may be diagnosed for the first time with chronic health problems such as arthritis, cardiovascular disease, cancer, diabetes, or asthma. In addition, women generally experience a decrease in estrogen and progesterone production and undergo menopause during their late 40s or early 50s, with ultimate cessation of menses. Men experience decreased testosterone production accompanied by longer erection time, and decreased sperm production during their late 50s and 60s.

Among the developmental tasks that must be achieved during late middle adulthood are to:

1. Manage life stresses accompanying change.
2. Maintain interest in current political, cultural, and scientific advances, trends, and issues.
3. Maintain affiliation with selected social, religious, professional, civic, and political organizations.
4. Adapt to physical and mental changes and health status accompanying aging.
5. Continue current and develop new interests and leisure activities that can be pursued consistent with changing abilities.
6. Adjust to more interaction and time spent with a life partner without the presence of children.
7. Develop supportive, interdependent relationships with adult children.
8. Help elderly parents and relatives cope with lifestyle changes (may include providing a home for them).
9. Adjust to possible or actual loss of parents, life partner, elder family members, and friends through their deaths or their decreasing abilities to maintain independent living and self-care.
10. Prepare for and adjust to changing roles, finances, and lifestyle resulting from retirement.

Developmental Tasks of Late Adulthood (70 Years to Death)

Although a loss of work-related status and social outlets, reduced income, decline in physical and in some cognitive capabilities, decreased resistance to illness, and decreased recuperative powers are inevitable during late adulthood, they are often adjusted to with equanimity.

One of the most important developmental tasks of late adulthood is conducting a life review (Levinson, Darrow, & Klein, 1986). A life review entails reviewing the experiences, relationships, and events of one's life as a whole, viewing successes and failures from the perspective of age and accepting one's life and accompanying life choices and outcomes in their entirety. Successful completion of the life review task provides a sense of having been a meaningful part of human history, provides a sense of integrity, and enables one to face death with equanimity. If one is unsuccessful in achieving the life review developmental task, however, hopelessness, resentment, futility, despair, fear of death, and clinical depression may result.

Among the other developmental tasks that must be achieved during late adulthood are to:

1. Maintain and develop new activities that help retain functional capacities.
2. Accept and adjust to changes in mental and physical strength and agility and in health status.
3. Maintain and develop activities that contribute to a continuing sense of usefulness and self-worth and that enhance self-image.
4. Develop new roles as eldest member in family.
5. Establish affiliation with own age group.
6. Accept and adjust to changing, and possibly restricted circumstances (social, financial, and lifestyle).
7. Adapt to loss of life partner, family members, and friends.
8. Work on life review.
9. Prepare for inevitability of own death.

REFERENCES

Aguilera, D. C. (1994). *Crisis intervention theory and methodology* (7th ed.). Baltimore: Mosby.

Erikson, E. (1974). *Dimensions of a new identity*. New York: W. W. Norton.

Freud, S. (1946). *The ego and the mechanism of defense*. New York: International Universities Press.

Grey, M. (1993). Stressors and children's health. *Journal of Pediatric Nursing, 8*(2), 85–91.

Kohlberg, L. (1981). *The philosophy of moral development: Moral stages and the idea of justice*. New York: Harper & Row.

Levinson, D. J., Darrow, C. N., & Klein, E. B. (1986). *The seasons of a man's life* (2nd ed.). New York: Ballantine.

Piaget, J. (1952). *The origins of intelligence in children*. New York: International Universities Press.

Wykle, M. L., Kahana, E., & Kowal, L. (Eds.). (1992). *Stress & health among the elderly*. New York: Springer.

5

Cultural Assessment

The racial, ethnic, and cultural diversification of American society is accelerating at an unprecedented rate. In 2004, an estimated 69.7% of the U.S. population was Euro-American (predicted to be only 52.8% by the year 2050), and 30.3% were members of ethnic and cultural minority groups: 12.3% African American, 13% Hispanic (the fastest growing minority group in the United States), 4.2% Asian and Pacific Islander, and 0.8% American Indian (U.S. Census Bureau, 2000). These changes in the demographic and ethnic composition of the population make it imperative that nurses be able to communicate effectively with a culturally diverse group of patients; make accurate cultural assessments; and plan, provide, and evaluate culturally competent care. Such care is based on awareness and utilization of knowledge and theories that explain patients' situations and responses within the context of their cultural, ethnic, gender, and sexual orientations (Meleis, 1999; St. Clair & McKenry, 1999; Rundle, Carvalho, & Robinson, 2002; Shearer & Davidhizar, 2003; Campinha-Bacote, 2003).

Culturally Competent Nursing Care

The U.S. health care system reflects the cultural diversity of the United States in that it consists of patients and health care providers from different combinations of ethnic (e.g., Hispanic), racial (e.g., Caucasian), national (e.g., Swiss), religious (e.g., Buddhist), generational (e.g., grandparent), marital (e.g., single), socioeconomic (e.g., middle class), and occupational (e.g., nurse) backgrounds and with different preferences in life partner (e.g., heterosexual), different health status (e.g., handicapped), and different cultural orientations. Nurses must develop a perspective of cultural relativity by viewing health beliefs and behaviors within the context of each patient's culture and by working to deliver culturally competent health care.

Culturally competent nursing care is provided by nurses who use cross-cultural nursing care (nursing care provided within the cultural context of patients who are members of a culture or subculture different from that of the nurse) models and research to identify health care needs and to plan and evaluate the care provided within the cultural context of patients.

Basic Concepts Associated with Culturally Competent Assessments

Culture and Subculture

Culture is a learned and socially transmitted orientation and way of life of a group of people. *Subculture* refers to membership in a smaller group within a larger culture. These smaller groups possess many of the values, beliefs, and customs of the larger culture but have unique characteristics such as age, education, marital status, preference in life partner, generational placement, occupation, socioeconomic level, health status, or religion.

Racial and Ethnic Groups

Race is defined as the classification of individuals based on shared traits, such as skin tone, facial features, and body build, that are inherited from biologic ancestors and are usually sufficiently obvious to warrant classification as a member of that racial group. Members of a given ethnic group share a unique national or regional origin and a unique social, cultural, and linguistic heritage. Five ethnic groups are usually recognized in the United States: whites (of European descent); blacks (of African, Haitian, Jamaican, and Dominican Republic descents); Hispanics (of Spanish-speaking descent); Asian and Pacific Islanders, and Native Americans (Office of the Director of the National Institutes of Health, 1998). Another ethnic group that is increasingly being recognized in the United States is Middle Easterners.

During the health assessment interview, you must avoid stereotyping the patient by depending too heavily on an "ideal" or normative racial, ethnic, or cultural characteristic or trait list. Table 5-1, Echols-Armstrong Cultural Assessment Tool (EACAT), will help you evaluate the patient's needs on the basis of the cultural underpinnings of the patient.

Self-Care Practices

All cultural groups employ a variety of self-care practices that may include the use of folk medicine and home remedies. Self-care includes practices in which persons engage on their own behalf to aid in health promotion and maintenance, disease or injury prevention or protection, and disease or injury treatment. When providing nursing care, be sure to ascertain what self-care and folk remedies are used by the patient and the patient's opinion of their effectiveness.

Assessing the Potential for Harm Associated with a Cultural Belief or Behavior

As a nurse, you are often faced with having to decide when it is appropriate for your cultural value orientation to take precedence over that of the patient.

TABLE 5-1 Echols-Armstrong Cultural Assessment Tool (EACAT)

Directions: **The questions in bold print are recommended for use during the initial contact with the patient.** The remaining items can be used during the initial contact if time permits or if examples are needed to prompt the patient's replies. If a long-term health care relationship or prolonged hospitalization and/or home care is anticipated, it is advisable to complete all remaining questions during subsequent encounters.

1. **ETHNIC GROUP AFFILIATION AND RACIAL BACKGROUND**
   a. **Would you tell me how long you have lived here in** _________?
   b. **Where are you from originally?** (or Where were you born? or Where were your parents or grandparents born and raised?)
   c. **With which particular ethnic group would you say you identify?** (African, Hispanic, English, Asian, Native American, and so forth) **How closely do you identify with this ethnic group or combination of ethnic groups?**
   d. **Where have you lived and when? What health problems did you experience or were you exposed to when you lived in each place? What helped you recover from each of the health problems identified?**

continues

TABLE 5-1 Echols-Armstrong Cultural Assessment Tool (EACAT) *continued*

2. MAJOR BELIEFS AND VALUES

a. What is your primary **time orientation**: past, present, future? What do you believe is the **basic nature of human beings**: basically good, evil but can be perfected, good and evil requiring self-control, or neither good nor evil? What is the **primary purpose of life**: just to be whatever one is; to be who one is while striving for self-improvement; or to exist to be constantly active and achieving, striving for excellence? What is the **purpose of human relations**? Whose goals should take precedence: the family, the community, or the individual? What should be the **relationship between human beings and nature**: humans dominate and control nature; live in harmony with nature; or be subjugated to nature with no control over it?

b. Do you practice any special activities that are part of your cultural traditions?

c. What are your values, beliefs, customs, and practices related to education, work, and leisure?

3. HEALTH BELIEFS AND PRACTICES

a. **What does being healthy mean to you?**

b. What do you believe promotes being healthy?

c. **What do you do to help you stay healthy?** (hygiene, immunizations, self-care practices such as over-the-counter drugs, herbal drinks, special foods, wearing charms)

d. **What does being ill or sick mean to you?**

e. What do you believe causes illness? What do you believe caused your illness?

f. **What do you usually do when you are sick or not feeling well?** (self-care and home remedies, herbal remedies, healing rituals, wearing medals or charms, prayers, relying on folk healers)

g. When you are sick or not feeling well, whom do you go to for help? How helpful are they, and for what type of problems?

h. Who determines when you are and when you are not sick? Who cares for you at home when you are sick? **Who do you want to be with when you are sick?** Who do you want to be with you when you are in the hospital?

i. **Who in your family is primarily responsible for making health care decisions** (such as when to go to someone outside the family for help, where to go, whom to see, what help to accept), **who should be taught how to deal with your** (or your loved one's) **specific health problems** (or what can be taught about how to prevent problems)?

j. What do you believe about mental illness, chronic disease, handicapping conditions, pain, dying, and death?

k. **Are there any cultural or ethnic sanctions or restrictions** (related to the expression of emotions and feelings, privacy, exposure of body parts, response to illness, certain types of surgery, or certain types of medical treatments) **that you want to or must observe?**

l. **By whom do you prefer to have your health and medical care provided: a nurse, physician, or other health care provider? Do you prefer they have the same cultural background** (or be the same age) **or gender as you?**

4. LANGUAGE BARRIERS AND COMMUNICATION STYLES

a. What language(s) or dialect(s) do you speak or read? Which one do you speak most frequently? Where? (home, work, with friends) **In which language are you most comfortable communicating?**

continues

TABLE 5-1 Echols-Armstrong Cultural Assessment Tool (EACAT) *continued*

b. How well do you understand spoken and written English? **Do you need an interpreter when discussing health care information and treatments?** Is there a relative or friend you would prefer to have interpret? Is there anyone you do not want to interpret?

c. Are there special ways of showing respect or disrespect in your culture?

d. Are there any cultural preferences or restrictions related to touching, social distance, making eye contact, or other verbal or nonverbal behaviors when communicating?

e. Are there culturally appropriate forms of greeting, parting, initiating or terminating an exchange, topic restrictions, or times to visit?

---

5. ROLE OF THE FAMILY, SPOUSAL RELATIONSHIP, AND PARENTING STYLES

a. What is the composition of your family? Who is considered to be a member of your family? (Include a genogram and an ecomap if needed.)

b. With what ethnic group(s) does your family as a whole (parents, aunts and uncles, cousins) **identify?** How do their ethnic identity and ethnic traditions affect the decision-making processes of your own family? **How does their ethnic identity and which of their ethnic traditions do you think most affect their health status?**

c. Which of your relatives live nearby? With which of your family members and relatives do you interact the most often?

d. How do each of your family members, relatives, and you and your significant other interact in relation to chores, mealtimes, child care, recreation, and other family-oriented responsibilities? Are you satisfied with these interactional patterns?

e. What are the major events that are most important to your family (marriage, birth, holidays, religious ceremonies), and how are they celebrated?

f. What are your family's goals for the health and well-being of the family as a group? What dreams do they have for the family's future? Do they work together as a family unit or individually to achieve these goals and dreams? What barriers do they see that might inhibit the accomplishment of these goals and dreams?

g. In what ways do your family members believe the nurse, physician, and other health care practitioners can help the family members achieve their goals and dreams for the health and well-being of the family?

h. With what social (church, community, work, recreation) groups does your family interact, and what is the nature of their social contact and social support?

i. Are there special beliefs and customs practiced by your family related to marriage, conception, pregnancy, childbirth, breastfeeding, baptism, child care (including attitude toward children, discipline, showing affection), puberty, separation, divorce, health, illness, and death?

j. What are the family members' health and social history including health habits, recent major stress events, work patterns, participation in religion, community activities, and recreation patterns?

---

6. RELIGIOUS INFLUENCES OR SPECIAL RITUALS (see Chapter 6)

---

7. DIETARY PRACTICES (see Chapter 7).

You must evaluate and decide when a patient's behavior is adaptive, harmful, or neutral. Sprott (1993) has suggested that nurses might make these judgments using Korbin's (1977) work on assessing whether an ethnic group's child-rearing practices constitute harm.

The conditions cited in Korbin's schema have relevance for evaluating the potential physical or psychological harm that health practices may have on a family member as perceived by health professionals or the agents of the family. When this schema is used, a practice would not be considered harmful if:

1. The practice actually reflects a practice that is sanctioned by that culture.
2. The practice is within the limits of deviations that are acceptable in that culture.
3. The practice is important for the acceptance of the patient as a member of that culture.
4. The patient on whom the practice will be carried out perceives that it is an appropriate practice in that situation.
5. The intent of the health care provider or agent of the family is consistent with the cultural "rules" that govern the practice.

For many situations, these five conditions can be quite helpful in clarifying the issues associated with evaluating whether an anticipated health practice is harmful.

REFERENCES

Campinha-Bacote, J. (2003). Many faces: Addressing diversity in health care. *Online Journal of Issues in Nursing, 8*(1). Retrieved March 15, 2004, from http://nursingworld.org/ojin/topic20/tcp20_2.htm

Korbin, J. (1977). Anthropological contributions to the study of child abuse. *Child Abuse and Neglect, 1*(1), 7–24.

Meleis, A. (1999). Culturally competent care. *Journal of Transcultural Nursing, 10,* 12.

Meleis, A. (2003). Egyptians. In P. Hill, J. G. Lipson, & A. I. Meleis (Eds.), *Caring for women cross-culturally* (pp. 123–141). Philadelphia: F. A. Davis.

Office of the Director of the National Institutes of Health. (1998). *Women of color health data book: Adolescents to seniors* (NIH Publication No. 98-4247). Bethesda, MD: National Institutes of Health, U.S. Department of Health and Human Services.

Rundle, A., Carvalho, M., & Robinson, M. R. (2002). *Cultural competence in healthcare: A practical guide.* San Francisco: Jossey-Bass.

Shearer, R., & Davidhizer, R. (2003). Using role-play to develop cultural competence. *Journal of Nursing Education, 42*(6), 273–276.

Sprott, J. E. (1993). The black box in family assessment: Cultural diversity. In S. L. Feetham, S. B. Meister, J. M. Bell, & C. L. Gilliss (Eds.), *The nursing of families: Theory, research, education, practice* (pp. 189–199). Norwalk, CT: Sage Publications.

St. Clair, A., & McKenry, L. (1999). Preparing culturally competent practitioners. *Journal of Nursing Education, 38*(5), 228–234.

U.S. Census Bureau, Population Division, Population Projections Branch. (2000). *Population projections of the United States by age, sex, race, Hispanic origin, and nativity: 1999 to 2100.* Retrieved December 23, 2004, from http://www.census.gov/population/www/projections/natsum-T7.html

6

Spiritual Assessment

Spiritual beliefs may be a factor in determining whether a patient will keep a clinic appointment, follow a diet, take medications, agree to surgery, or execute a living will. Further, recent studies have indicated that regular attendance at worship is positively associated with better health and longer life (Koenig & Cohen, 2002; Helm, Hays, & Koenig, 2000; Musick, Blazer, & Hays, 2000), and that prayer may positively influence a patient's outcome after surgery (Matthews & Clark, 1999; Koenig & Cohen, 2002). Patients' religious and spiritual beliefs can have an impact on their entrance into and response to health care. It is imperative to holistic nursing, that is, nursing that addresses all aspects of a patient's health and well-being, that spirituality and religion in patient care be addressed

Spirituality and Religion

Spirituality is the concern for the meaning and purpose of life. Spirituality integrates values and ultimate concern with oneself and one's relationship with a higher power and the surrounding environment. Spiritual beliefs help the individual define the self and the self's ultimate purpose in life. An example of spirituality is the belief that animals and human beings are both living beings that can feel pain and joy and that animals must therefore be treated with the same respect shown to humans.

By contrast, *religion* is an organized system of beliefs that is usually centered around the worship of a supernatural force or being and that in turn defines the self and the self's purpose in life. Religion exists in group form over time and is a tradition of shared beliefs. An example of a religion is Judaism. Followers of the Jewish faith worship Yahweh (God) and define humans as the special creations of God who must worship God.

A goal of nursing is to support the patient's spiritual well-being. Familiarity with various religions may help you as you work with patients. Table 6-1 describes certain religions and how they view sentinel events from birth to death.

Role of the Nurse in Spiritual Care

The nurse's role in the spiritual care of the patient includes:

1. Performing a spiritual assessment.
2. Making a nursing diagnosis based on the assessment.
3. Planning, implementing, and evaluating appropriate strategies for spiritual care.

Spiritual Assessment

1. The spiritual assessment should obtain the following information:
    a. The nature of the patient's spiritual beliefs
    b. The nature of the patient's spiritual support

TABLE 6-1 Religions and Health Care

RELIGION	JUDAISM	ISLAM	ROMAN CATHOLICISM
Description	A monotheistic religion that believes God has chosen the Jewish people and made a covenant with them to protect and preserve them if they follow God's laws.	A monotheistic religion following the teachings of the Prophet Mohammed.	A monotheistic religion and an offshoot of Judaism. Basis of belief is that God exists in three forms: God (Father), Jesus (Son), and the Holy Spirit. Jesus, as the Son of God, was sent to die on the cross for the sins of humanity and was subsequently resurrected from the dead.
Religious Leaders	Rabbi; cantor; mohel	Imam	Pope; archbishop; bishop; priest (father); monk (brother); nun (sister)
Sabbath	Sundown Friday to sundown Saturday	Friday	Sunday
Holy Books	Bible; Torah	Koran	Bible, including several books not found in the Hebrew or Protestant Bibles
Dietary Restrictions	Strict dietary laws, Kosher, prohibit shellfish and pork or any other meat from an animal with a cloven hoof. Meat must be ritualistically slaughtered. Meat and dairy products must not be taken together.	Pork and pork by-products, such as gelatin and lard, are forbidden. Alcohol and street drugs are also forbidden.	There is a tradition of not eating meat on Friday during Lent.

continues

TABLE 6-1 Religions and Health Care *continued*

RELIGION	JUDAISM	ISLAM	ROMAN CATHOLICISM
Withdrawal of Life Support	Active euthanasia and assisted suicide are forbidden. Termination of life support is allowed only to reduce suffering.	Active euthanasia and assisted suicide are forbidden. Termination of life support is allowed only to reduce suffering.	Active euthanasia and suicide are forbidden. Termination of life support is allowed only to reduce suffering.
Beliefs Associated with Death	Autopsies are controversial but permitted. Burial should be within 24 hours of death. Cremation is forbidden.	Relatives and friends are normally present. Men wash a man's body, and women wash a woman's body. Burial should be without delay.	Prayers are common "last rites." Burial or cremation is permitted. Autopsies are allowed.
Organ Donation	Organ donation and the receipt of transplanted organs are permitted.	Organ donation and the receipt of transplanted organs are permitted.	Organ donation is permitted.
Medical Treatment	Obligation to take care of oneself encourages medical treatment when needed.	Healing the sick is highly revered. Seeking medical treatment is encouraged.	Obligation to take care of oneself encourages medical treatment when needed.
Birth Control	Birth control is allowed within marriage.	Teachings appear contradictory, but in general, birth control within marriage is permitted.	Birth control is forbidden. Natural family planning is permitted.
Abortion	Reluctantly permits abortion to save the life of the mother.	Forbidden after the fetus is "ensouled," at either 40 or 120 days. Paternal permission is required.	Abortion is prohibited.
Birth Observances	Circumcision is performed on all males, traditionally at 8 days.	Upon birth, the closest male relative or the mother whispers the central tenet of Islam into the baby's ear.	Prayers and blessings are common. Baptism is a sacrament that should be performed shortly after birth.

continues

RELIGION	PROTESTANT	BUDDHISM	HINDUISM
Description	A monotheistic religion emphasizing the Bible and the individual's interpretation of it.	A varied, intellectual, and psychological religion originating with the teachings of Siddhartha Guatama (Buddha).	A complex religion embracing a variety of gods, practices, and spiritual paths.
Religious Leaders	Priest; minister; pastor	Monk; nun	Priest; guru; sadhu; yogi
Sabbath	Sunday	All days are holy.	No particular holy day
Holy Books	Bible	*Tibetan Book of the Dead; Buddha Dharma*	*Vedas; Upanishads; Bhagavad Gita*
Dietary Restrictions	There are no dietary restrictions.	Vegetarianism is common.	Cattle are sacred; no beef is taken. Dairy products are a staple.
Withdrawal of Life Support	Withdrawal of life support is permitted to reduce suffering.	Withdrawal of life support is permitted to reduce suffering.	Withdrawal of life support is permitted to reduce suffering.
Beliefs Associated with Death	Prayers are common. Anointing the sick and laying on of hands may be practiced.	Cremation is common. After death, the body should not be disturbed by movement, talking, or crying.	Holy water is poured into the mouth of the dying person. Autopsies are discouraged. The body should not be embalmed. Cremation is common, normally within 24 hours.

continues

TABLE 6-1 Religions and Health Care *continued*

RELIGION	PROTESTANT	BUDDHISM	HINDUISM
Organ Donation	Organ donation and the receipt of transplanted organs are permitted. Some sects are against donation.	Organ donation is controversial.	Organ donation is discouraged because it disturbs the body after death.
Medical Treatment	Same as for Roman Catholicism, although some sects emphasize prayer over medical treatment.	Medical treatment to enhance life is encouraged.	Obligation to take care of oneself encourages medical treatment when needed.
Birth Control	Birth control is permitted.	Birth control is discouraged.	Birth control is discouraged.
Abortion	Reluctantly permits abortion to save the life of the mother.	Permission for abortion is circumstantial.	Abortion is discouraged.
Birth Observances	Prayers and blessings are common.	The child is dedicated to Buddha.	A naming ceremony is performed on the 10th or 11th day.

   c. How the patient's spiritual beliefs affect the treatment of health and illness
   d. The patient's state of spiritual well-being or spiritual distress
2. Begin the interview with the physical history of the patient. Move on to the psychological history and end with the spiritual history.
3. Ask the patient whether he or she has an advance directive (Living Will or Durable Medical Power of Attorney) that states what should be done if the patient is too ill to self-direct medical care.
4. Ask the patient whether he or she has signed an organ donor card or given any thought to donating organs or tissue after death.
5. Ask the patient whether he or she holds any spiritual or religious beliefs that will affect the health care received.
6. While conducting the interview, observe the patient for clues about spiritual beliefs. Is the patient wearing any religious clothing or jewelry, such as a yarmulke, cross, or turban?
7. Ask the patient who should be notified in the event of a change in the patient's condition. After noting this, ask whether the patient also wants you to notify a place of worship or a specific religious leader.
8. Document the answers to these questions in the patient's chart. It is important to record in an easily accessible place whether the patient has an advance directive or is an organ donor. If the patient names a particular religion, you should ask whether he or she would like you to call that place of worship or a specific religious leader under certain circumstances, such as if the patient must be admitted to a hospital. Chart this information also.

Nursing Diagnosis

NANDA nursing diagnoses that address the spiritual care of the patient include *Spiritual distress, Risk for spiritual distress, Readiness for enhanced spiritual well-being, Impaired religiosity,* and *Readiness for enhanced religiosity.*

Planning and Implementation

Once a nursing diagnosis has been made, you can plan and implement nursing interventions for the patient. The following interventions are appropriate for all three spiritual nursing diagnoses:

1. Listen actively.
2. Project an empathetic, warm, interested response to the patient's concerns.
3. Show respect for the patient's spiritual beliefs.
4. Give the patient (and family) permission to practice their religion and spirituality if they wish to do so.
5. Make appropriate referrals to the hospital chaplain or the patient's own spiritual or religious leader.
6. Provide support for the patient's practice of religion.
7. Coordinate nursing care with respect to the patient's beliefs.

Several interventions you should avoid with regard to the patient's spirituality are as follows:

1. Do not proselytize your own spiritual beliefs.
2. Do not instruct the patient in religious or spiritual doctrine.
3. Do not perform the role of spiritual adviser to the patient.
4. Do not respond to the patient with clichés such as "there's always someone who's worse off than you" or "it's God's will." Such clichés are inappropriate and do not diminish the anguish of the patient (Linn, 1986).

Evaluation

Evaluate the effect of your nursing interventions by observing the patient. Signs that the patient's spiritual distress has decreased include:

1. Acceptance of spiritual support from the source with whom the patient feels most comfortable
2. Decrease in crying, restlessness, sleeplessness, and, possibly, complaints of pain or the severity of pain
3. Decrease in statements of worthlessness and hopelessness

4. Verbalization of satisfaction with spiritual beliefs and the support and comfort they provide

REFERENCES

Helm, H., Hays, J. C., & Koenig, H. G. (2000). Does private religious activity prolong survival? A six-year follow-up study of 3851 older adults. *Journal of Gerontology: Social Sciences, 55A*, M400–M405.

Koenig, H. G., & Cohen, H. J. (Eds.). (2002). *The link between religion and health: Psychoneuroimmunology and the faith factor.* New York: Oxford University Press.

Linn, E. (1986). *I know just how you feel: Avoiding the clichés of grief.* Incline Village, NV: The Publisher's Mark.

Matthews, D., & Clark, C. (1999). *The faith factor: Proof of the healing power of prayer.* Penguin University Press.

Musick, M. A., Blazer, D. G., & Hays, J. C. (2000). Religious activity, alcohol use and depression in a sample of elderly Baptists. *Research on Aging*, 22, 91–116.

BIBLIOGRAPHY

O'Brien, M. E. (2003). *Parish nursing: Health care ministry with the church.* Paulist Press.

Shelly, J. A. (2000). *Spiritual care: A guide for caregivers.* Intervarsity Press.

7

Nutritional Assessment

Nutrition, or the processes by which the body metabolizes and utilizes nutrients, affects every system in the body. Health care providers must understand how the body digests and absorbs nutrients, the importance of meeting daily nutritional requirements, the causes and results of an imbalance of nutrients, and how to assess nutritional imbalances. Psychological, social, and cultural issues must also be considered during the nutritional assessment.

Dietary Guidelines

Dietary guidelines are published by various government agencies to educate the general population regarding dietary needs. In 1997, the Food and Nutrition Board of the Institute of Medicine developed Dietary Reference Intakes (DRIs). DRIs are used to assess an individual's diet and are the basis on which nutritious, balanced diets are devised. DRIs have three components: Adequate Intake (AI), Tolerable Upper Intake Level (UL), and Recommended Dietary Allowances (RDA). AI is the intake value specific for each sex and various age groups that is estimated to provide adequate nutrition. UL is the maximum level of daily nutrients that is unlikely to pose health risks for most of the general population. Recommended dietary allowances (RDA) are the recommended amounts of nutrients that should be eaten daily by healthy individuals. Recommendations differ based on sex, age, and whether the patient is pregnant or lactating. These are recommendations, not requirements. Requirements are the amounts needed to prevent deficiencies. Recommendations exceed the required amounts in order to ensure that the entire population is considered.

The Dietary Guidelines Advisory Committee published the *Dietary Guidelines for Americans* in 2005. The U.S. Department of Health and Human Services and the U.S. Department of Agriculture use this information to formulate programs and policies for the American public. In 2005, the USDA published a new food guidance system entitled MyPyramid. The MyPyramid plan offers individuals a more personalized approach to nutrition that combines healthy eating with physical activity. For a description of the MyPyramid system, see Figure 7-1.

Nutrients

Nutrients are the substances found in food that are nourishing and useful to the body. Carbohydrates, proteins, fats, vitamins, minerals, and water are the nutrients essential for life. Carbohydrates, proteins, and fats supply the body with energy, which is measured in units called kilocalories (kcal). A kilocalorie (also called calorie) is the amount of heat required to raise 1 gram of water 1 degree centigrade.

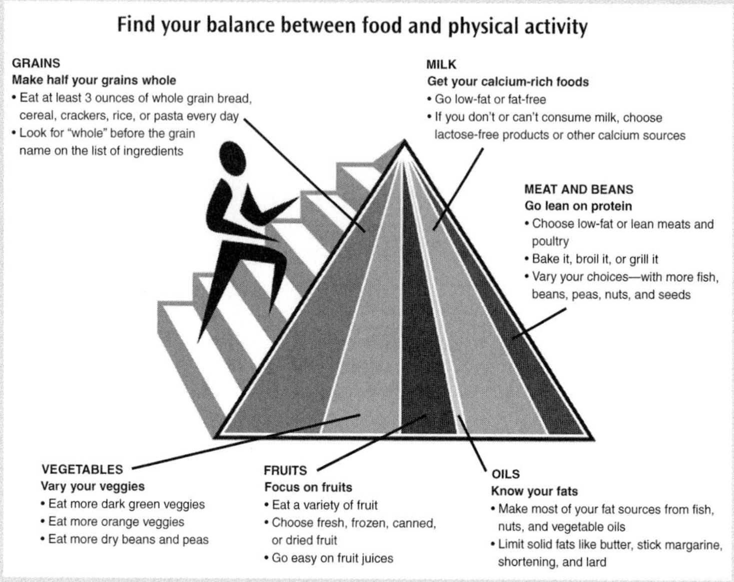
Find your balance between food and physical activity
GRAINS
Make half your grains whole
• Eat at least 3 ounces of whole grain bread, cereal, crackers, rice, or pasta every day
• Look for "whole" before the grain name on the list of ingredients
MILK
Get your calcium-rich foods
• Go low-fat or fat-free
• If you don't or can't consume milk, choose lactose-free products or other calcium sources
MEAT AND BEANS
Go lean on protein
• Choose low-fat or lean meats and poultry
• Bake it, broil it, or grill it
• Vary your choices—with more fish, beans, peas, nuts, and seeds
VEGETABLES
Vary your veggies
• Eat more dark green veggies
• Eat more orange veggies
• Eat more dry beans and peas
FRUITS
Focus on fruits
• Eat a variety of fruit
• Choose fresh, frozen, canned, or dried fruit
• Go easy on fruit juices
OILS
Know your fats
• Make most of your fat sources from fish, nuts, and vegetable oils
• Limit solid fats like butter, stick margarine, shortening, and lard

Note. *From* Inside MyPyramid, *by the U.S. Department of Agriculture, 2005, retrieved April 21, 2005, from http://www.mypyramid.gov/pyramid.*

Dietary Guidelines for Americans, 2005 serve as the U.S. federal nutrition policy (USDHHS and USDA, 2005). These guidelines form the basis for the MyPyramid food guidance system unveiled in April 2005. MyPyramid is applicable to Americans over age 2. By introducing all Americans to MyPyramid and its slogan, "Steps to a Healthier You," the USDA hopes to help people make informed and healthier food choices. These choices can lead to a decrease in major nutrition-related chronic diseases, such as anemia, diabetes mellitus, coronary heart disease, hypertension, and alcoholic cirrhosis.

MyPyramid is the former Food Guide Pyramid tipped on its side. The color bands in MyPyramid represent the types of foods that should be consumed, and the width of the band denotes the approximate relative quantity of each food that should be consumed. In addition, MyPyramid incorporates the concept of physical activity into its design. A person climbing the stairs denotes the importance of physical activity in one's daily life, just as the food groups denote daily food intake. Personalization of one's diet is easier to accomplish by accessing the MyPyramid.gov Web site, where age, gender, and physical activity can be keyed in and more specific nutrition guidelines are provided. Twelve different pyramids are available on the web site using these parameters. The 12 pyramids range from daily intake levels of 1,000 to 3,200 calories. By following the appropriate pyramid, the individual should be able to maintain a healthy body weight and decrease the risk of nutrition-related chronic diseases. Quantities are stated in household measures such as cups and ounces instead of the servings that were used in the Food Guide Pyramid.

Figure 7-1 Steps to a Healthier You: MyPyramid

Carbohydrates

Carbohydrates constitute the major source of energy for the various functions of the body. Each gram of carbohydrate contains 4 calories. Adults require 50 to 100 grams of carbohydrate per day to prevent carbohydrate deficiencies (ketosis and protein breakdown of muscles). This constitutes approximately 50% to 60% of daily caloric intake.

Carbohydrates help form adenosine triphosphate (ATP), which is needed to transfer energy within the cells. Carbohydrates supply fiber and assist in the utilization of fat. The primary sources of carbohydrates are bread, potatoes, pasta, corn, rice, dried beans, and fruits. A deficiency of carbohydrates in the diet may result in electrolyte imbalance, fatigue, and depression. An excess of carbohydrates may result in obesity and tooth decay and may adversely affect persons with diabetes mellitus.

Proteins

There are 4 calories in every gram of protein, and foods are usually a combination of protein and fat (meats, milk) or protein and carbohydrate (legumes). Adults require 0.8 g/kg/day of protein, or approximately 10% to 20% of daily caloric intake. Protein is required to give the body the nine essential amino acids, which are the amino acids that the body is unable to synthesize. These acids are needed to form the basis of all cell structures in the body. The major sources of protein are meat, poultry, fish, eggs, cheese, and milk. Legumes (dried beans and peas) are a good source of protein when eaten with cereal grains; for example, beans and rice provide a good source of protein.

Fats

Lipids, or fats, contain 9 calories per gram. The recommendation of many health care experts is to reduce fat intake to 20% to 30% of total calories consumed. Fats supply the essential fatty acids, which form part of the structure of all cells. They also help lower serum cholesterol. Essential fatty acids must be supplied by the diet. The food sources of fat are animal fat (butter, shortening, lard) and vegetable fat (vegetable oil, margarine, nuts). Saturated fats come from animal sources (butter, lard, fatty meats) and vegetable sources (coconut, palm, and partially hydrogenated oils, which are present in some processed foods). Saturated fats have been found to raise cholesterol levels. Monosaturated fats (olive and canola oils) lower low-density lipoproteins (LDLs) and do not lower high-density lipoproteins (HDLs). Cholesterol is a lipid found only in animal products. It is found in muscle, red blood cells, and cell membranes. Cholesterol is transported in the blood by HDLs and LDLs. The HDLs carry cholesterol toward the liver. The LDLs carry cholesterol toward the cells and the tissues and deposits it there. There is a strong association between high levels of LDLs and coronary artery disease (CAD); high levels of HDLs protect against CAD.

Triglycerides account for most of the lipids stored in the body's tissues. In the bloodstream, triglycerides produce energy for the body. An elevated triglyceride level occurs in hyperlipidemia, a risk factor for CAD.

A deficiency of fat in the diet can result in decreased weight, lack of satiety, and skin and hair changes. Excess fat in the diet contributes to obesity and is linked to CAD. There is also a correlation between a high-fat diet and certain cancers (colon, breast, and prostate cancers, in particular).

Vitamins

Vitamins are organic substances needed to maintain body function. They are not supplied by the body except in inadequate amounts and must therefore be obtained from dietary sources. Vitamins stored in dietary fat and absorbed in the fat portions of the body's cells are fat-soluble vitamins. These are vitamins A, D, E, and K. Water-soluble vitamins include vitamin C, thiamine (B_1), riboflavin (B_2), niacin, pyridoxine (B_6), folacin (folate), cobalamin (B_{12}), pantothenic acid, and biotin. They are not stored in the body and are excreted in the urine. Various disease conditions occur when a vitamin is lacking.

Minerals

Minerals are inorganic elements that build body tissue and regulate body processes such as fluid balance; acid-base balance; nerve impulse transmission; muscle contractions; and vitamin, enzyme, and hormonal activity. Minerals are divided into two classifications. Macrominerals are needed in large amounts by the body (>100 mg/day). Microminerals, or trace minerals, are needed in smaller amounts by the body (<15 mg/day).

Water

Water is essential to life; we cannot survive more than a few days without it. Water accounts for 50% to 60% of the body's weight. The daily amount needed depends on the size of the person, the climate, and the amount of activity. The average adult needs 6 to 8 cups of water per day; athletes and persons living in hot, dry climates require more. Thirst may not always be an adequate indicator of water intake needs; infants and very ill individuals, for example, may have poor thirst mechanisms, and persons who engage in intense physical activity may have a decreased thirst sensation.

> **Nursing Alert**
>
> **Signs and Symptoms of Dehydration**
>
> - Health history reveals inadequate fluid intake.
> - Decrease in urine output.
> - Urine specific gravity is >1.035.
> - Weight loss (% body weight): 3% to 5% for mild, 6% to 9% for moderate, and 10% to 15% for severe dehydration.
> - Eyes appear sunken, tongue has increased furrows and fissures.
> - Oral mucous membranes are dry.
> - Decreased skin turgor.
> - Sunken fontanels in infants.
> - Changes in neurological status may occur with moderate to severe dehydration.

Nutrition through the Life Cycle

The patient's developmental needs must always be assessed as part of the nutritional assessment. Nutrition needs change throughout the life cycle and are affected by both physical and developmental changes.

Children

Recommended daily requirements for children vary according to age group. An understanding of development with regard to physical, cognitive, and psychosocial changes is needed to properly assess the nutritional needs of children. In addition, the caregiver should be educated about these changes before they occur.

Infants

Humans grow more during the first 6 to 12 months of life than at any other time. Infancy is also characterized by many significant neurological changes. Proper nutrients are thus needed for growth and development. The American Academy of Pediatrics recommends the use of breast milk rather than formula for the first 6 to

> **Nursing Tip**
>
> **Nutritional Assessment of Infants**
>
> Ask whether the infant is ever put to bed with a bottle. If so, instruct the caregivers about infant bottle caries and the importance of not propping the bottle or placing it in the bed. (If the caregivers do not want to comply, try to get them to put only water in the bottle.)

Nursing Tip

Infant Feeding Guidelines

Birth to 6 months: breast milk or infant formula only. Increases gradually to 28 to 32 oz per day by the third to fourth month of life.

4 to 6 months: iron-fortified cereals. Rice cereal is the least allergenic and is usually introduced first. Wheat cereals are usually not added until after 6 months of age. Help the infant adjust to spoon-feeding. Offer only one new food every 3 to 4 days to observe for signs or allergic reactions. Do not use mixed foods that may have other ingredients added.

5 to 8 months: fruits and vegetables. Encourage parents to read the labels of all foods to determine what has been added. Fruit juices that are noncitrus may be introduced. It is helpful to use a cup. Using a cup prevents the infant from associating sweet fruit juices with a bottle and also limits the amount ingested. Do not add sugar or seasoning to foods. Introduce egg yolks, then gradually introduce meats last.

9 to 10 months: finger foods may be introduced. Small, bite-sized pieces that are cooked, mashed, and soft will allow the child independence and will provide increased texture that requires chewing. Gradually increase foods with texture as the child's chewing skills improve and teeth emerge.

12 months of life. Even a few weeks of breastfeeding is beneficial, except in cases in which the mother is HIV positive, because HIV disease can be transmitted via breast milk.

Toddlers

Toddlers have their own unique nutrition needs as their physical growth slows. As children experience increased independence and control over their body, some of this independence is demonstrated via their eating patterns. There is an increased problem with food refusal or the desire for only certain foods. This is a normal response to the developmental stage and should not be a problem unless it becomes excessive. To demonstrate they are in charge, toddlers may say "no" even to foods they desire.

Instruct caregivers to offer foods the toddler can self-feed in small portions and to offer only one new food at a time. A serving size should be approximately 1 to 2 tablespoons of food for each year of age. Toddlers are very good at imitating and often exhibit food dislikes that are shown at home (particularly if there is an older sibling). Provide the toddler with role models for developing good eating habits and encourage routine mealtimes that are enjoyed together.

Nursing Alert

Preventing Choking

Instruct caregivers to:

1. Avoid serving foods that may cause choking in infants and small children (up to 3 years old), such as corn, nuts, small candies, hot dogs, popcorn, raw peas, carrots, and celery, and any other small, hard foods.
2. Offer peanut butter only on bread or a cracker.
3. Stress the importance of sitting up while eating; prohibit running with food or objects in the mouth.

Preschoolers

Preschoolers continue to have food dislikes and become picky eaters. Giving choices, serving small amounts of foods children can easily eat (finger foods), and providing a routine and enjoyable eating environment help foster good eating habits by decreasing conflicts.

Preschoolers often have a smaller appetite than toddlers. This reduction in appetite may be caused by excessive beverage consumption (e.g., milk, juice, or Koolaid) and a slowing of growth. Preschoolers often are resistant to new foods and may eat only one food at a time. Encourage the offering of healthy snacks and discourage the offering of foods that are too high in sugar.

School-Age Children

School-age children tend to have erratic growth patterns that are reflected in equally erratic eating patterns. They also tend to continue having strong likes and dislikes. Encourage families to maintain a balanced diet and to limit highly sweetened snacks and foods. Caregivers should be encouraged to teach children proper nutrition and to show children how to read nutrition and ingredient labels. Advise caregivers and children that pubescent chubbiness is a normal part of growth and that it often precedes a rapid increase in height, but monitor for childhood obesity.

Adolescents

Adolescence is a period of rapid growth and change, and the nutritional needs of adolescents fluctuate accordingly. Adolescents typically are concerned with body image and often compare their bodies with those of their peers in an attempt to fit into an identity that is acceptable to them. A poor body image can lead to eating disorders such as anorexia nervosa, bulimia, and obesity. Although anorexia nervosa and bulimia can occur at any age, they are frequently seen in adolescents.

Young and Middle-Aged Adults

Growth and caloric needs usually stabilize in young and middle-aged adults. Eating habits may be altered by changes in activity levels and the effects of work and life stressors. The onset of obesity often occurs during young or middle adulthood.

Obesity is a weight greater than 120% of the ideal body weight (IBW). Obesity occurs when calories consumed are greater than calories expended and can result from an increase in food consumption, a decrease in activity level, or both. Many factors affect whether a person is prone to obesity, including genetic, physiological, psychological, and environmental factors. Obesity places a person at risk for hyperlipidemia, CAD, hypertension, diabetes mellitus, and chronic disorders.

Pregnant and Lactating Women

Promotion of a healthy pregnancy requires assessing and counseling the pregnant woman regarding nutrition. Proper nutrition for the mother from the time of conception is needed for the development of a healthy infant. The infant is at risk of being small for gestational age if the woman does not gain adequate weight, and the woman is at risk for gestational diabetes and hypertension if weight gain is excessive. Target weight gain is dependent on the woman's weight at conception. The woman at IBW should gain 24 to 28 pounds; the woman more than 20% over IBW should gain 15 to 20 pounds; and the woman 10% under IBW should gain 30 to 35 pounds. General knowledge of physical changes and their relationships to nutrition should be evaluated as part of the nutritional assessment of the pregnant woman. Some of the common complaints experienced during pregnancy (e.g., heartburn, constipation, nausea, and vomiting) can be alleviated via dietary changes such as small, frequent meals, increased fluid intake, and a well-balanced diet.

Iron supplements are given routinely during pregnancy because diet alone is not adequate in meeting the body's increased requirements. Prenatal vitamins are usually prescribed for all pregnant women. There is evidence that folic acid helps reduce the risk of neural tube defects, especially when the folic acid supplement is instituted 3 months before pregnancy. In fact, the U.S. Public Health Service recommends that all women of childbearing age consume 0.4 mg of folic acid per day. An additional 300 calories per day is recommended during pregnancy, and an additional 500 calories per day during lactation; also recommended is an increase in milk consumption, which increases both protein and caloric intake. Fluid intake is important, and pregnant women are thus encouraged to consume 6 to 8 glasses of fluid daily (in the form of water, fruit juices, and milk). Adequate fluid consumption helps decrease the risk of premature onset of labor caused by dehydration. Lactating women also need to increase fluid intake and may need 2 to 3 quarts of fluid daily to maintain adequate milk production.

Pica, or cravings for substances other than food, is a phenomenon documented primarily in pregnant women. It is the practice of eating dirt, clay, starch, or even ice cubes and may increase the risk of nutritional difficulties such as anemia.

Older Adults

Because of a reduction in basal metabolic rate, caloric needs decrease as a person ages. For older adults, stress the need to decrease portion size in proportion to reduced activity and caloric requirements.

Problems that may be noted when assessing the older adult include difficulty chewing (dentition problems), difficulty swallowing (possible stroke or Parkinson's disease), decreased appetite, decreased ability to feed self, and decreased taste and smell. There is also a decreased emptying time of the esophagus, making the older adult susceptible to aspiration. The older adult should eat in a sitting position to prevent aspiration. Constipation, resulting from a decrease in gastrointestinal motility, is a common problem that can be alleviated via adequate fluid intake and consumption of high-fiber foods.

Equipment

- Wall-mounted unit (stadiometer), rod attached to a scale that has a right-angle headboard
- Tape measure
- Scale (preferably a balance-beam scale or electronic scale)
- Skinfold calipers (ideally with a spring-loaded lever)

Nutritional Assessment

Table 7-1 illustrates a comprehensive nutritional assessment, including nutritional history, physical assessment, anthropometric measurements, and laboratory and diagnostic data. Table 7-2 outlines a diet history.

Physical Assessment

Certain physical signs may indicate poor nutrition. See Table 7-3 for a list of signs and symptoms of poor nutritional status.

Anthropometric Measurements

Anthropometric measurements are the various measurements of the human body, including height, weight, and body proportions. They measure growth patterns in children and changes in nutritional status in adults.

Height

A standing height is obtained for patients 3 years of age and older.

E 1. Have the patient stand erect and with the back and heels against the wall or measuring device.
2. Place the headboard at a right angle to the wall and along the crown of the patient's head.
3. Record height to the nearest ⅛ inch or 1 mm.

N **Compare with standardized growth charts and height at last visit. Note: Patients will reflect familial growth patterns.**

A Insufficient growth

P Chronic malnutrition

P Genetic disorder (dwarfism)

Nursing Tip

Measuring Height of the Bedridden Patient

When a patient is bedridden or immobile, use a rod or yardstick to measure recumbent length.

TABLE 7-1 Comprehensive Nutritional Assessment

NUTRITIONAL HISTORY (refer to Diet History format from Table 7-2)

PHYSICAL ASSESSMENT

1. General appearance
2. Skin
3. Nails
4. Hair
5. Eyes
6. Mouth
7. Head and neck
8. Heart and peripheral vasculature
9. Abdomen
10. Musculoskeletal system
11. Neurological system
12. Female genitalia

ANTHROPOMETRIC MEASUREMENTS

Height: ________ in or cm
Weight: ________ lb or kg
% Ideal Body Weight: ________
% Usual Body Weight: ________
% Weight Change: ________
Body Mass Index: ________
Waist/Hip Ratio: ________
Triceps Skinfold: ________ mm
Mid-Arm Circumference: ________ cm
Mid-Arm Muscle Circumference: ________ cm

LABORATORY DATA

Hematocrit (HCT): ________% Hemoglobin (HGB): ________ g/dl
Cholesterol: ________ mg/dl HDL: ________ mg/dl LDL: ________ mg/dl
Triglycerides: ________ mg/dl
Transferrin: ________ mg/dl
TIBC: ________ μg/dl
Iron: ________ μg/dl
Total Lymphocyte Count: ________ cells/mm^3
Antigen Skin Testing: ________
Prealbumin: ________ mg/dl Albumin: ________ g/dl
Glucose: ________ mg/dl
CHI: ________
Nitrogen Balance: ________ g

DIAGNOSTIC DATA

X-rays ________ DEXA Scan ________

TABLE 7-2 Diet History

PART 1: GENERAL DIET INFORMATION

Do you follow a particular diet?

What are your food likes and dislikes?

Do you have any especially strong cravings?

How often do you eat fast foods?

How often do you eat at restaurants?

Do you have adequate financial resources to purchase your food?

How do you obtain, store, and prepare your food?

Do you eat alone or with a family member or other person?

In the last 12 months, have you

- experienced any change in weight?
- had a change in your appetite?
- had a change in your diet?
- experienced nausea, vomiting, or diarrhea from your diet?
- changed your diet because of difficulty in feeding yourself, eating, chewing, or swallowing?

PART 2: FOOD INTAKE HISTORY (24-HOUR RECALL, 3-DAY DIARY, DIRECT OBSERVATION)

Time	Food/Drink	Amount	Method of Preparation	Eating Location

TABLE 7-3 Physical Signs and Symptoms of Poor Nutritional Status

	SUBJECTIVE	OBJECTIVE
1. General appearance	Fatigue, poor sleep, change in weight, frequent infections	Dull affect, apathetic, increased weight, decreased weight
2. Skin	Pruritus, swelling, delayed wound healing	Dry, rough, scaling, flaky, edema, lesions, decreased turgor, changes in color (pallor, jaundice), petechiae, ecchymoses, xanthomas (slightly elevated yellow nodules)
3. Nails	Brittle	Dry, splinter hemorrhages, spoon-shaped, pale
4. Hair	Easily falls out, brittle	Less shiny, dry, changes in color pigment
5. Eyes	Vision changes, night blindness, eye discharge	Hardening and scaling of cornea, conjunctiva pale or red
6. Mouth	Mouth sores	Lips: cracked, dry, swollen, fissures around corners Gums: recessed, swollen, bleeding, spongy Tongue: smooth, beefy red, magenta, pale, fissures, sores, increased or decreased in size, increased or decreased papillae Teeth: missing, caries
7. Head and neck	Headaches, decreased hearing	Xanthelasma, irritation and crusting of nares, swollen cheeks (parotid gland enlargement), goiter
8. Heart and peripheral	Palpitations, swelling	Cardiac enlargement, changes in blood pressure, vasculature tachycardia, heart murmur, edema
9. Abdomen	Tender, changes in appetite, nausea, changes in bowel habits	Edema, hepatosplenomegaly, vomiting, diarrhea
10. Musculoskeletal system	Weakness, pain, cramping, frequent fractures	Muscle tone is decreased, flabby muscles, muscle wasting, bowing of lower extremities
11. Neurological system	Irritable, changes in mood, numbness, paresthesia	Slurred speech, unsteady gait, tremors, decreased deep tendon reflexes, loss of position and vibratory sense, paresthesia, decreased coordination
12. Female genitalia	Changes in menstrual pattern	None

A Excessive growth
P Hormone abnormalities (acromegaly, giantism, precocious puberty)
A Decreased height
P Osteoporosis

Weight

E 1. Have patient stand on the scale and facing the weights.
2. Slide the weights until balanced.
3. Read and record the weight to the nearest 100 g or ¼ lb (10 g or ½ oz for infants).
4. Calculate the percentage of IBW.
5. Calculate the percentage of usual body weight.
6. Calculate the percentage of weight change.

N **Compare weight with standardized growth charts.**

A Mild obesity: 20% to 40% above IBW; moderate obesity: 40% to 100% above IBW; morbid obesity: more than 100% above IBW

P Steriod use; increased food intake or decreased activity level, or both; hypothyroidism; and genetic predisposition

A Undernutrition, weight under 90% of IBW; mild undernutrition, weight between 80% and 90% of IBW; moderate undernutrition, weight between 70% and 80% of IBW; severe undernutrition, weight below 70% of IBW

P Dental problems, depression, medications, alcoholism, anorexia nervosa, poverty, impaired absorption as is present in malabsorption diseases (e.g., celiac disease), small bowel disease, diarrhea, vomiting, diabetes mellitus, malignancies, fever, and hyperthyroidism

Body Mass Index

Body Mass Index (BMI) is a measurement that indicates body composition. The degree of overweight or obesity, as well as the degree of underweight, can be determined. The BMI can be associated with increased mortality at specific levels with patients with known chronic diseases and those without.

The BMI takes into account a person's height as well as his or her weight. The formula to determine BMI is:

$$\text{BMI} = \frac{\text{weight (in kg)}}{\text{m}^2}$$

The BMI can be difficult to calculate because few people know their height in meters squared. In this case, the BMI can be determined by two different methods:

E 1. Determine the BMI measurement by using the patient's height and weight.
2. Multiply the weight in lbs by 703.
3. Multiply the height in inches by the height in inches.
4. Divide the first number in 2 by the second number in 3.
5. The answer is the BMI.

For example: weight = 107 lbs; height = 60 inches

$$107 \times 703 = 75221$$
$$60 \times 60 = 3600$$
$$75221 \div 3600 = 20.9 \text{ or } 21$$

N **A BMI of 20 to 25 is considered within normal limits.**

A A BMI of 25 to 29.9 is considered overweight. A BMI of 30 to 34.9 is considered obese; 35 to 39.0 is moderately obese; and greater than 40 is extremely obese (Obesity Class III).

P A BMI greater than 25 is associated with an increased morbidity and mortality from cardiovascular disease, cancer, and other diseases.

A A BMI less than 20 is abnormal.

P A BMI less than 20 is underweight and can be associated with possible malnutrition. A BMI less than 18 is associated with definite malnutrition. The malnutrition can be self-induced (e.g., anorexia nervosa, bulimia), caused by illness (e.g., cancer, AIDS), or it can be from a lack of adequate nutrition.

Waist to Hip Ratio

Body fat distribution is linked to morbidity and mortality. This is frequently referred to as the "pears" and "apples" distribution. Women tend to deposit fat more in their hips and buttocks, giving them a pear shape appearance. Men, on the other hand, tend to deposit fat around the abdominal midline, thus giving them an apple appearance. The latter is usually connected more with the adverse effects associated with obesity. The waist to hip ratio is a simple method to determine one's body fat distribution.

E 1. Measure the waist in inches around the narrowest point of the waist between the 12th rib and the iliac crest.
2. Measure the hips at the widest point.
3. Divide the waist measurement by the hip measurement. This is the waist to hip ratio. For example:

waist = 25 inches, hips = 35 inches
$25 \div 35 = 0.71$

N **A waist to hip ratio less than 0.8 is normal in women. A waist to hip ratio less than 1.0 is normal in men.**

A A waist to hip ratio greater than 0.8 in women and 1.0 in men is abnormal.

P These measurements are associated with the adverse morbidity and mortality of obesity.

Skinfold Thickness

Skinfold thickness (Figure 7-2) is used to determine body fat stores and nutritional status. It is a more reliable indicator of body fat than is weight because more than one-half of the body's total fat is located in the subcutaneous tissue. The most common measurement site is the triceps skinfold (TSF). Measurements can also be performed on the subscapular and suprailiac skinfolds.

E 1. Place the patient in a sitting or standing position.
2. With the patient in a relaxed position, take the measurements on the nondominant arm.
3. Make a mark midway between the acromion process and the olecranon process on the posterior portion of the upper arm.

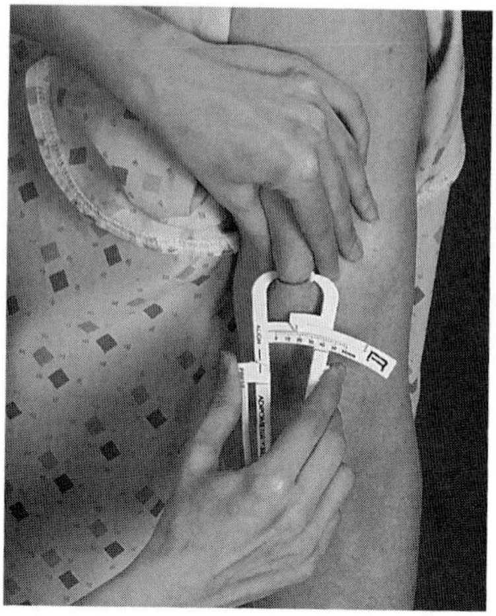

Figure 7-2 Skinfold Thickness

4. Using your nondominant hand, grasp the skin and pull it free from the muscle.
5. Using your dominant hand, apply the caliper and align the markers.
6. Note the measurement to the nearest 0.5 mm.
7. Release the skin and repeat 2 or 3 times.
8. Average the findings to determine the TSF.

N **See Table 7-4. Normal measurements fall between the 5th and 95th percentiles.**

A/P Refer to the second column of this page.

Mid-Arm and Mid-Arm Muscle Circumferences

The mid-arm circumference (MAC) provides information on skeletal muscle mass. This measurement alone is not of great significance, but it is used to calculate the mid-arm muscle circumference (MAMC).

E 1. Instruct the patient to flex the arm at the elbow.
2. Measure the circumference of the upper arm (MAC) midway between the acromion process and the olecranon process.
3. Calculate the MAMC (Table 7-5).

TABLE 7-4 Triceps Skinfold Percentiles (mm^2)*

Age	Males								Females							
(yr)	n	5	10	25	50	75	90	95	n	5	10	25	50	75	90	95
1–1.9	228	6	7	8	10	12	14	16	204	6	7	8	10	12	14	16
2–2.9	223	6	7	8	10	12	14	15	208	6	8	9	10	12	15	16
3–3.9	220	6	7	8	10	11	14	15	208	7	8	9	11	12	14	15
4–4.9	230	6	6	8	9	11	12	14	208	7	8	8	10	12	14	16
5–5.9	214	6	6	8	9	11	14	15	219	6	7	8	10	12	15	18
6–6.9	117	5	6	7	8	10	13	16	118	6	6	8	10	12	14	16
7–7.9	122	5	6	7	9	12	15	17	126	6	7	9	11	13	16	18
8–8.9	117	5	6	7	8	10	13	16	118	6	8	9	12	15	18	24
9–9.9	121	6	6	7	10	13	17	18	125	8	8	10	13	16	20	22
10–10.9	146	6	6	8	10	14	18	21	152	7	8	10	12	17	23	27
11–11.9	122	6	6	8	11	16	20	24	117	7	8	10	13	18	24	28
12–12.9	153	6	6	8	11	14	22	28	129	8	9	11	14	18	23	27
13–13.9	134	5	5	7	10	14	22	26	151	8	8	12	15	21	26	30
14–14.9	131	4	5	7	9	14	21	24	141	9	10	13	16	21	26	28
15–15.9	128	4	5	6	8	11	18	24	117	8	10	12	17	21	25	32

continues

TABLE 7-4 Triceps Skinfold Percentiles (mm^2)* *continued*

Age	Males								Females							
(yr)	*n*	*5*	*10*	*25*	*50*	*75*	*90*	*95*	*n*	*5*	*10*	*25*	*50*	*75*	*90*	*95*
16–16.9	131	4	5	6	8	12	16	22	142	10	12	15	18	22	26	31
17–17.9	133	5	5	6	8	12	16	19	114	10	12	13	19	24	30	37
18–18.9	91	4	5	6	9	13	20	24	109	10	12	15	18	22	26	30
19–24.9	531	4	5	7	10	15	20	22	1,060	10	11	14	18	24	30	34
25–34.9	971	5	6	8	12	16	20	24	1,987	10	12	16	21	27	34	37
35–44.9	806	5	6	8	12	16	20	23	1,614	12	14	18	23	29	35	38
45–54.9	898	6	6	8	12	15	20	25	1,047	12	16	20	25	30	36	40
55–64.9	734	5	6	8	11	14	19	22	809	12	16	20	25	31	36	38
65–74.9	1,503	4	6	8	11	15	19	22	1,670	12	14	18	24	29	34	36

**The Lange caliper was used in these studies.*

Note. *Reprinted with permission from "New Norms of Upper Limb Fat and Muscle Areas for Assessment of Nutrition Status," by A. R. Frisancho, 1981,* American Journal of Clinical Nutrition, *34, p. 2540, American Society for Clinical Nutrition.*

TABLE 7-5 MAC and MAMC Percentiles*

Age (yr)	ARM CIRCUMFERENCE (mm)						ARM MUSCLE CIRCUMFERENCE (mm)					
	5th	50th	95th	5th	50th	95th	5th	50th	95th	5th	50th	95th
	Males			Females			Males			Females		
1–1.9	142	159	183	138	156	177	110	127	147	105	124	143
2–2.9	141	162	185	142	160	184	111	130	150	111	126	147
3–3.9	150	167	190	143	167	189	117	137	153	113	132	152
4–4.9	149	171	192	149	169	191	123	141	159	115	136	157
5–5.9	153	175	204	153	175	211	128	147	169	125	142	165
6–6.9	155	179	228	156	176	211	131	151	177	130	145	171
7–7.9	162	187	230	164	183	231	137	160	190	129	151	176
8–8.9	162	190	245	168	195	261	140	162	187	138	160	194
9–9.9	175	200	257	178	211	260	151	170	202	147	167	198
10–10.9	181	210	274	174	210	265	156	180	221	148	170	197
11–11.9	186	223	280	185	224	303	159	183	230	150	181	223
12–12.9	193	232	303	194	237	294	167	195	241	162	191	220
13–13.9	194	247	301	202	243	338	172	211	245	169	198	240
14–14.9	220	253	322	214	252	322	189	223	264	174	201	247
15–15.9	222	264	320	208	254	322	199	237	272	175	202	244

continues

TABLE 7-5 MAC and MAMC Percentiles* *continued*

Age (yr)	ARM CIRCUMFERENCE (mm)						ARM MUSCLE CIRCUMFERENCE (mm)					
	5th	*50th*	*95th*	*5th*	*50th*	*95th*	*5th*	*50th*	*95th*	*5th*	*50th*	*95th*
	Males			*Females*			*Males*			*Females*		
16–16.9	244	278	343	218	258	334	213	249	296	170	202	249
17–17.9	246	285	347	220	264	350	224	258	312	175	205	257
18–18.9	245	297	379	222	258	325	226	264	324	174	202	245
19–24.9	262	308	372	221	265	345	238	273	321	179	207	249
25–34.9	271	319	375	233	277	368	243	279	326	183	212	264
35–44.9	278	326	374	241	290	378	247	286	327	186	218	272
45–54.9	267	322	376	242	299	384	239	281	326	187	220	274
55–64.9	258	317	369	243	303	385	236	278	320	187	225	280
65–74.9	248	307	355	240	299	373	223	268	306	185	225	279

**The Lange caliper was used in these studies.*

Note. *Reprinted with permission from "New Norms of Upper Limb Fat and Muscle Areas for Assessment of Nutrition Status," by A. R. Frisancho, 1981,* American Journal of Clinical Nutrition, *34, p. 2540. American Society for Clinical Nutrition.*

N **See Table 7-5. Normal measurements fall between the 5th and 95th percentiles.**

A Results less than the 5th percentile on the standard charts

P Malnutrition

A Results greater than the 95th percentile on the standard charts

P Obesity or edema

Laboratory Data

Laboratory analysis is used to screen for potential nutritional problems and to assist with diagnosis when problems are suspected after a thorough history and physical have been conducted.

Hematocrit and Hemoglobin

Hematocrit measures the percentage of red blood cells per volume of whole blood. It reflects the body's iron supply. Hemoglobin is the iron component of the blood and transports oxygen. Both values are obtained from a venous blood sample.

N **Hemoglobin and hematocrit results should fall within expected values as shown in Table 7-6. Hematocrit and hemoglobin may normally increase in people living at high altitudes, owing to the reduced partial pressure of oxygen in those areas.**

A Decreased hematocrit and hemoglobin

P Anemia, leukemia, cirrhosis, hyperthyroidism, hemorrhage, hemodilution, hemolytic reactions, decreased iron intake

A Increased hematocrit and hemoglobin

P Severe dehydration resulting in hemoconcentration; chronic hypoxia such as in cyanotic heart defects can result in polycythemia.

Lipids

In 2001, the Third Report of the National Cholesterol Education Program (NCEP) Expert Panel on Detection, Evaluation, and Treatment of High Blood Cholesterol in Adults (ATP III) published guidelines to assist health care providers in assessing and managing hyperlipidemia. Keep in mind that the laboratory values

TABLE 7-6 Normal Values for Hematocrit and Hemoglobin

	NORMAL VALUES	
Age	***Hematocrit (%)***	***Hemoglobin g/dl***
1 mo	33–55	10.7–17.1
12 mo	33–41	11.3–14.1
1–2 yr	32–40	11.0–14.0
12–14 yr		
Female	34–44	11.5–15.0
Male	35–45	12.0–16.0
18–44 yr		
Female	35–45	12.0–15.0
Male	39–49	13.0–17.0
45–64 yr		
Female	35–47	12.0–16.0
Male	39–50	13.0–17.0
65–74 yr		
Female	35–47	12.0–16.0
Male	37–51	13.0–17.0

are obtained from a fasting patient. The following values are drawn from ATP III:

N ***Total Cholesterol* (in mg/dl)**

<200	**Desirable**
200–239	**Borderline high**
>240	**High**

***HDL Cholesterol* (in mg/dl)**

<40	**Low**
>60	**High**

***LDL Cholesterol* (in mg/dl)**

<100	**Optimal**
100–129	**Near optimal/ above optimal**
130–159	**Borderline high**
160–189	**High**
>190	**Very high**

***Triglycerides* (in mg/dl)**

<150	**Normal**
150–199	**Borderline high**
200–499	**High**
>500	**Very high**

A Abnormal elevation of cholesterol, LDL, and triglycerides (hyperlipidemia and HDL less than 40 mg/dl)

P Excessive cholesterol, saturated fat, or calories; genetics; some medications (e.g., cyclosporin); diabetes; alcohol; hypothyroidism; chronic renal failure; anorexia nervosa

Transferrin, Total Iron-Binding Capacity (TIBC), and Iron

Transferrin is a protein that regulates iron absorption. Transferrin can be measured by the total iron-binding capacity (TIBC), or the amount of iron with which it can bind. Serum iron is the amount of transferrin-bound iron. These data are obtained from a venous blood sample.

N **Normal adult levels are:**
Transferrin: 170–250 mg/dl
TIBC: 240–450 μg/dl
Serum iron (women): 65–165 μg/dl
Serum iron (men): 75–175 μg/dl

A Transferrin >400 mg/dl

P Inadequate dietary iron, iron-deficiency anemia, hepatitis, oral contraceptive use, late pregnancy

A Transferrin <200 mg/dl

P Pernicious anemia, sickle cell anemia, anemia associated with infection or chronic disease, cancer, malnutrition

A Serum iron levels <65 μg/dl in women and <75 μg/dl in men

P Hemolytic anemias, lead poisoning

A Serum iron levels <65 μg/dl in women and <75 μg/dl in men

P Iron deficiency, chronic disease, third-trimester pregnancy, severe physiological stress

Total Lymphocyte Count

Total lymphocyte count (TLC) is assessed as part of the complete blood count with differential and measures immune function and visceral protein status. When the white blood cell count is abnormally elevated or decreased, such as in bacterial infections or AIDS, the TLC is not always a reliable indicator of nutritional status.

N **Normal adult levels are 1500–1800 cells/mm³.**

A Moderate protein deficiency: TLC >1500; severe protein deficiency: TLC <900

P Malnourished state as occurs in an immunocompromised state such as HIV infection

Antigen Skin Testing

Antigen skin testing is another test of immune function. Intradermal injections of various antigens can be used. Antigens commonly used are PPD tuberculin skin tests, mumps virus, *Candida albicans*, streptokinase, *Streptococcus*, *coccidioidin*, and *Trichophyton*. Results are read at 24 and 48 hours postinjection.

N **A negative skin reaction (no induration or erythema) after being tested with various antigens is normal. These are antigens to which most**

people have been exposed and have developed an antibody response.

A A positive reaction to antigens placed intradermally is abnormal, which is indicated by a red area or induration 5 mm or more around the test site 24 hours or more after the injection. A negative reaction to only one of the antigens tested or a delayed positive reaction may occur with malnutrition.

P Poor antibody response occurs in patients who are immunocompromised. They have a decreased ability to fight infection and build antibodies. Protein malnutrition has been shown to decrease immune function. This diminished reaction to antigens is called anergy. Antigen skin testing is often called anergy panels.

Prealbumin

Prealbumin (also called thyroxine-binding prealbumin) is the transport protein for thyroxine and retinol-binding protein. The half-life is 24 to 48 hours so it is an excellent value to monitor the effects of recent nutritional support and changes in nutritional status.

N **The normal range for prealbumin is 10–40 mg/dl.**

A Liver disease, such as cirrhosis and hepatitis, as well as severe stress from infection, burn injury, and sepsis, prolonged surgery, hyperthyroidism, and cystic fibrosis can all lead to decreased prealbumin levels.

P Severe acute conditions where severe catabolism occurs tend to lower the prealbumin level. In the case of liver disease, the levels are lower because of decreased hepatic synthesis of proteins.

Albumin

Albumin is formed in the liver. It transports nutrients, blood, and hormones and helps maintain osmotic pressure. Albumin must have functioning liver cells and an adequate amount of amino acids in order to be synthesized. It is an indicator of visceral protein status. Because albumin has a long half-life (i.e., approximately 20 days), it is not an indicator of subtle or early changes in nutritional status. It is measured via a venous blood sample.

N **The normal range for serum albumin is 3.5–5 g/dl.**

A Albumin <3.5 g/dl

P Malnutrition (a decrease in visceral protein stores, or the amount of protein stored in organs), massive hemorrhage, burns, kidney disease

Glucose

Serum glucose tests the body's ability to metabolize glucose. It is best assessed after a fasting period and via a venous blood sample.

N **Normal serum glucose levels are:**

Adult:	**Fasting**	**70–110 mg/dl**
	Nonfasting	**85–125 mg/dl**
Child:	**60–100 mg/dl**	

A An increase in glucose level (hyperglycemia)

P Diabetes mellitus, impaired glucose tolerance, vitamin B_1 deficiency, convulsive states

A A decrease in glucose level (hypoglycemia)

P Pancreatic disorders, liver disease, insulin overdose

Creatinine Height Index (CHI)

Creatinine is a substance normally excreted in the urine; it is dependent on the amount of skeletal muscle mass, and it measures protein reserves. Urine creatinine is tested after collecting a 24-hour urine sample. A table that shows the ideal urine creatinine level by height is used to establish the denominator in the equation used to calculate CHI.

N **Normal CHI values are greater than 90%.**

deficiency, CHI between 70% and 80%; severe protein deficiency, CHI less than 70%

P Loss of lean body mass as can occur in severe trauma, prolonged fever, and stress

Nitrogen Balance

Nitrogen is usually taken into the body in the form of protein in food. It is one of the compounds of amino acids. Nitrogen is incorporated into protein and excreted in urine and feces. Nitrogen balance is a comparison of the amount of nitrogen consumed with the amount excreted, usually measured via a 24-hour urine sample.

N **A zero balance is normal. A positive balance indicates tissue formation, found in growing children and pregnant women.**

A A negative nitrogen balance

P Catabolic state (more nitrogen excreted than consumed) as seen in malnutrition, burns, severe stress, trauma, and surgery

Diagnostic Data

Radiographic studies are used to assess bone formation and bone development. Rickets and scurvy are examples of long-term nutritional deficiencies that have radiographic manifestations. Rickets is a deficiency of vitamin D, and scurvy is a deficiency of vitamin C; both are characterized by softening and deformity of the bones. Osteoporosis, which can be linked to nutrition, can show up on a DEXA scan.

REFERENCES

Frisancho, A. R. (1981). New norms of upper limb fat and muscle areas for assessment of nutrition status. *American Journal of Clinical Nutrition, 34*, 2540.

National Heart, Lung, and Blood Institute, National Institutes of Health. (2001). *Third report of the National Cholesterol Education Program (NCEP) expert panel on detection, evaluation, and treatment of high blood cholesterol in adults (Adult Treatment Panel III), Executive summary* (NIH Publication No. 01-3670). Bethesda, MD: Authors.

U.S. Department of Agriculture. (2005). *MyPyramid food intake pattern calorie levels.* Retrieved April 21, 2005, from http://www.mypyramid.gov/professionals/pdf_calorie_levels.html

U.S. Department of Health and Human Services and U.S. Department of Agriculture. (2005). *Dietary guidelines for Americans, 2005* (6th ed.). Washington, DC: U.S. Government Printing Office.

BIBLIOGRAPHY

Krauss, R. M., Eckel, R. H., Howard, B., Appel, L. J., Daniels, S. R., Deckelbaum, R. J., et al. (2000). ADA Dietary Guidelines. Revision 2000: A statement for health care professionals from the Nutrition Committee of the American Heart Association. *Circulation, 102*, 2296.

Unit 3 Physical Assessment

8

Physical Assessment Techniques

Inspection, palpation, percussion, and auscultation are the techniques used by the nurse to assess patients during a physical examination. This chapter introduces the assessment techniques and equipment used to conduct physical examinations.

Aspects of Physical Assessment

Physical assessment of a patient serves many purposes:

1. Screening of general well-being. The findings will serve as baseline information for future assessments.
2. Validation of the complaints that brought the patient to seek health care.
3. Monitoring of current health problems.
4. Formulation of diagnoses and treatments.

The need for physical assessment depends on, among other factors, the patient's health status and concept of health care and on the accessibility to health care. For example, a brittle diabetic with arthritis and glaucoma who has access to health care is likely to enter the health care delivery system more often than is a healthy college student.

Role of the Nurse

The professional nurse plays a vital role in the assessment of patient problems. Educational preparation and clinical setting in part determine the extent to which the nurse participates in the assessment process. For example, a primary care nurse may perform a comprehensive physical assessment of patients, whereas a critical care nurse may only conduct selected patient assessments to monitor and evaluate current health problems.

Standard Precautions and Transmission-Based Precautions

The transmission of hepatitis, human immunodeficiency virus (HIV), and other infectious diseases is a primary concern for you and the patient. Standard precautions, formerly known as universal precautions, were developed by the Centers for Disease Control and Prevention (CDC) to protect health care professionals

Nursing Alert

Latex Allergies

In accordance with standard precautions, nurses use gloves frequently when dealing with patients' body fluids. Be alert to the possible presence of latex allergies in yourself as well as in your patients. Reactions range from eczematous contact dermatitis to anaphylactic shock. Ask patients whether they have any known allergy to latex products before touching patients with latex products, and using other latex products.

and patients. The primary goal of standard precautions is to prevent the exchange of blood and body fluids. Standard precautions should be practiced with every patient and throughout the entire encounter. Figure 8-1 illustrates the standard precautions recommended by the CDC.

The CDC has developed another level of precautions called transmission-based precautions. These precautions are to be used in conjunction with standard precautions. Contact, droplet, and airborne transmissions of microorganisms that are known to exist in a patient or are

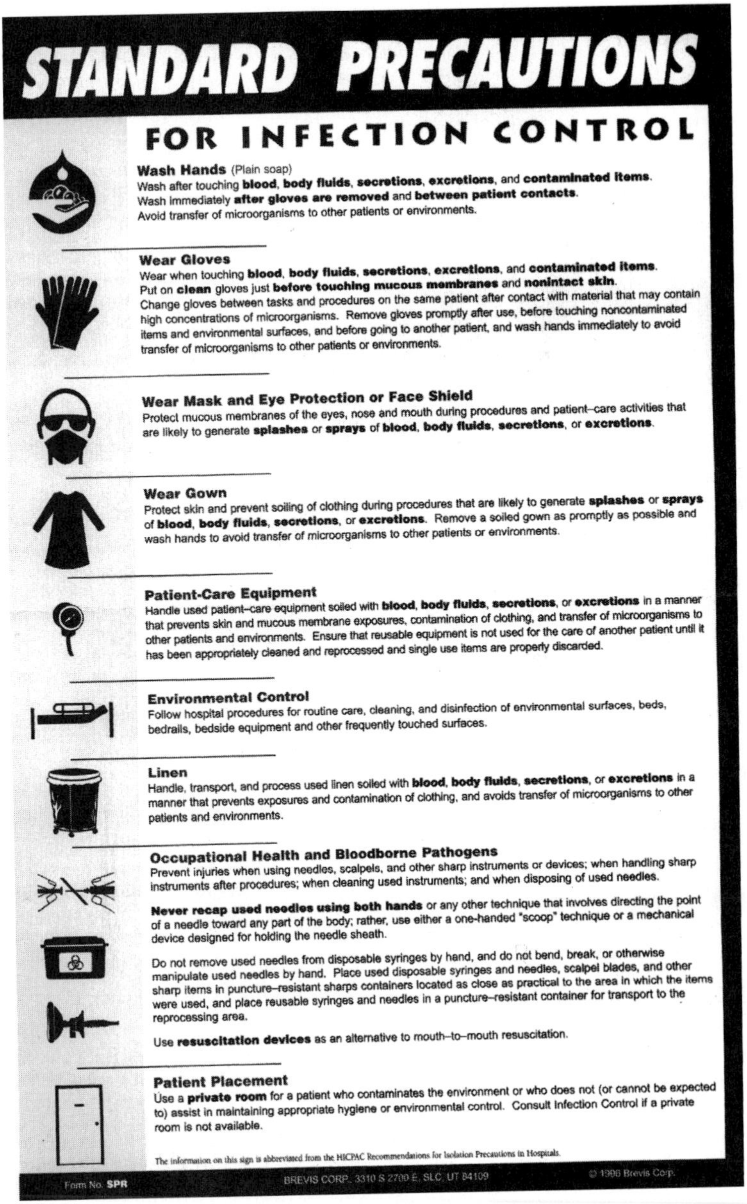
STANDARD PRECAUTIONS
FOR INFECTION CONTROL
Wash Hands (Plain soap)
Wash after touching blood, body fluids, secretions, excretions, and contaminated items.
Wash immediately after gloves are removed and between patient contacts.
Avoid transfer of microorganisms to other patients or environments.
Wear Gloves
Wear when touching blood, body fluids, secretions, excretions, and contaminated items.
Put on clean gloves just before touching mucous membranes and nonintact skin.
Change gloves between tasks and procedures on the same patient after contact with material that may contain high concentrations of microorganisms. Remove gloves promptly after use, before touching noncontaminated items and environmental surfaces, and before going to another patient, and wash hands immediately to avoid transfer of microorganisms to other patients or environments.
Wear Mask and Eye Protection or Face Shield
Protect mucous membranes of the eyes, nose and mouth during procedures and patient–care activities that are likely to generate splashes or sprays of blood, body fluids, secretions, or excretions.
Wear Gown
Protect skin and prevent soiling of clothing during procedures that are likely to generate splashes or sprays of blood, body fluids, secretions, or excretions. Remove a soiled gown as promptly as possible and wash hands to avoid transfer of microorganisms to other patients or environments.
Patient-Care Equipment
Handle used patient–care equipment soiled with blood, body fluids, secretions, or excretions in a manner that prevents skin and mucous membrane exposures, contamination of clothing, and transfer of microorganisms to other patients and environments. Ensure that reusable equipment is not used for the care of another patient until it has been appropriately cleaned and reprocessed and single use items are properly discarded.
Environmental Control
Follow hospital procedures for routine care, cleaning, and disinfection of environmental surfaces, beds, bedrails, bedside equipment and other frequently touched surfaces.
Linen
Handle, transport, and process used linen soiled with blood, body fluids, secretions, or excretions in a manner that prevents exposures and contamination of clothing, and avoids transfer of microorganisms to other patients and environments.
Occupational Health and Bloodborne Pathogens
Prevent injuries when using needles, scalpels, and other sharp instruments or devices; when handling sharp instruments after procedures; when cleaning used instruments; and when disposing of used needles.
Never recap used needles using both hands or any other technique that involves directing the point of a needle toward any part of the body; rather, use either a one-handed "scoop" technique or a mechanical device designed for holding the needle sheath.
Do not remove used needles from disposable syringes by hand, and do not bend, break, or otherwise manipulate used needles by hand. Place used disposable syringes and needles, scalpel blades, and other sharp items in puncture–resistant sharps containers located as close as practical to the area in which the items were used, and place reusable syringes and needles in a puncture–resistant container for transport to the reprocessing area.
Use resuscitation devices as an alternative to mouth–to–mouth resuscitation.
Patient Placement
Use a private room for a patient who contaminates the environment or who does not (or cannot be expected to) assist in maintaining appropriate hygiene or environmental control. Consult Infection Control if a private room is not available.
The information on this sign is abbreviated from the HICPAC Recommendations for Isolation Precautions in Hospitals.
Form No. SPR
BREVIS CORP. 3310 S 2700 E, SLC, UT 84109
© 1996 Brevis Corp.

Figure 8-1 Standard Precautions. *Courtesy of BREVIS Corporation*

suspected in a patient are targeted. Contact transmissions, such as in impetigo, scabies, and varicella zoster virus, are spread directly from person to person. They can also be spread indirectly from a contaminated inanimate object to a person. Droplet transmission occurs when microorganisms are deposited on susceptible body parts via sneezing and coughing. Suctioning a patient can also transmit droplets. Pertussis and *Haemophilus influenzae* are examples of this mode of transmission. Airborne transmission spreads microorganisms by air currents and inhalation. They can also be passed through ventilation systems. Measles and the varicella virus can spread in this mode.

Handwashing

The most important infection control practice is handwashing. You must begin every physical assessment with a thorough handwash. Some nurses wash their hands in the assessment area and with the patient present.

The CDC in 2002 issued *Guideline for Hand Hygiene in Health-Care Settings* (Boyce & Pittet, 2002). These handwashing guidelines recommend the use of an alcohol-based hand rub, an antimicrobial soap and water, or a nonantimicrobial soap and water when the hands are visibly contaminated with body fluids. Your institution may provide some or all of these methods of handwashing; regardless, the most important factor is that you use them with every patient interaction.

Legal Issues

In today's litigious society, you must be ever vigilant when engaging in nursing practice. Documentation must be complete and accurate. Equally important is how you execute the nursing assessment. Establishing a trusting and caring relationship is the primary element in avoiding malpractice claims. Before performing each step in the physical assessment process, you must inform the patient of what to expect, where to expect it, and how it will feel. Protests by the patient must be addressed before continuing the examination; otherwise, the patient may claim insufficient informed consent, sexual abuse, or physical harassment.

All assessments and procedures, including any injury that was caused during the physical assessment, must be completely documented. The institutional policy regarding patient injury in the workplace must be followed.

Assessment Techniques

Physical assessment findings, or objective data, are obtained through the use of four specific diagnostic techniques: inspection, palpation, percussion, and auscultation. These assessment techniques are usually performed in this order when body systems are assessed. An exception is in the assessment of the abdomen, when auscultation is performed before percussion and palpation, because the latter two can alter bowel sounds. These four techniques validate information provided by a patient in the health history, or they can verify a suspected physical diagnosis.

Inspection

Inspection is an ongoing process used throughout the physical assessment. Inspection is the use of one's visual and olfactory senses to consciously observe the patient.

Vision

Use of sight can reveal many facts about a patient. Visual inspection of a patient's respiratory status, for example, might reveal cyanotic nailbeds and a respiratory rate of 38 breaths per minute. This tachypneic and possibly hypoxic patient would need a more thorough respiratory assessment. The process of visual inspection necessitates full exposure of the body part being inspected, adequate overhead lighting, and, when necessary, tangential lighting (lighting shone at a right angle to the patient in order to accentuate shadows and highlight subtle findings).

Smell

The olfactory sense can provide the nurse with vital information about a patient's health status. For example, the patient may have a fruity breath odor, which may indicate diabetic ketoacidosis.

Palpation

The second assessment technique is palpation, which is the act of touching a patient in a therapeutic manner to elicit specific information. Before palpating a patient, you must observe some basic principles. Your fingernails should be kept short to prevent injury to the patient as well as to yourself. Also, you should warm your hands before placing them on the patient; cold hands can cause the patient to tense muscles, an action that can distort assessment findings. Encourage the patient to breathe normally throughout the palpation process. If pain is experienced during the palpation, discontinue the palpation immediately. Most significantly, inform the patient where, when, and how the touch will occur, especially when the patient cannot see what you are doing. In this way, the patient is made aware of what to expect in the assessment process.

Your hands are the tools used to perform palpation. Different sections of the hands are best used for assessing certain areas of the body. The dorsum of the hand is most sensitive to temperature changes in the body. Thus, placing the dorsum of the hand on the patient's forehead to assess body temperature will yield a more accurate result than will using the palmar surface of the hand. The palmar surfaces of the fingers as well as the ulnar surface of the hand best discriminate vibrations such as a cardiac thrill. The finger pads are the most frequently used portion of the hand for purposes of palpation. The finger pads are useful in assessing skin moisture, texture, and temperature; the shape, size, position, mobility, and consistency of organs; and the presence of masses, fluid, and crepitus. Observe standard precautions when you are performing palpation. Gloves must be worn when examining any open wounds, skin lesions, discharge, and the mouth, rectum, or genitalia.

There are two distinct types of palpation: light palpation and deep palpation.

Light Palpation

Light palpation is used more frequently than deep palpation and is always performed before deep palpation. As the name implies, light palpation is superficial, delicate, and gentle. In light palpation, the finger pads are used to obtain information by exploring the skin's surface to a depth of approximately 1 cm. Light palpation reveals information on skin texture and moisture; overt, large, or superficial masses; fluid; muscle guarding; and superficial tenderness. To perform light palpation:

1. Keeping the fingers of your dominant hand together, place the finger pads lightly on the skin area to be palpated. The hand and forearm will be on a plane parallel to the area being assessed.
2. Using light, gentle, circular motions, depress the skin 1 cm.
3. Keeping the finger pads on the skin, let the depressed body surface rebound to its natural position.
4. If the patient is ticklish, lift the hand off the skin before moving it to another area.
5. Using a systematic approach, move the fingers to an adjacent area and repeat the process.
6. Continue to move the finger pads until the entire area being examined has been palpated.
7. If the patient complains of tenderness in any given area, palpate this area last.

See Figure 8-2 for an illustration of how light palpation is performed.

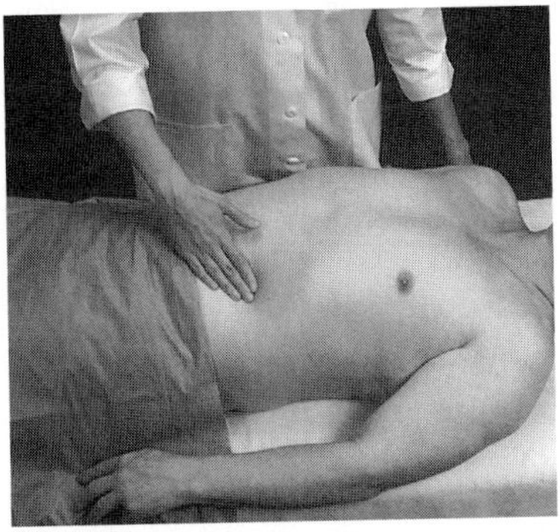

Figure 8-2 Technique of Light Palpation

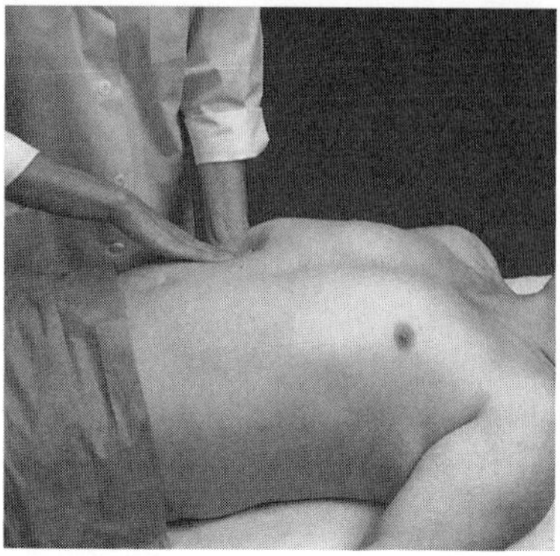

Figure 8-3 Technique of Deep Palpation

Deep Palpation

Deep palpation can reveal information about the position, size, shape, mobility, and consistency of organs, masses, and areas of discomfort. Deep palpation uses the hands to explore the body's internal structures to a depth of 4 to 5 cm or more (Figure 8-3). This technique is most often performed for the abdominal assessment and assessment of the male and female reproductive systems. Variations on this technique are single-handed palpation and bimanual palpation (discussed in Chapter 17). If the abdomen or genitalia are to be palpated, the patient should be given the opportunity to void before the examination.

Percussion

Percussion is the technique of striking one object against another to cause vibrations that produce sound. The density of underlying structures produces characteristic sounds. These sounds are diagnostic of normal and abnormal findings. The presence of air, fluid, or solids can be confirmed, as can organ size, shape, and position. The thorax and abdomen are the most frequently percussed body areas.

Percussion sound can be analyzed according to its intensity, duration, pitch (frequency), quality, and location. Intensity, or amplitude, refers to the relative loudness or softness of the sound. Duration refers to the time period over which a sound is heard when elicited. Frequency, or pitch, is caused by a sound's vibrations and refers to the highness or lowness of the sound. Fast vibrations have a higher pitch than do slow vibrations. The quality of a sound refers to the sound's timbre, or how one perceives the sound musically. Location refers to the area where the sound is produced and heard.

The process of percussion can produce five distinct sounds: flatness, dullness, resonance, hyperresonance, and tympany. Specific parts of the body elicit distinct percussable sounds.

Table 8-1 lists each of the five percussable sounds along with its intensity, duration, pitch, quality, location, and relative density. In addition, examples are provided of normal and abnormal locations of percussed sounds.

Sound waves are conducted better through a solid medium than through an air-filled medium because of the higher concentration of molecules. The basic premises underlying percussed sounds are:

1. The more solid a structure, the higher the pitch, the softer the intensity, and the shorter the duration.
2. The more air-filled a structure, the lower the pitch, the louder the intensity, and the longer the duration.

There are four types of percussion techniques: immediate, mediate, direct fist, and indirect fist. It is important to keep in mind that the sounds produced by percussion are generated from body tissue up to 5 cm below the surface of the skin.

Immediate Percussion

Immediate, or direct, percussion is the striking of an area of the body directly. To perform immediate percussion:

1. Spread the index or middle finger of the dominant hand slightly apart from the rest of the fingers.
2. Lightly tap the finger pad of the index or middle finger against the body part being percussed.

TABLE 8-1 Characteristics of Percussion Sounds

SOUND	INTENSITY	DURATION	PITCH	QUALITY	NORMAL LOCATION	ABNORMAL LOCATION	DENSITY
Flatness	Soft	Short	High	Flat	Muscle (thigh) or bone	Lungs (severe pneumonia)	Most dense ↓
Dullness	Moderate	Moderate	High	Thud	Organs (liver)	Lungs (atelectasis)	
Resonance	Loud	Moderate-long	Low	Hollow	Normal lungs	No abnormal location	
Hyperresonance	Very loud	Long	Very low	Boom	No normal location in adults; normal lungs in children	Lungs (emphysema)	
Tympany	Loud	Long	High	Drum	Gastric air bubble	Lungs (large pneumothorax)	Least dense

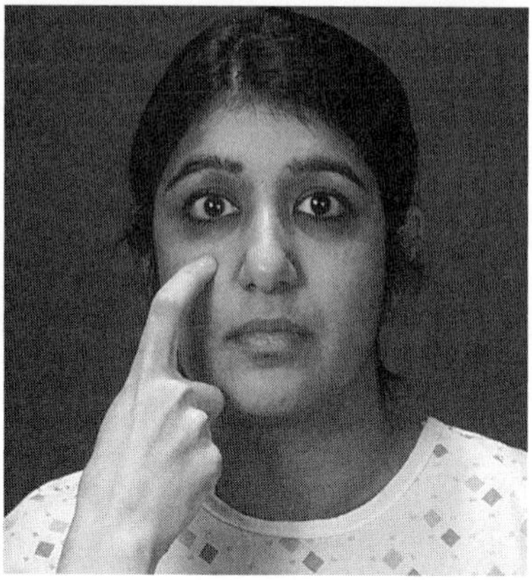

Figure 8-4 Technique of Immediate Percussion

Percussion of the sinuses (Figure 8-4) illustrates the use of immediate percussion in the physical assessment.

Mediate Percussion

Mediate percussion is also referred to as indirect percussion. To perform mediate percussion (Figure 8-5):

1. Lightly place the nondominant hand on the surface to be percussed.
2. Extend the middle finger of this hand, known as the pleximeter, and press its distal phalanx and distal interphalangeal joint firmly on the location where percussion is to begin. The pleximeter will remain stationary while percussion is performed in this location.
3. Spread apart the other fingers of the nondominant hand and raise them slightly off the surface. This position prevents interference and, thus, dampening of vibrations during the actual percussion.
4. Flex the middle finger of the dominant hand, called the plexor. The other fingers on this hand should be fanned.
5. Flex the wrist of the dominant hand and place the hand directly over the pleximeter finger.
6. The plexor should be perpendicular to the pleximeter. With a sharp, crisp, rapid movement from the wrist of the dominant hand, use the plexor to strike the pleximeter. The blow to the pleximeter should fall between the distal interphalangeal point and the fingernail. Use the finger pad rather than the fingertip of the plexor to deliver the blow. Concentrate on the movement to create the striking action from the dominant wrist only.
7. As soon as the plexor strikes the pleximeter, withdraw the plexor to prevent dampening of the resulting vibrations. Do not move the pleximeter.
8. Note the sound produced by the percussion.
9. Repeat the percussion process one or two times in this location to confirm the sound.
10. Move the pleximeter to a second location, preferably the contralateral location from where the previous percussion took place. Repeat the percussion process in this manner until the entire body surface area being assessed has been percussed.

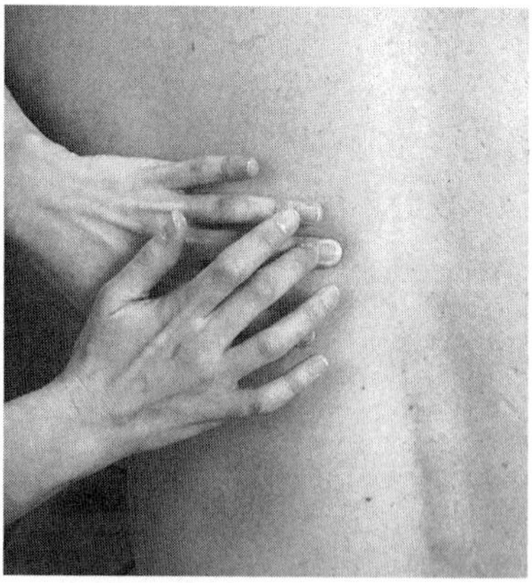

Figure 8-5 Technique of Mediate Percussion

Recognizing Percussed Sounds

When mediate and immediate percussion are being used, the change from resonance to dullness is more easily recognized by the human ear than is the change from dullness to resonance. This concept has implications for patterns of percussion in areas of the body where known locations have distinct percussable sounds. For example, the techniques of diaphragmatic excursion and liver border percussion can each proceed in a more defined pattern because percussion can be performed from an area of resonance to an area of dullness.

Direct Fist Percussion

Direct fist percussion is used to assess the presence of tenderness in internal organs such as the liver and the kidneys. To perform direct fist percussion (Figure 8-6):

1. Explain the technique thoroughly so the patient does not think you are hitting him or her.
2. Make a fist of the dominant hand.
3. With the ulnar aspect of the closed fist, directly hit the area where the organ is located. The strike should be of moderate force, and it may take some practice to achieve the right intensity.

The presence of pain in conjunction with direct fist percussion indicates either inflammation of the organ or a strike too high in intensity.

Indirect Fist Percussion

The purpose of indirect fist percussion is the same as that of direct fist percussion. The indirect method, however, is preferred over the direct method. To perform indirect fist percussion (Figure 8-7):

1. Place the nondominant hand over the organ to be percussed, palmar side down. Place the fingers adjacent to one another and in straight alignment with the palm.
2. Make a fist of the dominant hand.
3. With the ulnar aspect of the closed fist, use moderate intensity to hit the dorsum of the outstretched nondominant hand.

The nondominant hand absorbs some of the force of the striking hand. The resulting force should be of sufficient intensity to produce pain in the patient if organ inflammation is present.

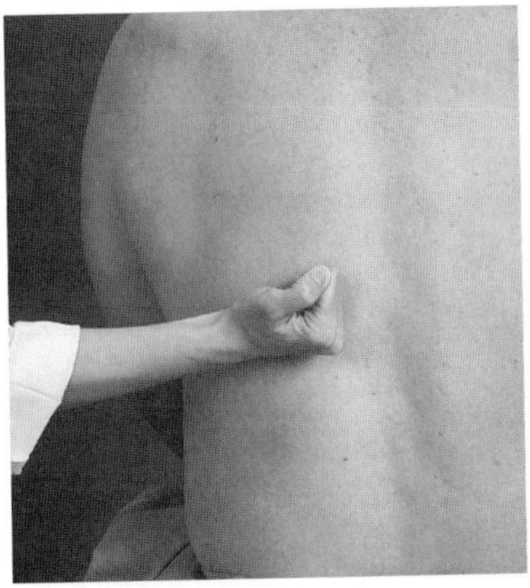

Figure 8-6 Technique of Direct Fist Percussion: Left Kidney

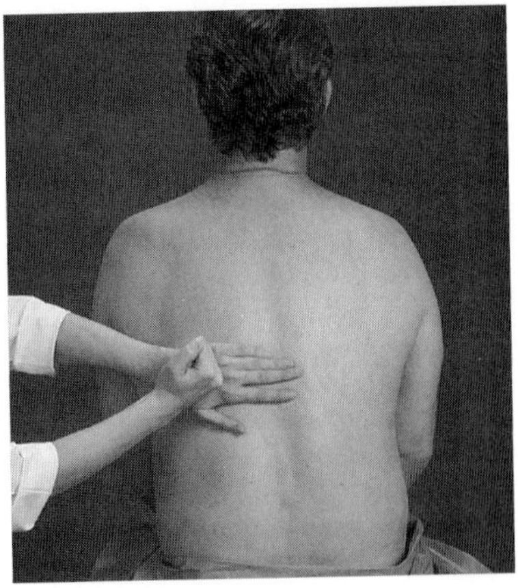

Figure 8-7 Technique of Indirect Fist Percussion: Left Kidney

Auscultation

Auscultation is the art of actively listening to body organs to gather information about the patient's clinical status. Auscultation involves listening to voluntarily as well as involuntarily produced body sounds. A quiet environment is necessary for auscultation. Auscultated sounds should be analyzed with regard to relative intensity, pitch, duration, quality, and location. There are two types of auscultation: direct and indirect.

Direct Auscultation

Direct, or immediate, auscultation is the process of listening with the unaided ear.

This can encompass listening to the patient from some distance away or placing your ear directly on the patient's skin surface and listening.

Indirect Auscultation

Indirect, or mediate, auscultation is the process of listening with the aid of some amplification or mechanical device. The nurse most often performs mediate auscultation using an acoustical stethoscope, which does not amplify body sounds but, rather, blocks out environmental sounds. Amplification of body sounds can also be achieved using a Doppler ultrasonic transducer. The text following describes the use of an acoustical stethoscope.

Acoustical stethoscopes come with earpieces in various sizes. Choose an earpiece sized to fit snugly in the ear canal without causing pain. The earpieces and binaurals should be angled toward the nose. By angling the earpieces and binaurals in this manner, sound will follow the natural direction of the ear canal and thus be directed toward the adult tympanic membrane. The rubber or plastic tubing should be between 30.5 and 40 cm (12 and 18 in.). Longer tubing will diminish auscultated body sounds.

The acoustical stethoscope has two listening heads: the bell and the diaphragm. The diaphragm is flat, and the bell is a concave cup. The diaphragm best transmits high-pitched sounds, and the bell best transmits low-pitched sounds. Breath sounds and normal heart sounds are examples of high-pitched sounds; bruits and some heart murmurs are examples of low-pitched sounds. The single-sided, dual-frequency listening head stethoscope has a single chestpiece. The nurse applies different pressures on the chestpiece to auscultate high- and low-pitched sounds.

Prior to using the stethoscope, use your hands to warm the headpieces, because patient shivering and movement can obscure body sounds. To use the diaphragm, place it firmly against the skin surface to be auscultated. If the patient has a large quantity of hair in this area, a grating sound may be heard; it may be necessary to wet the hair to prevent it from interfering with the sound being auscultated. To use the bell, place it lightly on the skin surface to be auscultated. If it is pressed too firmly on the skin, the bell will stretch the skin and act like a diaphragm, transmitting high-pitched rather than low-pitched sounds.

Equipment

Equipment needed to perform a complete physical examination of the adult patient includes the following:

- Pen and paper
- Marking pen
- Tape measure
- Clean gloves
- Penlight or flashlight
- Scale (You may have to walk the patient to a central location if a scale cannot be brought to the patient's room.)
- Thermometer
- Sphygmomanometer
- Gooseneck lamp
- Tongue depressor
- Stethoscope
- Otoscope
- Nasal speculum
- Ophthalmoscope
- Transilluminator
- Visual acuity charts
- Tuning forks
- Reflex hammer
- Cotton balls
- Sterile needle
- Odors for cranial nerve assessment (e.g., coffee, lemon, flowers)
- Small objects for neurological assessment (e.g., paperclip, door key, pen)
- Water-soluble lubricant
- Various-sized vaginal speculums
- Cervical brush
- Cotton-tipped applicator
- Cervical spatula
- Slide and fixative
- Guaiac material
- Specimen cup
- Goniometer

The use of these items is discussed in the chapters describing the assessments for which they are used.

NURSING CHECKLIST

Preparing for a Physical Assessment

- Always dress in a clean, professional manner; make sure your name pin or workplace identification is visible.
- Remove all jewelry that can interfere with the physical assessment, such as bracelets and rings.
- Be sure that your fingernails are short and your hands are warm for maximum patient comfort.
- Be sure your hair will not fall forward and touch the patient.
- Arrange for a well-lit, warm, and private room.
- Assemble and arrange all needed equipment.
- Introduce yourself to the patient: "My name is Mary Gill. I am a nurse, and I will be performing a physical assessment on you."
- Instruct the patient to undress; the patient's underpants can be left on until the end of the assessment; provide the patient with a gown and drape and explain how to use them.
- Allow the patient to undress privately; inform the patient of when you will return to start the assessment.
- Have the patient void before the assessment.
- Wash your hands in front of the patient to show your concern for cleanliness.
- Observe standard precautions and transmission-based precautions, as indicated.
- Ensure that the patient is accessible from both sides of the examination bed or table.
- If a bed is used, raise the height so that you do not have to bend over to perform the assessment.
- Position the patient as dictated by the body system being assessed; see Figure 8-8 for positioning and draping techniques.
- Enlist the patient's cooperation by explaining what you are about to do, where it will be done, and how it may feel.
- Use your hands or warm water to warm all instruments before use.
- If the patient complains of fatigue, continue the assessment later (if possible).
- Avoid making crude or negative remarks; be cognizant of your facial expressions when dealing with malodorous or dirty patients or with disturbing findings (e.g., infected wounds or disfigurement).
- Conduct the assessment in a systematic fashion every time. (Consistency decreases the likelihood of forgetting to perform a particular assessment.)
- Thank the patient when the physical assessment is concluded; inform the patient of what will happen next.
- Document assessment findings in the appropriate section of the patient record.

REFERENCE

Boyce, J. M., & Pittet, D. (2002). Guideline for hand hygiene in health-care settings. Recommendations of the Healthcare Infection Control Practices Advisory Committee and the HICPAC/SHEA/ADIC/IDSA Hand Hygiene Task Force. *Morbidity and Mortability Weekly Report*, *51*(RR16), 1–44.

POSITION	SYSTEM ASSESSED
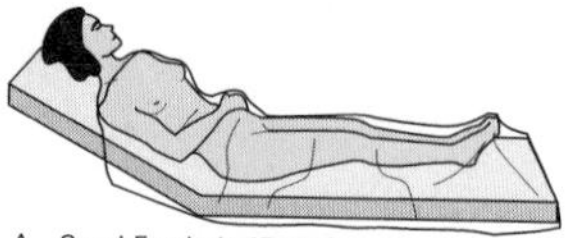 A. Semi-Fowler's 45 angle	Skin; head, and neck; eyes, ears, nose, mouth, and throat; thorax and lungs; heart and peripheral vasculature; musculoskeletal; neurological; patients who cannot tolerate sitting up at a 90 angle
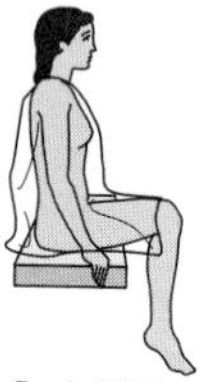 B. Sitting (High Fowler's) 90 angle	Skin; head, and neck; eyes, ears, nose, mouth, and throat; back; posterior thorax and lungs; anterior thorax and lungs; breast; axillae; heart; peripheral vasculature; musculoskeletal; neurological
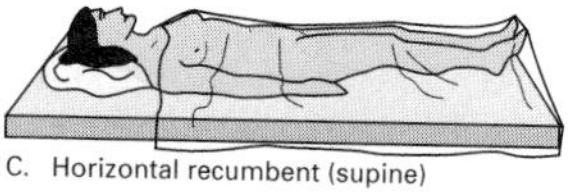 C. Horizontal recumbent (supine)	Breasts; heart and peripheral vasculature; abdomen; musculoskeletal
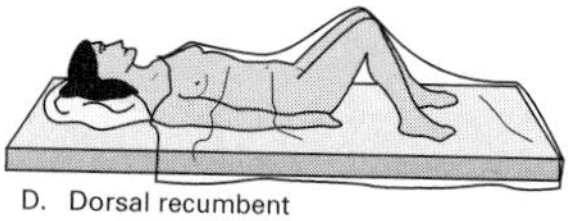 D. Dorsal recumbent	Female genitalia; patients who cannot tolerate knee flexion
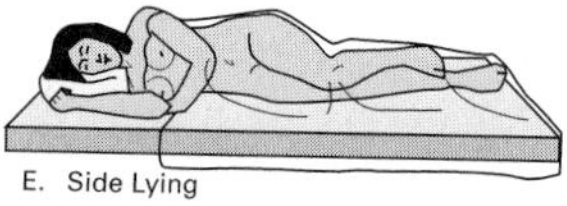 E. Side Lying	Skin; thorax and lungs; bedridden patients who cannot sit up
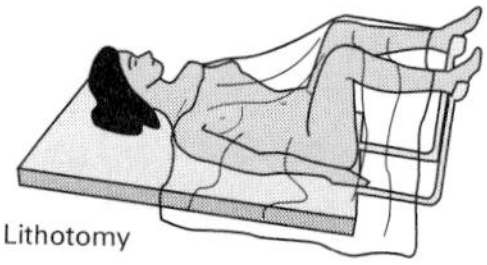 F. Lithotomy	Female genitalia and rectum
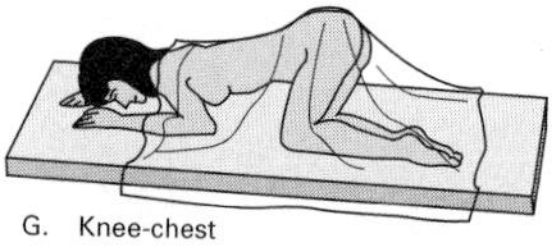 G. Knee-chest	Rectum and prostate
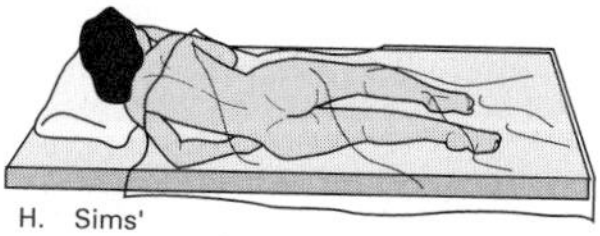 H. Sims'	Rectum and female genitalia
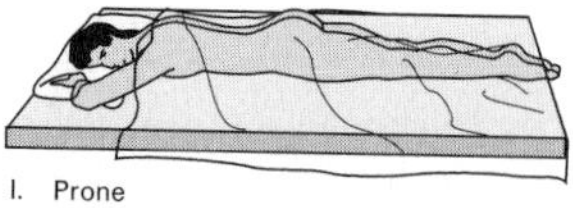 I. Prone	Skin; posterior thorax and lungs; hips

Figure 8-8 Positioning and Draping Techniques

9

General Survey, Vital Signs, and Pain

A complete physical assessment is initiated by performing general observations of the patient, obtaining the patient's vital signs, and assessing a patient for pain. Vital signs include the patient's respirations, pulse, temperature, and blood pressure (BP). These observations and measurements provide information about the patient's basic physiological status.

Equipment

- Stethoscope
- Watch with a second hand
- Thermometer (gloves and lubricant, if using a rectal thermometer)
- Sphygmomanometer

General Survey

Initial observations involve collecting information about the patient's physical presence, psychological presence, and signs and symptoms of distress.

Physical Presence

E Observe the patient's:

1. Stated age versus apparent age. The patient's stated chronological age should be congruent with the apparent age.

2. General appearance. The patient should exhibit body symmetry, no obvious deformity, and a well appearance.

3. Body fat. Body fat should be evenly distributed. Body fat composition is difficult to estimate accurately without the use of immersion tanks or calipers.

4. Stature. Limbs and trunk should appear proportional to body height; posture should be erect.

5. Motor activity. Walking gait as well as other body movements should be smooth and effortless. All body parts should demonstrate controlled, purposeful movement.

6. Body and breath odors. Normally, the patient should emit no apparent odor. It is normal for some people to have bad breath related to the types of foods ingested or to individual digestive processes.

Psychological Presence

E Observe the patient's:

1. Dress, grooming, and personal hygiene. The patient should appear clean and neatly dressed. Clothing choice should be appropriate to the weather. Norms and standards for dress and cleanliness may vary between cultures.

2. Mood and manner. The patient should be generally cooperative and pleasant.

3. Speech. The patient should respond to questions and commands

easily, and the patient's speech should be clear and understandable. Pitch, rate, and volume should vary normally.
4. Facial expressions. The patient should appear awake and alert. Facial expressions should be appropriate to what is happening in the environment. Facial expression should change naturally.

Distress

E Observe for:
1. Labored breathing or speech; wheezing or coughing. Breathing should be effortless and without coughing or wheezing.
2. Painful facial expression, sweating, or physical protection of a painful area. Speaking should not leave the patient breathless. The patient's face should be relaxed, and the patient should be willing to move all body parts freely.
3. Serious or life-threatening occurrences such as seizure activity, active and severe bleeding, gaping wounds, and open fractures. There should be no life-threatening conditions.
4. Signs of emotional distress or anxiety, which may include but are not limited to tearfulness, nervous tics or laughter, lack of eye contact, excessive nail biting, inability to pay attention, autonomic responses such as diaphoresis, changes in breathing patterns, or cold, clammy hands. The patient should not be perspiring excessively or showing signs of emotional distress, such as nail biting or avoiding eye contact.

Vital Signs

Respiration

Respiration is the act of breathing. Breathing supplies oxygen to the body and occurs in response to changes in the concentration of oxygen (O_2), carbon dioxide (CO_2), and hydrogen ($H+$) in the arterial blood. Inspiration occurs when the diaphragm and intercostal muscles contract, thus moving the abdomen and chest upward and outward. Expiration occurs when the external intercostal muscles and diaphragm relax, allowing the abdomen and chest to return to a resting position. Respiratory rate is measured in breaths per minute. One respiratory cycle consists of one inspiration and one expiration. A complete discussion of respiratory assessment is found in Chapter 15.

E To assess respiratory rate:
1. Stand in front of or to the side of the patient.
2. Discreetly observe the patient's breathing (the rise and fall of the chest).
3. Discreetly count the number of respiratory cycles that occur in 1 minute.

N **Table 9-1 lists the normal respiratory rates for different ages. Respiratory rate decreases with age and may vary with excitement, anxiety, fever, exercise, medications, and altitude.**

TABLE 9-1

Respiratory Rate

AGE	RESTING RESPIRATORY RATE (Breaths/Minute)	AVERAGE
Newborn	30–50	40
1 Year	20–40	30
3 Years	20–30	25
6 Years	16–22	19
10 Years	16–20	18
14 Years	14–20	17
Adult	12–20	18

Pulse

As the heart contracts, blood is ejected from the left ventricle (stroke volume) and into the aorta. A pressure wave is created as the blood is carried to the peripheral vasculature. This palpable pressure is the pulse. Pulse assessment can determine heart rate and rhythm and the estimated volume of blood being pumped by the heart.

Rate

Pulse rate is the number of pulse beats counted in 1 minute. Several factors influence pulse rate and heart rate. These include:

- The SA node, which fires automatically at a rate of 60 to 100 times/minute and is the primary controller of pulse rate and heart rate.
- Parasympathetic, or vagal, stimulation of the autonomic nervous system, which can result in decreased heart rate.
- Sympathetic stimulation of the autonomic nervous system, which results in increased heart rate.
- Baroreceptor sensors, which can detect changes in blood pressure and influence heart rate. Elevated blood pressure can decrease heart rate, whereas low blood pressure can increase heart rate.

Other factors influencing heart rate include:

- Age: heart rate generally decreases with age.
- Gender: the average female's heart rate is higher than that of the average male.
- Activity: heart rate increases with activity. Athletes have a low resting heart rate owing to increased cardiac strength and efficiency.
- Emotional status: heart rate increases in response to anxiety.
- Pain: heart rate increases in response to pain.
- Environmental factors: temperature and noise level can alter heart rate.
- Stimulants: caffeinated beverages and tobacco elevate heart rate.
- Medications: drugs such as digoxin decrease heart rate, and drugs such as amphetamines increase heart rate.

Rhythm

Pulse rhythm refers to the pattern of pulses and the intervals between pulses. Pulses can be regular or irregular. An irregular pulse can be regularly irregular or irregularly irregular.

Volume

Pulse volume (also called pulse strength or amplitude) reflects the stroke volume and the peripheral vasculature resistance (afterload). It can range from absent to bounding. Table 9-2 displays the two most commonly used scales: a 3-point scale and a 4-point scale. In reports of pulse volume, 2+/4+ indicates that the pulse is normal (2+) using a 4-point scale (4+), whereas 2+/3+ indicates pulse is normal (2+) using a 3-point scale (3+).

Site

Peripheral pulses can be palpated where the large arteries are close to the skin's surface. There are nine common sites for assessment of pulse, as indicated in

TABLE 9-2

Scales for Measuring Pulse Volume Systems

3-POINT SCALE

Scale	*Description of Pulse*
0	Absent
1+	Thready/weak
2+	Normal
3+	Bounding

4-POINT SCALE

Scale	*Description of Pulse*
0	Absent
1+	Thready/weak
2+	Normal
3+	Increased
4+	Bounding

Figure 9-1. When routine vital signs are assessed, the pulse is generally measured in one of two sites: radial or apical.

Radial Pulse

E To palpate the radial pulse:

1. Select the pulse point. Place the pads of your first, second, or third finger on the site of the radial pulse. The radial pulse can be palpated where the radial artery runs along the radial bone on the thumb side of the inner wrist.

2. Gently press your finger pad against the artery, using enough pressure to feel the pulse. Pressing too hard will obliterate the pulse.

3. Using the second hand of a watch, count the pulse rate. If the pulse is regular, count for 30 seconds and multiply by 2 to obtain the pulse rate per minute. If the pulse is irregular, count for 60 seconds.

4. Identify the pulse rhythm (regular or irregular) as you palpate.

5. Using the scales from Table 9-2, identify the pulse volume as you palpate.

Apical Pulse

E To assess the apical pulse:

1. Place the diaphragm of the stethoscope on the apical pulse site. The apex is on the left side of the chest, to the left of the sternum and between the fourth and sixth intercostal spaces. Remember to warm the diaphragm in your hand before placing the diaphragm on the patient.

2. Count the pulse rate for 30 seconds, if regular, or for 60 seconds, if irregular.

3. Identify the pulse rhythm and volume.

4. Identify a pulse deficit (apical pulse rate greater than radial pulse rate) by listening to the apical pulse and palpating the radial pulse simultaneously.

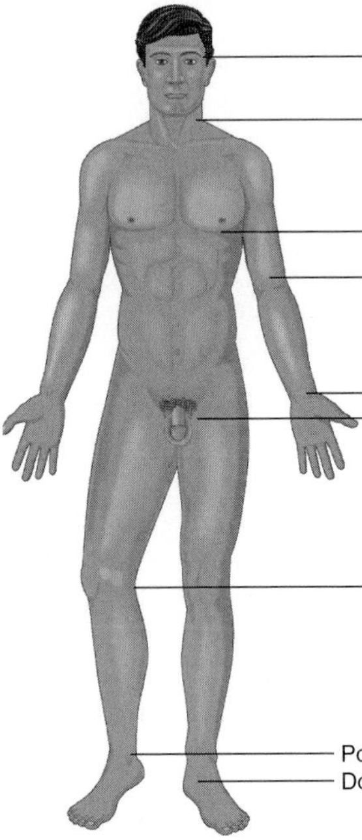

Figure 9-1 Pulse Sites

Rate

N **Normal pulse rate varies with age. Table 9-3 shows ranges for normal pulse rate according to age. Pulse rate normally increases during periods of exertion. Athletes commonly have a resting heart rate less than 60.**

Rhythm

N **Normal pulse rhythm is regular, with equal intervals between beats.**

Volume

N **The pulse volume is normally the same with each beat. A normal pulse volume can be felt with the fingers using a moderate amount of pressure and can be obliterated by the use of too great a pressure.**

A complete discussion of cardiovascular assessment is found in Chapter 16.

TABLE 9-3 Pulse Rate: Normal Range According to Age

AGE	RESTING PULSE RATE (Beats/Minute)	AVERAGE
Newborn	100–170	140
1 year	80–160	120
3 years	80–120	110
6 years	70–115	100
10 years	70–110	90
14 years	60–110	85–90
Adult	60–100	72

A Tachycardia: pulse rate faster than 100 beats per minute in an adult

P Trauma, blood volume losses, anemias, infection, fear, fever, pain, hyperthyroidism, shock, anxiety

A Bradycardia: pulse rates below 60 beats per minute in an adult

P Use of medications such as cardiotonics (digoxin) and beta blockers, eye surgery, increased intracranial pressure, myocardial infarction, hypothyroidism, prolonged vomiting

A Asystole: absence of a pulse

P Cardiac arrest, hypovolemia, pneumothorax, cardiac tamponade, or acidosis

A Dysrhythmias, or arrhythmias: pulse rhythms that are not regular

P Cardiac dysrhythmias that are atrial and ventricular in origin cause abnormal rhythms, such as atrial fibrillation and premature ventricular contractions

A Small, weak pulses

P Decreased cardiac stroke volume caused by heart failure, hypovolemic shock, and cardiogenic shock

P Aortic stenosis, constrictive pericarditis, dysrhythmias

A Bounding pulses

P Exercise, fever, anemia, anxiety, hyperthyroidism, early stages of septic shock

Temperature

Both the Celsius scale and the Fahrenheit scale are commonly used to measure temperature, which is the indicator of core body heat. To convert temperatures between the two scales, use the following formulas:

$$\left(\frac{9}{5} \times \text{temperature in Celsius}\right) + 32° = \text{temperature in Fahrenheit}$$

$$\frac{5}{9} \times (\text{temperature in Fahrenheit} - 32°) = \text{temperature in Celsius}$$

Variables Affecting Body Temperature

There are physiological variables that affect body temperature. These include circadian rhythm patterns, hormones, age, exercise, stress, and environmental extremes of hot and cold.

Measurement Routes

There are four basic routes by which temperature can be measured: oral, rectal, axillary, and tympanic. Each route has advantages and disadvantages. The advantages and disadvantages of each route are summarized in Table 9-4.

TABLE 9-4 Advantages and Disadvantages of Four Routes for Body Temperature Measurement

ROUTE	NORMAL RANGE	ADVANTAGES	DISADVANTAGES
Oral Average 37.0°C or 98.6°F	36.0°–38.0°C 96.8°–100.4°F	Convenient; accessible	**Safety:** Glass thermometers with mercury can be bitten and broken, causing patient injury. Patients need to be alert and cooperative and cognitively capable of following instructions for safe use. **Physical abilities:** Patients need to be able to breathe through the nose and be without oral pathology or recent oral surgery; route not applicable for comatose or confused patients, or for infants and toddlers. **Accuracy:** Oxygen therapy by mask and ingestion of hot or cold drinks immediately before oral temperature measurement affect accuracy of the reading.
Rectal Average 0.4°C or 0.7°F higher than oral	36.7°C–38.0°C 98.0°F–100.4°F	Considered most accurate	**Safety:** Contraindicated after rectal surgery. Risk of rectal perforation in children less than 2 years of age. Risk of stimulating valsalva maneuver in cardiac patients. **Physical aspects:** Invasive and uncomfortable.
Axillary Average 0.6°C or 1°F lower than oral	35.4°C–37.4°C 95.8°F–99.4°F	Safe; noninvasive	**Accuracy:** Glass thermometer must be left in place for 5 minutes to obtain accurate measurement. Placement and position of thermometer tip affect reading.
Tympanic Calibrated to oral or rectal scales	See oral or rectal	Convenient; fast; safe; noninvasive. Does not require contact with any mucous membrane.	**Accuracy:** Research is inconclusive as to accuracy of readings and correlations with other body temperature measurements. Technique affects reading. Tympanic membrane is thought to reflect the core temperature.

Oral Method

E **1.** Place the thermometer at the base of the patient's tongue and to the right or left of the frenulum, and instruct the patient to close the lips around the thermometer, and to avoid biting the thermometer. Ensure that the patient has not consumed food or beverage 15 minutes prior to monitoring the temperature.

2. Leave the thermometer in the mouth for the time recommended by your institution (usually 3 to 10 minutes).

3. Read the thermometer and record the temperature.

Rectal Method

E **1.** Position the patient with the buttocks exposed. Adults may be more comfortable lying on the side facing away from you and with the knees slightly flexed or lying prone.

2. Don clean gloves.

3. Lubricate the tip of the thermometer with a water-soluble lubricant.

4. Ask the patient to take a deep breath. Insert the thermometer into the anus 0.5 to 1.5 inches, depending on the patient's age.

5. Do not force the insertion of the thermometer or insert into feces.

6. Hold the thermometer in place for 3 to 5 minutes or the time recommended by your institution.

Note: Never interchange a thermometer used rectally for one used orally.

Axillary Method

E **1.** Place the thermometer into the middle of the axilla and fold the patient's arm across the chest to keep the thermometer in place.

2. Leave the thermometer in place 5 to 10 minutes, depending on your institution's protocol.

Electronic Thermometer

E **1.** Remove the electronic thermometer from its charging unit.

2. Attach a disposable cover to the probe.

3. Using a method previously described (oral, rectal, or axillary), measure the patient's temperature.

4. Listen for the sound or look for the symbol that indicates maximum body temperature has been reached.

5. Observe and record the reading.

6. Remove and discard the probe cover.

7. Return the electronic thermometer to the charging unit.

Tympanic Thermometer

E **1.** Attach the probe cover to the nose of the thermometer.

2. Gently place the probe of the thermometer over the entrance to the ear canal. If the patient is under 3 years old, pull the pinna down and aim the probe toward the opposite eye. If the patient is over 3 years old, grasp the pinna, gently pull it up and back, and aim the probe toward the opposite ear. Make sure there is a tight seal.

3. Press the start button on the thermometer handle.

4. Wait for the beep, remove the probe from the ear, and read the temperature.

5. Discard the probe cover.

6. Return the tympanic thermometer to the charger unit.

N **Normal body temperatures are described in Table 9-4.**

A Hyperthermia, pyrexia, or fever: body temperature exceeding 38.5°C, or 101.5°F; associated clinical signs of hyperthermia: increased respiratory rate and pulse, shivering, pallor, thirst

P Infection resulting from an increased basal metabolic rate and environmental exposure

A Hypothermia: body temperature below 34°C, or 93.2°F; associated clinical signs of hypothermia: decreased body temperature, initial shivering that ceases as drowsiness and coma ensue, hypotension, decreased urinary output, lack of muscle coordination, disorientation

P Prolonged exposure to cold, such as immersion in cold water, administration of large volumes of unwarmed blood products, induced hypothermia to decrease the tissue's need for oxygen (as during cardiac surgery)

Blood Pressure

Blood pressure (BP) is the measurement (in millimeters of mercury [mm Hg]) of the force exerted by the flow of blood pumped into the large arteries. There is a diurnal variation in BP characterized by a high point in the early evening and a low point during the early, deep stage of sleep.

Korotkoff Sounds

Korotkoff sounds are generated when the flow of blood through an artery is altered by inflating a blood pressure cuff that is wrapped around the corresponding extremity. Korotkoff sounds may be heard by listening over a pulse site that is distal to the BP cuff. As the air is released from the bladder of the cuff, the pressure on the artery changes from that which completely occludes blood flow to that which allows free flow. As the pressure against the artery wall decreases, five distinct sounds occur. They are as follows:

Phase I: The first audible sound heard as the cuff pressure is released; sounds like clear tapping and is correlated with systolic pressure (the force needed to pump the blood out of the heart).

Phase II: Sounds like swishing or a murmur; created as the blood flows through blood vessels narrowed by the inflation of the BP cuff.

Phase III: Sounds like clear, intense tapping; created as blood flows through the artery but cuff pressure is still great enough to occlude flow during diastole.

Phase IV: Sounds are muffled and are heard when cuff pressure is low enough to allow some blood flow during diastole. The change from the tapping sound of Phase III to the muffled sound of Phase IV is referred to as the first diastolic reading.

Phase V: No sounds are heard; occurs when cuff pressure is released enough to allow normal blood flow. This is referred to as the second diastolic reading.

Measuring Blood Pressure

Systolic pressure represents the pressure exerted on the arterial wall during systole, when the ventricles are contracting. Diastolic pressure represents the pressure in the arteries when the ventricles are relaxed and filling. Blood pressure is recorded as a fraction, with the top number representing systole and the bottom number(s) representing diastole. If first and second diastolic sounds are recorded, the first diastolic sound is written over the second. For example, 120/90/80 indicates that 120 mm Hg is the systolic pressure, 90 mm Hg is the first diastolic sound, and 80 mm Hg is the second diastolic sound. Pulse pressure is the difference between diastolic and systolic blood pressures.

Measurement Sites

There are several potential sites for BP measurement. The preferred site is the brachial pulse site, where the brachial artery runs across the antecubital fossa. The posterior thigh, where the popliteal artery runs behind the knee joint, can also be used. A site should not be used if there is pain or injury around or near the site; for instance, a postmastectomy patient should have BP assessed on the unaffected side. Surgical incisions; intravenous, central venous, or arterial lines; or areas with poor perfusion should be avoided when measuring BP. Patients with arteriovenous (AV) fistulas or AV shunts should not have BP measured in the affected extremities.

Equipment

Blood pressure is measured indirectly with a stethoscope or Doppler ultrasonic transducer and a sphygmomanometer, which consists of a BP cuff, connecting tubes, air pump, and manometer. Blood pressure cuffs come in several sizes. The size of the cuff bladder should be 80% of the limb width (Chobanian et al., 2003). The cuff should completely encircle the limb.

E **1.** Ensure that the patient has not had any caffeine or tobacco products in the past 30 minutes. Allow the patient to rest for 5 minutes before the blood pressure is taken.

2. Select an appropriately sized cuff.

3. Position the patient. The patient may be sitting, standing, or supine. At the first encounter, all three positions are recommended.

4. To prevent an inaccurate reading, position the arm or leg to be used so that the extremity is at a level equal to or lower than the heart.

5. Apply the deflated BP cuff:

- **a.** Upper arm: wrap the BP cuff snugly around the bare upper arm. The bottom of the BP cuff should be 1 to 2 inches above the antecubital fossa. The center of the bladder should be directly above the brachial artery (Figure 9-2).
- **b.** Leg: wrap the BP cuff around the bare thigh, with the bottom of the BP cuff slightly above the knee. The popliteal artery below the cuff is used for BP measurement.

6. Establish the baseline systolic BP (palpating the BP), if needed:

- **a.** Use the finger pads of your nondominant hand to palpate the brachial or radial artery distal to the BP cuff.
- **b.** Inflate the BP cuff and note when the arterial pulsation is no longer palpable.

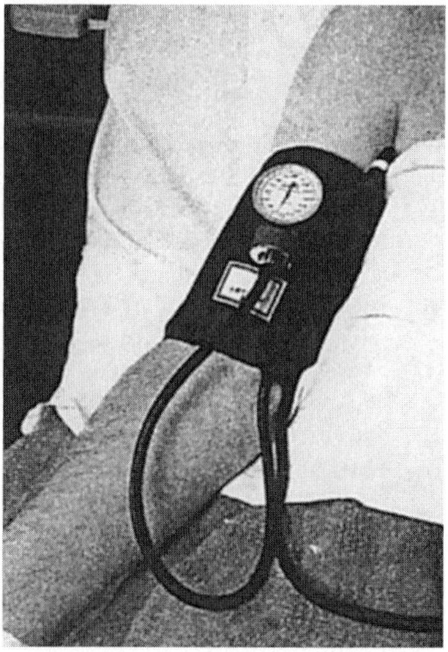

Figure 9-2 Appropriate Cuff Placement on Arm

- **c.** Release the air from the BP cuff and wait 1 to 2 minutes.

7. Palpate the pulse distal to the BP cuff.

8. Place the diaphragm of the stethoscope over the BP site:

- **a.** If a Doppler ultrasonic transducer is to be used, apply conducting gel to the site where the pulse was palpated.
- **b.** Place the Doppler transducer over the site.

9. Inflate the BP cuff to approximately 20 mm Hg above the previously established baseline BP, or 20 mm Hg above where the Korotkoff sounds disappear.

10. Slowly open the valve and release the pressure at a rate of 2 to 3 mm Hg/second.

11. Listen for the Korotkoff sounds:

- **a.** Onset of Korotkoff sounds is correlated with systolic pressure.
- **b.** Muffling or disappearance of Korotkoff sounds is correlated with diastolic pressure.

12. Completely deflate the BP cuff.

13. Record the BP reading(s). The extremity used and the position of the patient are important data to record along with the BP reading.

N **Normal BP varies with age. As a person ages, BP generally increases. Table 9-5 shows ranges for normal BP at different ages. Pulse pressure is normally 30 to 40 mm Hg.**

A Hypertension, or high BP in an adult patient: blood-pressure measures above 140 mm Hg systolic and 90 mm Hg diastolic on two consecutive checks after an initial screening. See Table 9-6 for recommendations on detection, evaluation, and treatment of hypertension. The cause of hypertension in 90% of patients who have it is unknown; such hypertension is known as primary or essential hypertension.

P Primary hypertension may be caused by abnormal functioning of the heart, kidneys, nervous system, or renin-angiotensin-aldosterone system.

A The remaining 10% of patients with high BP have secondary hypertension.

P Etiologies of secondary hypertension include arteriosclerosis, hypercholesterolemia resulting in decreased lumen size and increased BP, increased cardiac output, increased blood viscosity (sickle cell crisis), kidney disease resulting in decreased production of antidiuretic hormone, adrenal gland tumor, pheochromocytoma, fluid overload resulting from poor renal function, indiscriminant intravenous fluid administration (particularly in children), stress, and stimulation of the sympathetic nervous system.

TABLE 9-5 Blood Pressure: Normal Range According to Age and Gender*

AGE (FEMALE)	SYSTOLIC (MM HG)	DIASTOLIC (MM HG)
1	97–103	52–56
5	103–109	66–70
10	112–118	73–76
15	120–127	78–81
≥18	<120	<80
AGE (MALE)	**SYSTOLIC (MM HG)**	**DIASTOLIC (MM HG)**
1	94–103	49–54
5	104–112	65–70
10	111–119	73–78
15	122–131	76–81
≥18	<120	<80

**The National Heart, Lung, and Blood Institute of the National Institutes of Health developed pediatric blood pressure guidelines based on gender, age, and height percentiles. The measurements listed for pediatric patients are consolidated for ease in reporting. Normal blood pressure is defined as the systolic (SBP) and diastolic (DBP) blood pressures that are below the 90th percentile for age and gender. High-normal blood pressure is defined as the SBP or DBP being at the 90th percentile and above, but not including, the 95th percentile. Hypertension is defined as a SBP or DBP greater than or equal to the 95th percentile on three different occasions. Refer to the Bibliography for the National High Blood Pressure Education Program, which offers more detailed information.*

TABLE 9-6 Classification and Management of Blood Pressure for Adults 18 Years or Older

			MANAGEMENT		
				INITIAL DRUG THERAPY**	
BP CLASSIFICATION	SBP* (MM HG)	DBP* (MM HG)	LIFESTYLE MODIFICATION	WITHOUT COMPELLING INDICATIONS	WITH COMPELLING INDICATIONS
Normal	<120	and <80	Encourage	N/A	N/A
Prehypertension	120–139	or 80–89	Yes	No antihypertensive drug indicated	Drug(s) for the compelling indications**
Stage 1 hypertension	140–159	or 90–99	Yes	Thiazide-type diuretics for most. May consider ACEI, ARB, BB, CCB, or a combination	Drug(s) for the compelling indications** Other antihypertensive drugs (diuretics, ACEI, ARB, BB, CCB) as needed
Stage 2 hypertension	≥160	or ≥100	Yes	Two-drug combination for most*** (usually thiazide-type diuretic and ACEI, ARB, BB, or CCB)	Drug(s) for the compelling indications** Other antihypertensive drugs (diuretics, ACEI, ARB, BB, CCB) as needed

**BP, blood pressure; SBP, systolic BP; DBP, diastolic BP; ACEI, angiotensin-converting enzyme inhibitor; ARB, angiotensin receptor blocker; BB, β-blocker; CCB, calcium channel blocker, Treatment determined by highest BP category.*

***Treat patients with chronic kidney disease or diabetes to BP goal of less than 130/80 mm Hg.*

****Initial combined therapy should be used cautiously in those at risk for orthostatic hypotension.*

Note. *From "The seventh report of the Joint National Committee on Prevention, Detection, Evaluation, and Treatment of High Blood Pressure," by A. V. Chobanian, G. L. Bakris, H. R. Black, W. C. Cushman, L. A. Green, J. L. Izzo, Jr., et al., 2003,* Journal of the American Medical Association, *289(19), p. 2560–2571.*

> **Nursing Tip**
>
> **Documenting Blood Pressure**
>
> The position of the patient during the blood pressure measurement should be recorded. Use the following symbols to depict patient position:
>
> 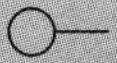 supine 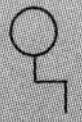 sitting 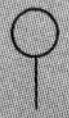 standing
>
> Also record where the blood pressure was taken. Use the following abbreviations:
>
> RA = right arm LA = left arm
> RL = right leg LL = left leg
>
> Examples of blood pressure readings are:
>
> 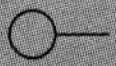 160/122 LL (left leg, supine)
>
> 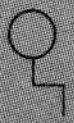 98/52 RA (right arm, sitting)
>
> 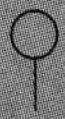 118/85 LA (left arm, standing)

A Hypotension, or low BP, results in inadequate tissue perfusion and oxygenation.

P Etiologies of hypotension include hypovolemic shock, use of nitroglycerin or antihypertensives, and anaphylactic shock.

A A difference of greater than 10 to 15 mm Hg between the BP in each arm

P Coarctation of the aorta, aortic aneurysm, atherosclerotic obstruction, subclavian steal syndrome

A Systolic BP greater in the arms than in the legs

P Increased stroke volume ejection velocity, increased cardiac output, peripheral vasodilation, aortic constriction resulting from decreased distensibility of the aorta and major arteries

A Decreased pulse pressure

P Decreased stroke volume (cardiac tamponade, shock, tachycardia) or increased peripheral resistance (aortic stenosis, coarctation of the aorta, mitral stenosis or mitral regurgitation, cardiac tamponade)

A Increased pulse pressure

P Increased stroke volume (aortic regurgitation) or increased peripheral vasodilatation (fever, anemia, heat, exercise, hyperthyroidism, arteriovenous fistula)

Pain

Pain is "an unpleasant sensory or emotional experience associated with actual or potential tissue damage, or described in terms of such damage" (IASP, 1979). It is a complex sensory experience. Pain has become the focus of many clinical research projects as a single clinical phenomenon, not just a symptom of clinical pathology.

Nociceptive Pain

Nociceptive pain arises from somatic or visceral stimulation. Nociception, or pain perception, is a multistep process that involves the nervous system as well as other body systems. A noxious stimulus occurs, which stimulates the nociceptors (receptive neurons of pain sensation that are located in the skin and various viscera). The noxious stimulus can be many things (e.g., trauma, burn, chemical exposure, internal body inflammation, internal body growth of tissue).

Neuropathic Pain

Neuropathic pain can result from lesions in the central nervous system (CNS) or peripheral nervous system (PNS). It is often characterized as a severe burning or tingling, such as that experienced with herpes zoster. Neuropathic pain may be difficult to treat clinically.

Types of Pain

Pain can be grouped by its origin as well as its duration. Cutaneous, somatic, visceral, and referred pain are the types of pain grouped by origin. Cutaneous pain arises from the stimulation of cutaneous nerves. This pain usually has a burning quality. Somatic pain originates from bone, tendons, ligaments, muscles, and nerves and is frequently caused by musculoskeletal injury. Visceral pain arises from the organs. Diseased organs can change size, usually resulting in stretching of the organ, leading to pain. Acute appendicitis is an example of visceral pain. Referred pain is perceived in a location other than where the pathology is occurring. The location of the referred pain is in the dermatome of the spinal cord that is innervating the affected viscera and where the organ was located in its embryonic stage. An example of referred pain is the pain of pancreatitis felt on the left shoulder.

Acute, chronic malignant, and chronic nonmalignant pain are examples of pain grouped by their duration. Acute pain has a sudden onset, is of short duration, and is self-limiting. It ranges in intensity from mild to severe. It usually has an identifiable cause, such as surgery or trauma. Chronic malignant pain is pain of more than 6 months' duration, for example, in a patient with cancer. This persistent pain can be due to a tumor, inflammation, blocked ducts, pressure on other body parts, and necrosis. Chronic nonmalignant pain also lasts more than 6 months. It can occur with and without an identifiable cause. The pain can remain even after an initial injury is healed. Back pain and fibromyalgia are examples of chronic nonmalignant pain.

Variables Affecting Pain

Gender, age, previous experience with pain, and cultural expectations can affect an individual's response to pain. Studies have shown that females have a lower pain tolerance or threshold than males and report pain more frequently.

Regarding the effect of age on pain, typically, young children become sensitized to pain and may be greatly affected by the pain experience. As they reach adolescence, children may become more stoic about pain. Older adults, especially those who have chronic pain, may also not complain about their pain until it becomes debilitating. Lastly, cultural norms can help determine what the patient's pain experience will be.

Effects of Pain on the Body

Pain affects everyone in different ways. Acute pain usually manifests itself differently from chronic pain although there are some common elements. Physiological responses to pain include tachycardia, tachypnea, hypertension, diaphoresis, dilated pupils, and an altered immune response. Additional responses to pain include complaints of pain, crying, moaning, frowning, anger, fear, anxiety, depression, suicidal ideation, decreased appetite, sleep deprivation, altered concentration, pacing, rubbing the affected body part, and protecting or splinting the affected body part.

Assessing Pain

Many pain intensity rating scales are available to assess the severity of a patient's pain experience. The Pain Intensity Scale (Figure 9-3) is a quick assessment tool that is easily understood. The Wong-Baker FACES Pain Rating Scale (Figure 9-4) is recommended for children over the age of 3. The Oucher Pain Assessment Tool (Figure 9-5) is used with children 3–12 years old. Caucasian, Hispanic, and African American versions of this tool are available.

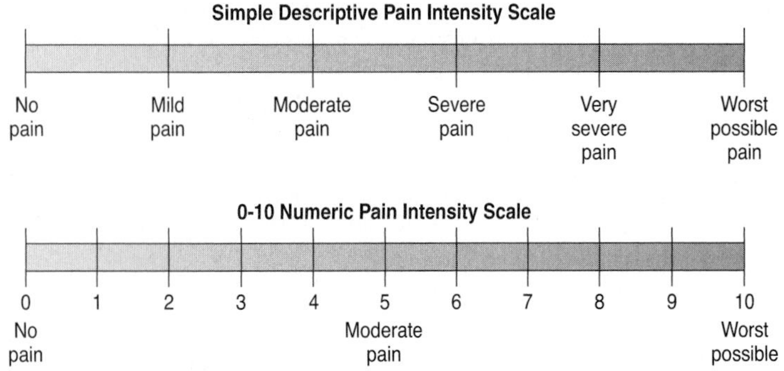

Figure 9-3 Pain Intensity Scale. Note. *From* Acute Pain Management: Operative or Medical Procedures and Trauma. *Clinical Practice Guideline (AHCPR Publication No. 92-0032), by the Acute Pain Management Guideline Panel, 1992, Rockville, MD: Agency for Health Care Policy and Research.*

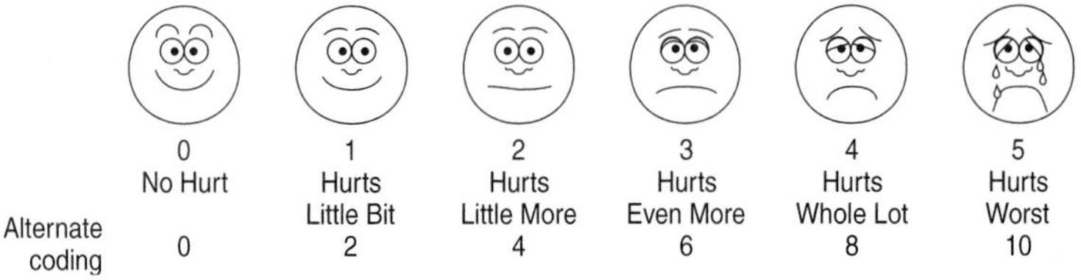

Figure 9-4 Wong-Baker FACES Pain Rating Scale. Note. *From M. Hockenberry, D. Wilson, M. Winkelstein:* Wong's Essentials of Pediatric Nursing, *7th ed., St. Louis, MO, 2005, p. 663. Copyrighted by Mosby, Inc. Reprinted by permission.*

REFERENCES

Acute Pain Management Guideline Panel. (1992). *Acute pain management: Operative or medical procedures and trauma. Clinical practice guideline* (AHCPR Publication No. 92-0032). Rockville, MD: Agency for Health Care Policy and Research. (Telephone: 800-358-9295 or 301-495-3453; or write Acute Pain Management Guideline, AHCPR Publications Clearinghouse, P.O. Box 8547, Silver Spring, MD 20907)

Beyer, J. (1983). *The Caucasian version of the Oucher.* Developed and copyrighted by Judith E. Beyer, RN, PhD, 1983.

Chobanian, A. V., Bakris, G. L., Black, H. R., Cushman, W. C., Green, L. A., Izzo, Jr., J. L., et al. (2003). The seventh report of the Joint National Committee on Prevention, Detection, Evaluation, and Treatment of High Blood Pressure. *Journal of the American Medical Association, 289*(19), 2560–2571.

Hockenberry, M., Wilson, D., Winkelstein, M., & Kline, N. (2003). *Wong's nursing care of infants and children* (7th ed.). St. Louis, MO: Mosby.

International Association for the Study of Pain. (1979). *IASP pain terminology.* Retrieved December 23, 2004, from http://www.iasp-pain.org/terms-p.html

BIBLIOGRAPHY

National High Blood Pressure Education Program Working Group on High Blood Pressure in Children and Adolescents. (2004). The Fourth Report on the Diagnosis, Evaluation, and Treatment of High Blood Pressure in Children and Adolescents. *Pediatrics, 114,* 555–576. Retrieved December 23, 2004, from http://nhlbi.nih.gov/health/prof/heart/hbp/hbp_ped.htm

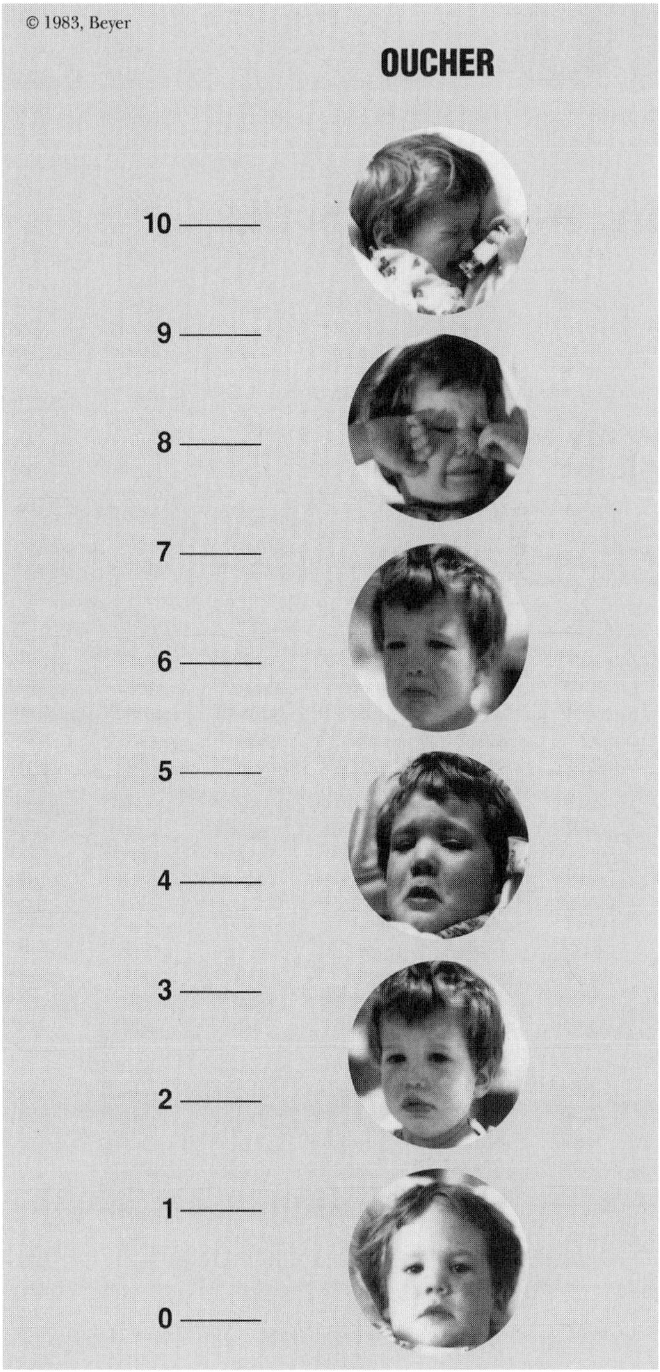

Figure 9-5 Oucher Pain Assessment Tool. Note. *From* The Caucasion version of the Oucher, *developed and copyrighted by Judith E. Beyer, RN, PhD, 1983.*

10

Skin, Hair, and Nails

Anatomy and Physiology

Skin

The surface area of the skin covers approximately 20 square feet in the average adult. Skin thickness varies from 0.2 to 1.5 mm, depending on the region of the body and the person's age. The skin can be divided into three main layers: the epidermis, the dermis, and the subcutaneous tissue, or hypodermis (Figure 10-1).

The skin serves as a protective barrier against invasion, provides boundaries for fluids and mobile tissues within the body, regulates temperature through perspiration and vasoconstriction, contains receptors for pain, touch, pressure, and temperature, and acts as an organ of excretion for substances such as water, salts, and nitrogenous wastes.

Glands of the Skin

There are two main groups of glands in the skin: the sebaceous glands and the sweat glands.

The sebaceous glands are sebum-producing glands found almost everywhere in the dermis except for the palmar

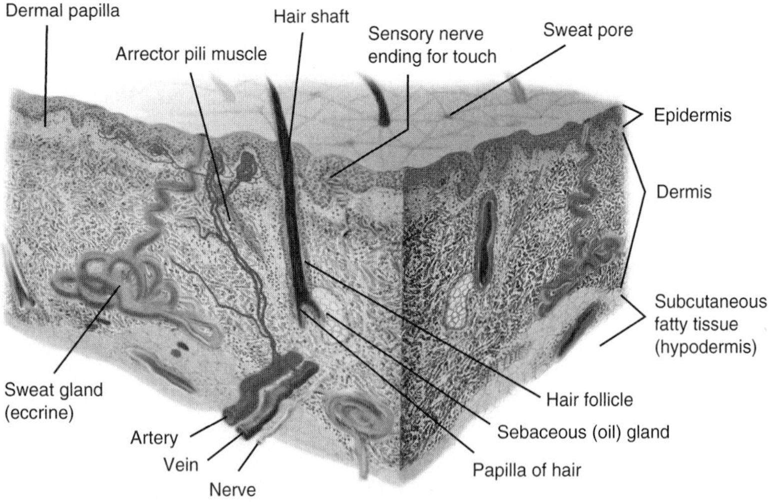

Figure 10-1 Structures of the Skin

and plantar surfaces. The ducts of the sebaceous glands open into the upper part of the hair follicles and are responsible for producing sebum, an oily secretion thought to retard evaporation and water loss from the epidermal cells. Sebaceous glands are most prevalent in the scalp, forehead, nose, and chin.

The two main types of sweat glands are apocrine glands, which are associated with hair follicles, and eccrine glands, which are not associated with hair follicles. Apocrine glands appear after puberty and are associated with body odor. They are found primarily in the axillae, genital and rectal areas, nipples, and navel. Eccrine glands open directly onto the skin's surface and are widely distributed throughout the body. Both types of gland are located in the subcutaneous tissue.

Hair

With few exceptions (the palmar and plantar surfaces, lips, nipples, and glans penis), hair is distributed over the entire body surface. Vellus, or fine, faint hair covers most of the body. Terminal hair is the coarser, darker hair of the scalp, eyebrows, eyelashes, and axillary and pubic areas. Hair color is determined by the melanocytes produced in the cells at the base of each hair follicle; an abundance of pigment produces dark hair color, whereas smaller amounts of pigment produce light hair color.

Nails

Nails are composed of keratinized, or horny, layers of cells that arise from undifferentiated epithelial tissue called the matrix.

The nail plate (the tissue that covers the distal portion of the digits and provides protection) is approximately 0.5 to 0.75 mm thick. The nails consist of the nail root, which lies posteriorly to the cuticle and is attached to the matrix; the nailbed, which is the vascular bed located beneath the nail plate; and the periungual tissues, which surround the nail plate and the free edge of the nail (Figure 10-2). The normally translucent nail plate is given a pinkish cast by the underlying vascular bed in light-skinned individuals and a brownish cast in dark-skinned individuals.

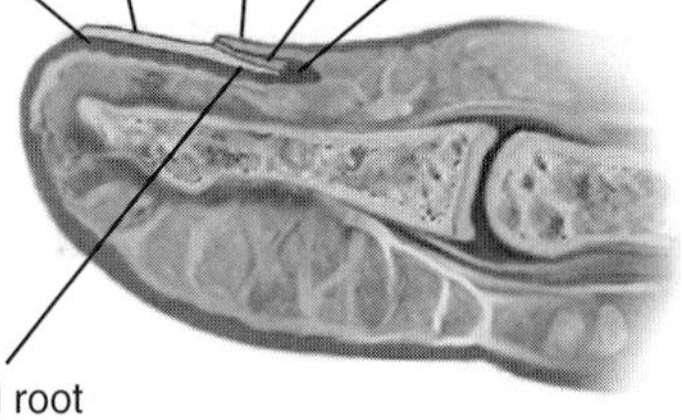

Figure 10-2 Structures of the Nail

HEALTH HISTORY

Medical History

Skin specific: allergies, eczema, atopic dermatitis, melanoma, albinism, vitiligo, psoriasis, skin cancer, athlete's foot, bacterial or fungal infections of the skin, birthmarks, tattoos

Hair specific: allergies, alopecia, lice, bacterial or fungal infections of the scalp, brittle hair, rapid hair loss, trichotillomania, trauma, congenital anomalies

Nail specific: allergies, psoriasis, bacterial or fungal infections, trauma, brittle nails, nail biting, congenital anomalies

Surgical History

Keloid and scar formation, plastic surgery, skin grafts, reconstructive surgery, excision biopsy, piercing, hair plugs

NURSING CHECKLIST

Specific Health History Questions Regarding the Skin, Hair, and Nails

Skin Care Habits

- Do you use lotions, perfumes, cologne, cosmetics, soaps, oils, shaving cream, after shave lotion, or an electric or standard razor?
- What type of home remedies do you use for skin lesions and rashes?
- How often do you bathe or shower?
- Do you use a tanning bed or salon?
- What type of sun protection do you use?
- Have you ever had a reaction to jewelry that you wore?
- Do you wear hats, visors, gloves, long sleeves, pants, or sunscreen when exposed to the sun?
- How much time do you spend in the sun?

Hair Care Habits

- Do you use shampoo, conditioner, hair spray, or setting products?
- Do you color, dye, bleach, frost, or relax your hair?
- What products do you use?
- Do you wear a wig or hair piece?
- Do you have graying or hair loss?
- Do you use a hair dryer, heated curlers, or curling iron?
- Do you perform tight hair braiding?

Nail Care Habits

- Do you have manicures or pedicures?
- What type of nail care do you perform (trimming, clipping, use of polish, nail tips, acrylics)?
- Do you bite your nails?
- Do you suffer from nail splitting or discoloration?

NURSING CHECKLIST

General Approach to Skin, Hair, and Nail Assessment

1. Ensure that the room is well lit. Daylight is the best source of light, especially when determining skin color. If daylight is unavailable, however, overhead fluorescent lights should be used.
2. Use a handheld magnifying glass to aid in inspection when simple visual inspection is not adequate.
3. Explain to the patient each step of the assessment process before initiating the assessment.
4. Ensure patient privacy by providing drapes.
5. Ensure patient comfort by keeping the room at an appropriate temperature.
6. Warm hands by washing them in warm water before the assessment.
7. Gather equipment on a table before initiating the assessment.
8. Ask the patient to undress completely and to put on a gown, leaving the back untied.
9. Perform the assessment in a cephalocaudal fashion.
10. For episodic illness, the skin examination is incorporated into the regional physical exam.

Equipment

- Magnifying glass
- Good source of natural light
- Penlight
- Clean gloves
- Microscope slide
- Small centimeter ruler

For Advanced Techniques:
- Wood's lamp
- No. 15 scalpel blade
- Microscope slide with cover slips
- Mineral oil
- Microscope

Assessment of the Skin, Hair, and Nails

Inspection of the Skin

E In each area, observe for color, bleeding, ecchymosis, erythema, vascularity, lesions, moisture, temperature, texture, turgor, and edema.

1. Facing the patient, inspect the color of the skin of the face, eyelids, ears, nose, lips, and mucous membranes.

2. Inspect the anterior and lateral aspects of the neck, then behind the ears.

3. Inspect the arms and the dorsal and palmar surfaces of the hands. Pay special attention to the webs between the fingers.

4. Have the patient assume a supine position, with the arms placed over the head.

5. Lower the patient's gown to uncover the chest and breasts.

6. Inspect the intramammary folds and ridges. Pendulous breasts may need to be raised to perform this inspection.

7. Assess the axillae and re-cover the chest and breasts with the gown.

8. Raise the gown to uncover the abdomen and the anterior aspects of the lower extremities; place a sheet over the genital area.

9. Inspect the abdomen, anterior aspects of the lower extremities, dorsal and plantar surfaces of the feet, and toe webs.

10. Don gloves and uncover the genital area.

11. Inspect the inguinal folds and genitalia.

12. Remove gloves.

13. Have the patient assume a side-lying position on the examination table, so that the patient's back is facing you.

14. Inspect the back and the posterior neck and scalp. Specifically look for nevi or other lesions.

15. Inspect the posterior aspects of the lower extremities.

16. Don clean gloves, raise the gluteal cleft, and inspect the gluteal folds and perianal area; remove and discard gloves.

17. Cover the patient and assist back to a sitting position. Wash hands.

Color

E Assess for coloration.

N **The skin is normally a uniform whitish pink or brown color, depending on the race of the patient. Dark-skinned persons may normally have freckling on the gums, tongue borders, and lining of the cheeks; the gingiva may appear blue or variegated in color.**

A Cyanosis: dusky blue fingers, lips, or mucous membranes; bluish tint to skin in light-skinned individuals; ashen-gray to pale tint (including on the lips and tongue) in dark-skinned individuals

P Greater than 5 g/dl of deoxygenated hemoglobin in the blood; central cyanosis secondary to marked heart and lung disease; peripheral cyanosis secondary to systemic disease or vasoconstriction stimulated by cold or anxiety

A Jaundice: yellow-green to orange cast or coloration of skin, sclera, mucous membranes, fingernails, and palmar and/or plantar surfaces in light-skinned individuals; yellow staining in the sclera, hard palate, and palmar or plantar surfaces in dark-skinned individuals

P Increased serum bilirubin, liver disease, hemolytic disease

A Carotenemia: orange-yellow coloration of palmar and plantar surfaces and forehead but no involvement of the mucous membranes

P Elevated levels of serum carotene from excessive ingestion of carotene-rich foods such as carrots

A Grayish cast to the skin

P Seen in renal patients, associated with chronic anemia in conjunction with retained urochrome pigments

A Sustained bright-red or pink coloration (hyperemia) in light-skinned individuals; possibly no underlying change in coloration in dark-skinned individuals; may use palpation to ascertain signs of warmth, swelling, or induration

P Dilated superficial blood vessels, increased blood flow, febrile states, local inflammatory condition, excessive alcohol intake

A Polycythemia: bright-red to ruddy sustained appearance evident on the integument, mucous membranes, palmar or plantar surfaces

P Increased number of red blood cells

A Generalized or discrete brown cast to the skin

P Genetic predisposition, pregnancy, Addison's disease (deficiency in cortisol leading to enhanced melanin production), café au lait spots, exposure to sunlight

A Albinism: white cast to the skin, including the hair and eyebrows

P Congenital inability to form melanin

A Vitiligo: patchy, symmetrical areas of white on the skin

P Loss of melanin, trauma

A An erythematous, confluent eruption in a butterfly-like distribution over the face

P Systemic lupus erythematosus, a connective tissue disorder, is the most likely etiology.

Bleeding, Ecchymosis, and Vascularity

E Inspect the skin for evidence of bleeding, ecchymosis, and increased vascularity.

N **There are normally no areas of bleeding, ecchymosis, or increased vascularity.**

A Spontaneous bleeding from the mucous membranes, previous venipuncture sites, or lesions

P Clotting disorders, trauma, use of anti-thrombolytic agents

A Petechiae: violaceous discoloration of less than 0.5 cm in diameter, which does not blanch; in dark-skinned individuals, evaluate for petechiae in the mucous membranes and axillae

P Increased bleeding tendency, embolism, intravascular defects, infections

A Purpura: confluent petechiae or confluent ecchymosis over any part of the body

P Decreased platelet formation, pigmentation changes may become permanent

A Ecchymosis: violaceous discoloration of varying size, also called a black and blue mark; deeper in color in dark-skinned individuals

P Extravasation of blood into the skin as the result of trauma, heparin or coumadin use, or liver dysfunction

A Venous stars: linear or irregularly shaped blue vascular patterns that do not blanch

P Increased venous pressure in the superficial veins

A Cherry angiomas: bright-red circumscribed areas that may darken with age

P Unknown, are pathologically not significant

A Port-wine stain or nevus flammeus: burgundy, red, or purple macular vascular patch located along the course of a peripheral nerve

P Patches composed of mature but thin-walled capillaries usually present at birth and located on the face can indicate Sturge-Weber syndrome

A Gas gangrene or clostridial myonecrosis: dark-brown or blackened areas of skin that are edematous and painful and that may drain a thin liquid having a sweet, foul odor

P Gram-positive infection that affects skeletal muscles having decreased oxygenation; secondary to circulatory compromise, such as in diabetes mellitus, arterial insufficiency, trauma, constricting casts, or contaminated wounds

A Spider angiomas: bright-red or star-shaped with central pulsation

P Causes include pregnancy, liver disease, hormone therapy

> **Nursing Alert**
>
> **Signs of Abuse**
>
> Areas of ecchymosis are often signs of trauma that could be the result of physical abuse. Ecchymotic areas on the base of the skull, the face, buttocks, breasts, or abdomen should warrant a high index of suspicion for abuse, especially if found in children or pregnant women. Burns (e.g., from cigarettes or an iron) and belt buckle and bite marks should also be highly suspect. Any signs of abuse should be further investigated and referred as necessary.

Lesions

E 1. Inspect the skin for any lesions, noting anatomic location. Lesions can be localized, regionalized, or generalized.
2. Note the grouping or arrangement of any lesions: discrete, grouped, confluent, linear, annular, polycyclic, generalized, or zosteriform (Figure 10-3).
3. Inspect any lesions for elevation (e.g., flat or raised).
4. Use a ruler to measure the size of any lesions.
5. Describe the color of any lesions.
6. Note the color and odor of any exudate.
7. Note the morphology of any skin lesions. Skin lesions can be primary, originating from previously normal skin, or secondary, originating from primary lesions. For specific descriptions of primary lesion morphology, see Figure 10-4. For specific descriptions of secondary lesion morphology, see Figure 10-5.

N **No skin lesions should be present except for freckles, birthmarks, or moles (nevi), which may be flat or elevated.**

A/P See Figures 10-3, 10-4, and 10-5.

> **Nursing Tip**
>
> **ABCDE Mnemonic for Evaluating Skin Lesions**
>
> **A** (asymmetric): Is the lesion asymmetric?
> **B** (borders): Are the borders of the lesion irregular?
> **C** (color): Is the color of the lesion uneven, irregular, or multicolored?
> **D** (diameter): Has the lesion's diameter changed recently?
> **E** (elevation): Has the lesion become elevated?

Nursing Alert

Danger Signs in Potentially Cancerous Lesions

- Rapid change in size
- Change in color
- Irregular border or butterfly-shaped border
- Elevation in a previously flat mole
- Multiple colors in a lesion
- Change in surface characteristics, such as oozing
- Change in sensation, such as pain, itching, or tenderness
- Change in surrounding skin, such as inflammation or induration
- Bleeding or ulcerative appearance of a mole

Because of the risk of basal cell or squamous cell carcinoma, patient referral is required for any of the above-mentioned abnormal findings.

Nursing Alert

Stages of Pressure Ulcers

Uniform standards for staging pressure ulcers are used on patients having pressure sores on any portion of the body.

Stage 1: In light-skinned individuals, the area is reddened but the skin is not broken; in dark-skinned individuals, pigmentation is enhanced.

Stage 2: The epidermal and dermal layers have sustained injury.

Stage 3: The subcutaneous tissues have sustained injury.

Stage 4: Muscle tissue and, perhaps, bone have sustained injury.

Nursing Tip

Identifying Burns

Burn patients frequently have varying degrees of injury to the body. Some parts of the body may have first-degree burns, while others have second- or third-degree burns. The following descriptions will help you identify degree of burn:

First-Degree Burn: the epidermis is injured or destroyed; there may be some damage to the dermis; the hair follicles and sweat glands are intact; the skin is red and dry; the burn is painful.

Second-Degree Burn: the epidermis and upper layers of the dermis are destroyed; the deeper dermis is injured; the hair follicles, sweat glands, and nerve endings are intact; the skin is red and blistery with exudate; the burn is painful; also called partial-thickness burns.

Third-Degree Burn: the epidermis and dermis are destroyed; the subcutaneous tissue may be injured; the hair follicles, sweat glands, and nerve endings are destroyed; the skin is white, red, black, tan, or brown and leathery in appearance; the burn is painless because nerve endings have been destroyed; also called full-thickness burns.

Fourth-Degree Burn: the epidermis and dermis are destroyed; the subcutaneous tissue, muscle, and bone may be injured; the hair follicles, sweat glands, and nerve endings are destroyed; the skin is white, red, black, tan, or brown with exposed and damaged subcutaneous tissue, muscle, or bone; the hair follicles, sweat glands, and nerve endings are destroyed; the burn is painless.

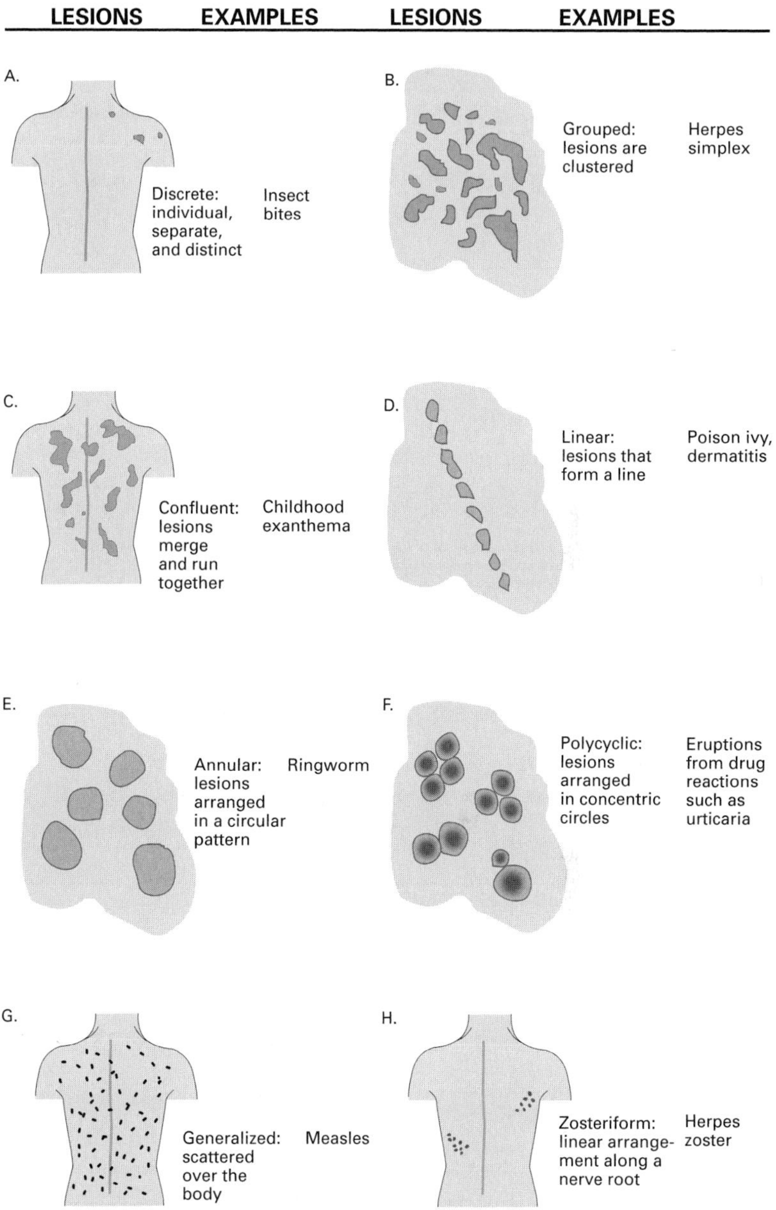
LESIONS
EXAMPLES
LESIONS
EXAMPLES
A.
Discrete: individual, separate, and distinct
Insect bites
B.
Grouped: lesions are clustered
Herpes simplex
C.
Confluent: lesions merge and run together
Childhood exanthema
D.
Linear: lesions that form a line
Poison ivy, dermatitis
E.
Annular: lesions arranged in a circular pattern
Ringworm
F.
Polycyclic: lesions arranged in concentric circles
Eruptions from drug reactions such as urticaria
G.
Generalized: scattered over the body
Measles
H.
Zosteriform: linear arrangement along a nerve root
Herpes zoster

Figure 10-3 Arrangement of Lesions

NONPALPABLE

A.

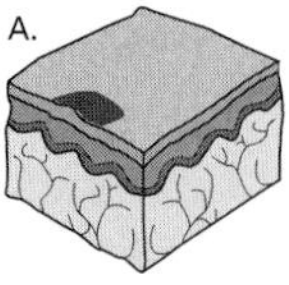

MACULE:
Localized changes in skin color of less than 1 cm in diameter
Example:
Freckle

B.

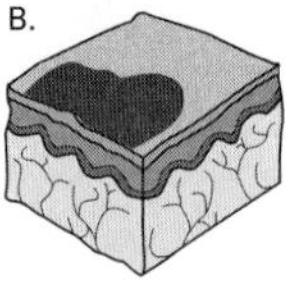

PATCH:
Localized changes in skin color of greater than 1 cm in diameter
Example:
Vitiligo, stage 1 of pressure ulcer

PALPABLE

C.

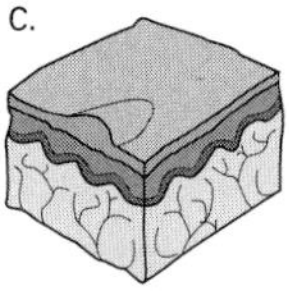

PAPULE:
Solid, elevated lesion less than 0.5 cm in diameter
Example:
Warts, elevated nevi

D.

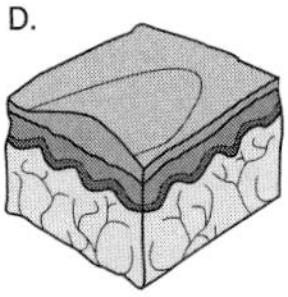

PLAQUE:
Solid, elevated lesion greater than 0.5 cm in diameter
Example:
Psoriasis

E.

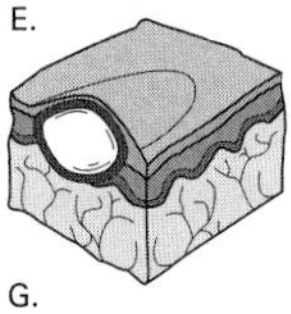

NODULES:
Solid and elevated; however, they extend deeper than papules into the dermis or subcutaneous tissues, 0.5-2.0 cm
Example:
Lipoma, erythema nodosum, cyst

F.

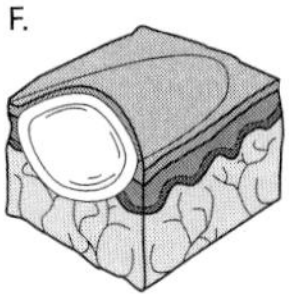

TUMOR:
The same as a nodule only greater than 2 cm
Example:
Carcinoma (such as advanced breast carcinoma); not basal cell or squamous cell of the skin

G.

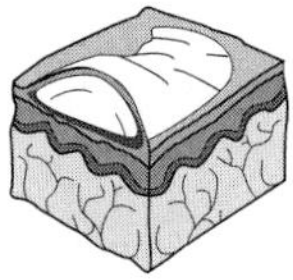

WHEAL:
Localized edema in the epidermis causing irregular elevation that may be red or pale
Example:
Insect bite or a hive

FLUID-FILLED CAVITIES WITHIN THE SKIN

H.

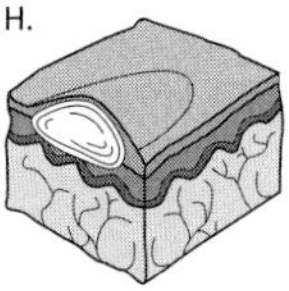

VESICLE:
Accumulation of fluid between the upper layers of the skin; elevated mass containing serous fluid; less than 0.5 cm
Example:
Herpes simplex, herpes zoster, chickenpox

I.

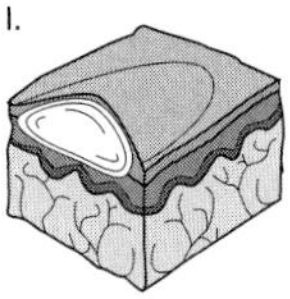

BULLAE:
Same as a vesicle only greater than 0.5 cm
Example:
Contact dermatitis, large second-degree burns, bullous impetigo, pemphigus

J.

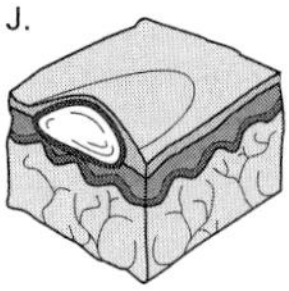

PUSTULE:
Vesicles or bullae that become filled with pus, usually described as less than 0.5 cm in diameter
Example:
Acne, impetigo, furuncles, carbuncles, folliculitis

K.

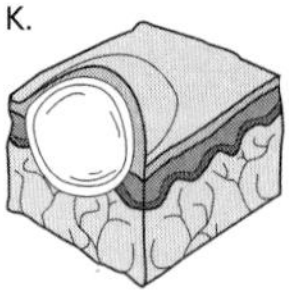

CYST:
Encapsulated fluid-filled or a semi-solid mass in the subcutaneous tissue or dermis
Example:
Sebaceous cyst, epidermoid cyst

Figure 10-4 Morphology of Primary Lesions

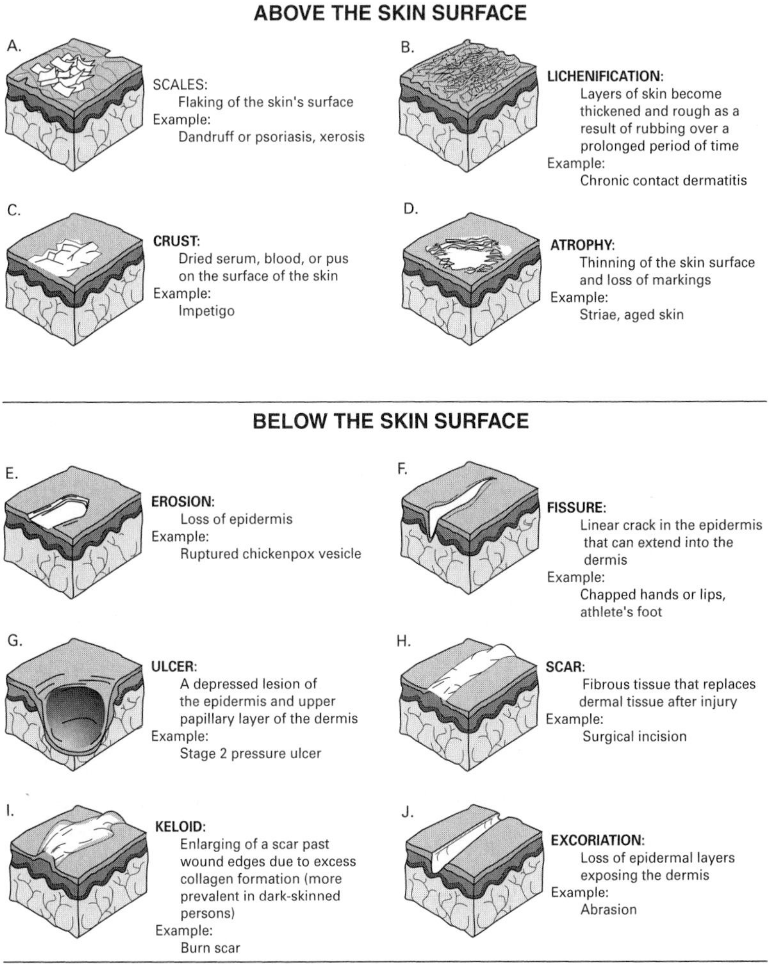
ABOVE THE SKIN SURFACE
A.
SCALES:
Flaking of the skin's surface
Example:
Dandruff or psoriasis, xerosis
B.
LICHENIFICATION:
Layers of skin become thickened and rough as a result of rubbing over a prolonged period of time
Example:
Chronic contact dermatitis
C.
CRUST:
Dried serum, blood, or pus on the surface of the skin
Example:
Impetigo
D.
ATROPHY:
Thinning of the skin surface and loss of markings
Example:
Striae, aged skin
BELOW THE SKIN SURFACE
E.
EROSION:
Loss of epidermis
Example:
Ruptured chickenpox vesicle
F.
FISSURE:
Linear crack in the epidermis that can extend into the dermis
Example:
Chapped hands or lips, athlete's foot
G.
ULCER:
A depressed lesion of the epidermis and upper papillary layer of the dermis
Example:
Stage 2 pressure ulcer
H.
SCAR:
Fibrous tissue that replaces dermal tissue after injury
Example:
Surgical incision
I.
KELOID:
Enlarging of a scar past wound edges due to excess collagen formation (more prevalent in dark-skinned persons)
Example:
Burn scar
J.
EXCORIATION:
Loss of epidermal layers exposing the dermis
Example:
Abrasion

Figure 10-5 Morphology of Secondary Lesions

Palpation of the Skin

Moisture

E Using the dorsal surfaces of the hands and fingers, palpate all nonmucous membrane skin surfaces for moisture.

N **The skin is normally dry, with a minimum of perspiration. Moisture on the skin will vary from one body area to another, with perspiration normally present on the hands, axillae, and face, and between the skin folds. Moisture also varies with changes in environment, muscular activity, body temperature, stress, and activity levels. Body temperature is regulated by the skin's production of perspiration, which evaporates to cool the body.**

A Xerosis: excessive dryness of the skin

P Hypothyroidism, exposure to extreme cold and dry climates
A Diaphoresis: profuse perspiration
P Hyperthyroidism, increased metabolic rate, sepsis, anxiety, pain

Temperature

E Using the dorsal surfaces of the hands and fingers, palpate all nonmucosal skin surfaces for temperature.
N **Skin surface temperature should be warm and equal bilaterally. The hands and feet may be slightly cooler than the rest of the body.**
A Hypothermia: generalized or localized cooling of the skin
P Generalized hypothermia: shock; localized hypothermia: arterial insufficiency in the affected area
A Hyperthermia: generalized or localized excessive warming of the skin
P Generalized hyperthermia: febrile state, hyperthyroidism, increased metabolic function; localized hyperthermia: infection, trauma, sunburn, windburn

Tenderness

E Palpate skin surface for tenderness using the dorsal surfaces of the hands and fingers.
N **Skin surfaces should be nontender.**
A Tenderness over the skin structures can be discrete and localized or generalized.
P Discrete tenderness may indicate a localized infection such as cellulitis, or generalized tenderness can indicate systemic illness such as lymphoma or allergic reaction.

Texture

E 1. Use the finger pads to evaluate the texture of the skin.
2. Evaluate surfaces such as over the abdomen and the medial surfaces of the arms first.
3. Compare these with areas that are covered with hair.
N **Skin should normally feel smooth, even, and firm, except where there is significant hair growth. A certain amount of roughness can be normal.**
A Roughness
P Wool clothing, cold weather, use of soap, scleroderma, hypothyroidism, amyloidosis, lichenification, occupational exposures
A Soft, silk-like texture
P Hyperthyroidism secondary to elevated metabolism

Turgor

E Palpate skin turgor, or elasticity, which reflects the skin's state of hydration.
1. Between your thumb and forefinger, pinch a small section of the patient's skin. The anterior chest, under the clavicle, and the abdomen are optimal areas to assess.
2. Slowly release the skin.
3. Observe the speed with which the skin returns to its original contour when released.
N **When the skin is released, it should rapidly return to its original contour.**
A Decreased skin turgor: skin remains pinched when initially released and slowly returns to its original contour.
P Dehydration, the aging process, scleroderma
A Increased turgor: skin returns to its original contour too quickly.
P Connective tissue disease

Edema

E Palpate the skin for edema, or accumulation of fluid in the intercellular spaces.
1. Firmly imprint your thumb against a dependent portion of the body, such as the arm, hand, leg, foot, ankle, or sacrum.
2. Release the pressure.
3. Observe for indentation on the skin.

4. Rate the degree of edema. Pitting edema is rated on a 4-point scale:
+0 — no pitting
+1 — 0" to ¼" pitting (mild)
+2 — ¼" to ½" pitting (moderate)
+3 — ½" to 1" pitting (significant)
+4 — greater than 1" pitting (severe)

5. Check for symmetry by measuring the circumference of affected extremities.

N **Edema is not normally present.**

A Edema: puffy, tight skin; localized or generalized (Table 10-1)

P Localized edema: dependency (Figure 10-6); generalized or bilateral edema: increased hydrostatic pressure, decreased capillary osmotic pressure, increased capillary permeability, obstruction to lymph flow

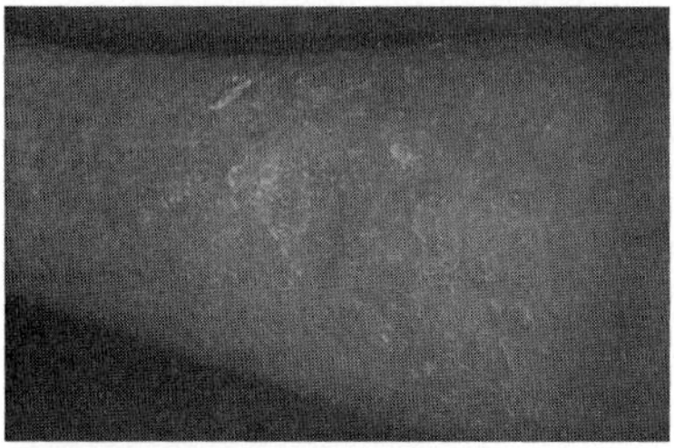

Figure 10-6 Pitting Edema

Inspection of the Hair

Color

E Inspect the scalp hair, eyebrows, eyelashes, and body hair for color.

N **Hair varies from dark black to pale blonde, depending on the amount of melanin present. As melanin production diminishes, hair turns gray. Hair color may also be chemically changed.**

A Patches of gray hair that are isolated or occur in conjunction with scarring

P Nerve damage, trauma

Distribution

E Evaluate hair distribution on the body, eyebrows, face, and scalp.

N **The body is covered in vellus hair. Terminal hair is found in the eyebrows, eyelashes, and scalp, and, after puberty, in the axillae and pubic areas. Males may experience a**

TABLE 10-1 Types of Edema

TYPE	LOCATION
Pitting	Edema that is present when an indentation remains on the skin after applying pressure
Nonpitting	Edema that is firm with discoloration or thickening of the skin; results when serum proteins coagulate in tissue spaces
Angioedema	Recurring episodes of noninflammatory swelling of skin, brain, viscera, and mucous membranes; onset may be rapid with resolution requiring hours to days
Dependent	Localized increase of extracellular fluid volume in a dependent limb or area
Inflammatory	Swelling due to an extracellular fluid effusion into the tissue surrounding an area of inflammation
Noninflammatory	Swelling or effusion due to mechanical or other causes not related to congestion or inflammation
Lymphedema	Edema due to the obstruction of a lymphatic vessel

certain degree of normal balding and may also develop terminal facial and chest hair.

A Absence of pubic hair, unless purposefully removed

P Endocrine disorders, such as anterior pituitary adenomas or chemotherapy

A Male or female pattern baldness (alopecia areata): circumscribed bald area

P Genetic predisposition, androgenetic effects on the hair follicle, chemotherapy, radiation, infection, stress, drug reactions, lupus, traction

A Total scalp baldness, or alopecia totalis

P Autoimmune diseases, emotional crisis, stress, heredity

A Hair loss in linear formations reflecting hair style

P Traction alopecia, common in conjunction with hair style known as "cornrows"

A Hirsutism: excess facial and body hair

P Endocrine disorders such as hypersecretion of adrenocortical androgens, side effects of medications

A Trichotillomania: areas of broken-off hairs in irregular patterns accompanied by scaliness but no infection

P Manipulation of the hair via twisting and pulling, leading to reduced hair mass

A Tinea capitis (ringworm): broken-off hairs accompanied by scaliness and follicular inflammation

P Fungal infection caused by dermatophytic trichomycosis

Lesions

E **1.** Don gloves and lift the scalp hair by segments.
2. Evaluate the scalp for lesions and signs of infestation.

N **The scalp should be pale white to pink in light-skinned individuals and light brown in dark-skinned individuals. There should be no signs of infestation or lesions. Seborrhea, commonly known as dandruff, may be present.**

A Head lice (pediculosis capitis): white dandruff-looking areas that are attached to the hair shaft and are difficult to remove; associated itching

P Lice larvae

Palpation of the Hair

Texture

E **1.** Between your fingertips, palpate the hair.
2. Note the condition of the hair, from the scalp to the end of the hair.

N **Hair may feel thin, straight, coarse, thick, or curly. It should be shiny and resilient when traction is applied and should not come out in clumps in your hands.**

A Brittle hair that easily breaks off

P Malnutrition, hyperthyroidism, use of chemicals such as permanents, infections secondary to damage of the hair follicle

Inspection of the Nails

Color

E **1.** Inspect the fingernails and toenails, noting the color of the nails.
2. Check capillary refill by depressing the nail until blanching occurs.
3. Release the nail and evaluate the time required for the nail to return to its previous color.
4. Perform a capillary refill check on all four extremities.

N **The nails normally have a pink cast in light-skinned individuals and a brown cast in dark-skinned individuals. Capillary refill is an indicator of peripheral circulation. Normal capillary refill may vary by age, but color should return to normal within 2 to 3 seconds.**

A Leukonychia: white striations or dots

P Trauma, infection, vascular diseases, psoriasis, anemia, cirrhosis, hypercalcemia

A Melanochyia: brown nail plate (Figure 10-7A)

P Addison's disease, malaria

A Splinter hemorrhage: red or brown linear streaks (Figure 10-7B)

P Subacute bacterial endocarditis, mitral stenosis

A A yellow or white hue in a hyperkeratotic nailbed

P Onychomycosis, a fungal infection of the nail

Shape and Configuration

E **1.** Assess the fingernails and toenails for shape, configuration, and consistency.
2. View the profile of the middle finger and evaluate the angle of the nail base.

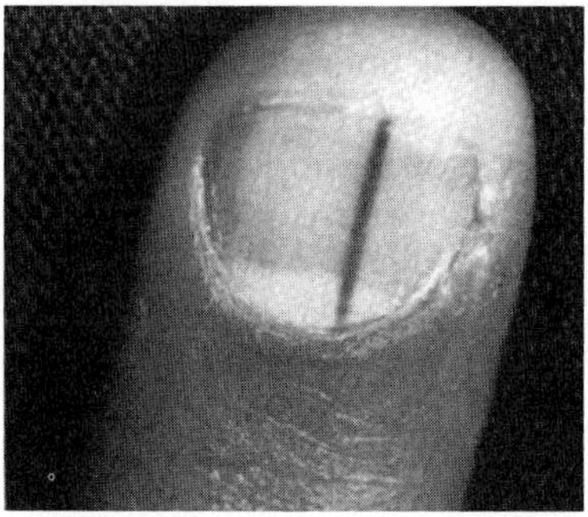

A. Longitudinal Melanochyia. *Courtesy of Robert A. Silverman, M.D., Clinical Associate Professor, Department of Pediatrics, Georgetown University*

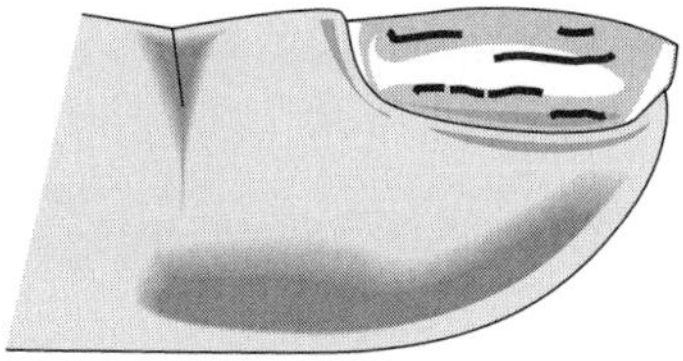

B. Splinter Hemorrhages

Figure 10-7 Abnormal Color Changes of the Nailbed

N **The nail surface should be smooth and slightly rounded to flat. Curved nails are a normal variant. Nail thickness should be uniform throughout, with no splintering or brittle edges. The angle of the nail base should be approximately 160° (Figure 10-8). Longitudinal ridging is a normal variant.**

A Clubbing: nail base angle greater than 160°

P Hypoxia, lung cancer

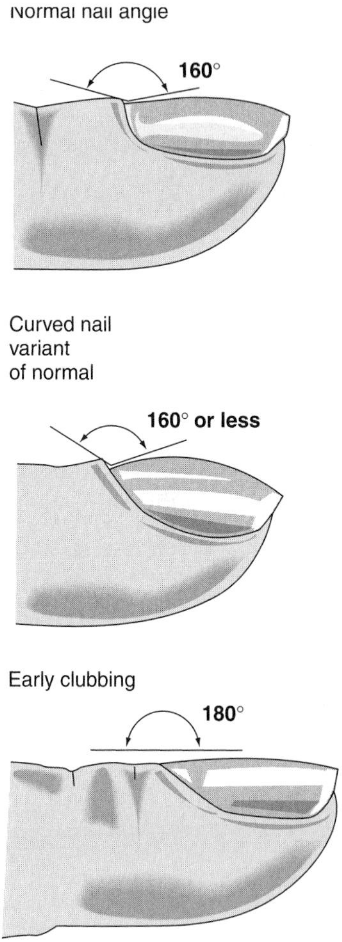

Figure 10-8 Nail Angles

Palpation of the Nails

Texture

E 1. Between your thumb and index finger, palpate the nail base.

2. Note the consistency.

N **The nail base should be firm to palpation.**

A Spongy nail base indicative of clubbing

P Chronic bronchitis, emphysema, heart disease, or impaired tissue oxygenation over a prolonged period

Advanced Technique

Skin Scraping for Scabies

1. Place a drop of mineral oil on a sterile no. 15 scalpel blade.
2. Scrape the suspected papule or known scabies burrow vigorously in order to excavate the top of the papule or burrow. Flecks of blood will mix with the oil.
3. Place some of the oil and skin scrapings onto a microscope slide and cover with a cover slip.
4. Examine the slide for mites, ova, or feces.

11

Head, Neck, and Regional Lymphatics

Anatomy and Physiology

The skull is a complex bony structure that rests on the superior end of the vertebral column (Figure 11-1). The skull protects the brain from direct injury and provides a surface for the attachment of the muscles that assist with mastication and produce facial expressions.

Cranial bones of the skull are connected by immovable joints called sutures.

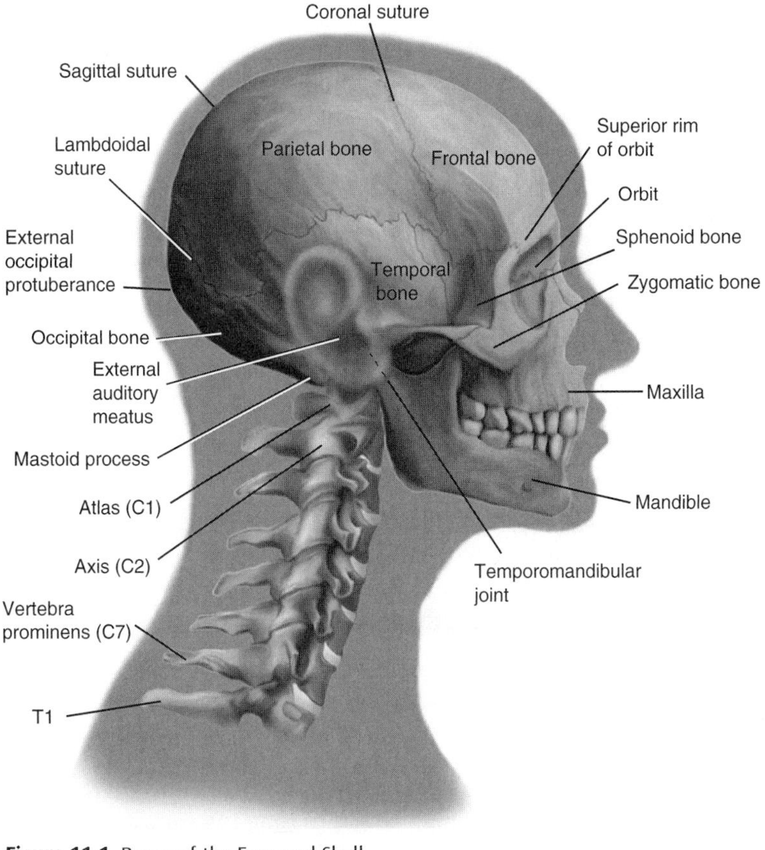

Figure 11-1 Bones of the Face and Skull

The most prominent sutures are the coronal suture, the sagittal suture, and the lambdoidal suture. The junction of the coronal and sagittal sutures is called the bregma.

Facial characteristics are influenced by factors such as race, state of health, emotions, and environment. Facial structures such as the eyes, eyebrows, nose, mouth, nasolabial folds, and palpebral fissures are symmetrical.

The neck is made up of seven flexible cervical vertebrae that both support the head and allow it maximum mobility. The major muscles of the neck are the sternocleidomastoids and the trapezii. The anterior triangle is formed by the mandible, the trachea, and the sternocleidomastoid muscles and contains the anterior cervical lymph nodes, the trachea, and the thyroid gland. The posterior triangle, formed by the sternocleidomastoid, the trapezius, and the clavicle, contains the posterior cervical lymph nodes (Figure 11-2).

The trapezii extend from the occipital bone, down the neck to insert at the outer third of the clavicles at the acromion process of the scapula, and along the spinal column to the level of T_{12}.

The thyroid gland, the largest endocrine gland in the body, secretes thyroxine (T_4) and triiodothyronine (T_3), which regulate the rate of cellular metabolism. The gland, a flattened, butterfly-shaped structure with two lateral lobes connected by the isthmus, is slightly larger in females than in males (Figure 11-3). The isthmus rests on top of the trachea, inferior to the cricoid cartilage.

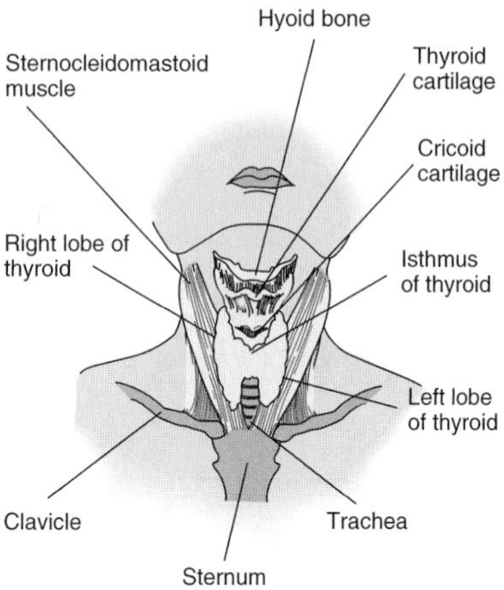

Figure 11-3 Thyroid Gland and Surrounding Structures

Lymphatic tissue in the nodes is responsible for the filtering and sequestration of pathogens and other harmful substances and drains the head and neck

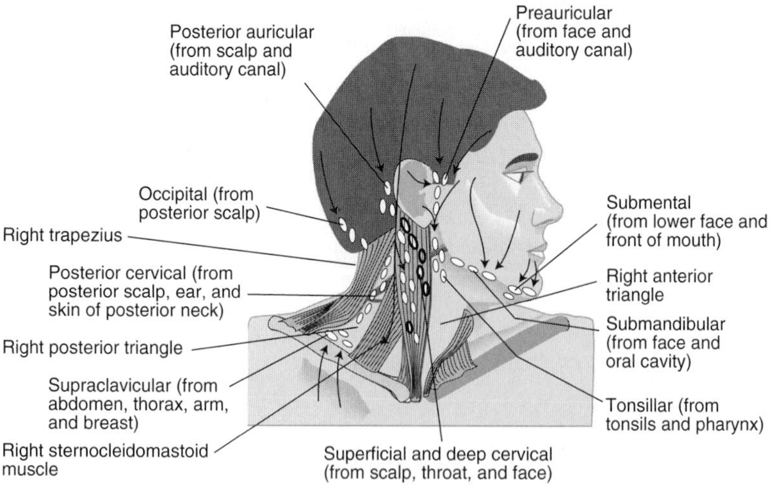

Figure 11-2 Lymph Nodes of the Head and Neck: Drainage Patterns and Anterior and Posterior Cervical Triangles

(see Figure 11-2). Lymph nodes are usually less than 1 cm round or ovoid in shape and smooth in consistency. When nodes are enlarged or tender, it is important to assess for infection or other causes in the area they drain, such as malignancy.

Major vessels carrying blood to the head and neck include the internal and external carotids, the internal and external jugulars, and the subclavian veins and arteries.

HEALTH HISTORY

Medical History (see also Table 11-1)
Hypo- or hyperthyroidism, sinus infections, migraine headache, cancer, closed head injury or skull fracture, stiff neck, masses, hoarseness

Surgical History
Thyroidectomy, facial reconstruction, cosmetic surgery, neurosurgery, other surgery related to the head or neck

NURSING CHECKLIST

General Approach to Head and Neck Assessment

1. Place the patient in an upright sitting position on the examination table or, for the patient who cannot tolerate the sitting position, gain access to the supine patient's head by removing nonessential equipment or bedding.
2. Ask the patient to remove any wigs and headpieces.
3. Always compare the right and left sides of the head, neck, and face.

Equipment

- Stethoscope
- Cup of water

Assessment of the Head and Neck

Inspection of the Shape of the Head

E 1. Have the patient sit in a comfortable position.
2. Face the patient, with your head at the same level as the patient's head.
3. Inspect the head for shape and symmetry.

N **The head should be normocephalic and symmetrical.**

A Hydrocephalus: enlargement of the head without enlargement of the facial structures

P Abnormal accumulation of cerebrospinal fluid within the skull

A Acromegaly: abnormal enlargement of the skull and bony facial structures

P Excessive secretion of growth hormone from the pituitary gland

A Craniosynostosis: characterized by abnormal shape of the skull or bone growth at right angles to suture lines, exophthalmos, and drooping eyelids

P Premature closure of one or more sutures of the skull before brain growth is complete

Palpation of the Head

E 1. Place your finger pads on the patient's scalp and palpate all of its surface, beginning in the frontal area and continuing over the parietal, temporal, and occipital areas.
2. Assess for contour, masses, depressions, and tenderness.

TABLE 11-1 Classification of Headaches

VASCULAR ETIOLOGIES
Migraine headaches
Cluster headaches
Subarachnoid hemorrhage
Subdural hematoma
Infarction
Cerebral aneurysm
Temporal arteritis
Vasculitis

MUSCLE CONTRACTION
Tension headache

INTRACRANIAL ETIOLOGIES
Brain tumors
Increased intracranial pressure from hydrocephalus, pseudotumor cerebri
Intracranial infection (e.g., meningitis, encephalitis, abscess)
Ischemic cerebrovascular disease

SYSTEMIC ETIOLOGIES
Infection
Post-lumbar puncture
Hypertension
Exertion from coitus, cough, exercise
Postictal
Pheochromocytoma
Premenstrual syndrome

FOOD-RELATED ETIOLOGIES
Nitrites (e.g., hot dogs, bacon)
Tyramine (e.g., red wine, cheese, chocolate)
Monosodium glutamate (e.g., Chinese food)
Food allergy

FACIAL OR CERVICAL ETIOLOGIES
Sinusitis
Temporomandibular joint dysfunction
Dental lesions
Trigeminal neuralgia
Cervical spine radiculopathies

OCULAR-RELATED ETIOLOGIES
Narrow-angle glaucoma
Uveitis
Extraocular muscle paralysis
Eye strain

METABOLIC ETIOLOGIES
Hypoxia
Hypercapnia
Hypoglycemia

DRUG ETIOLOGIES
Alcohol and alcohol withdrawal
Caffeine withdrawal
Nitrates
Oral contraceptives
Estrogen

ENVIRONMENTAL ETIOLOGIES
Change in barometric pressure (from weather or altitude)
Carbon monoxide poisoning
Tobacco smoke
Glaring or flickering lights
Odors

MISCELLANEOUS ETIOLOGIES
Fever
Influenza
Head trauma
Otitis media
Parotitis
Pregnancy
Fatigue and decreased sleep
Psychogenic disorders

N **The normal skull is smooth, nontender, and without masses or depressions.**

A Hard or soft masses in the cranial bones

P Carcinomatous metastasis from other regions of the body, resulting from lymphomas, multiple myeloma, or leukemia

A Osteomyelitis: localized edema over the bony frontal portion of the skull

P Acute or chronic sinusitis if the infection infiltrates the surrounding bone

A Craniotabes: softening of the outer bone layer

P Hydrocephalus or demineralization of the bone due to rickets, hypervitaminosis A, or syphilis

Inspection and Palpation of the Scalp

E 1. Part the patient's hair repeatedly all over the scalp and inspect the scalp for lesions and masses.
2. Place your finger pads on the scalp and palpate for lesions and masses.
3. Palpate the superficial temporal artery, which is located anterior to the tragus of the ear.

N **The scalp should be shiny, intact, and without lesions or masses. The temporal pulse is weaker than other peripheral pulses ($1^+/4^+$), such as the brachial or radial pulse.**

A Laceration or laceration with bleeding

P May indicate trauma resulting from a compound skull fracture

A Hematomas: localized, easily movable accumulation of blood in the subcutaneous tissue

P Direct trauma to the skull

A Sebaceous cysts: single or multiple masses that are easily movable, round, firm, and nontender and that arise from either the skin or subcutaneous tissue

P Retention of secretions from sebaceous glands

A Lipomas: nonmobile, fatty masses with smooth, circular edges

P Benign fatty tumors

A Hard tender temporal artery

P Temporal arteritis

Inspection of the Face

Symmetry

E Observe the patient's face for expression, shape, and symmetry of the following structures: eyebrows, eyes, nose, mouth, and ears.

N **The facial features should be symmetrical. The two palpebral fissures should be equal, and the nasolabial fold should present bilaterally. It is important to remember that slight variations in symmetry are common. Slanted eyes with inner epicanthal folds are normal findings in patients of Asian descent.**

A Facial structures are absent, deformed, or asymmetrical

P Stroke, Bell's palsy (Figure 11-4), congenital defects, damage to cranial nerve VII

Shape and Features

E 1. Observe the shape of the patient's face.
2. Note any swelling, abnormal features, unusual movement, or changes in shape.

N **The face can be oval, round, or slightly square in shape. There should be no edema, disproportionate structures, or involuntary movements.**

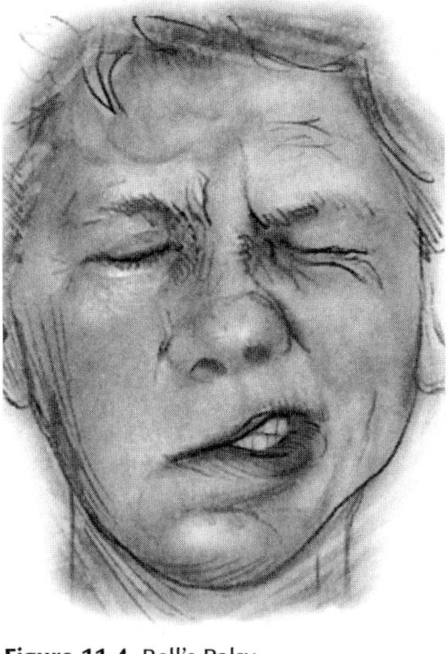

Figure 11-4 Bell's Palsy

A Down syndrome: slanted eyes with inner epicanthal folds; a short, flat nose; and a thick, protruding tongue

P Chromosomal aberration

A Graves' disease: thin face with sharply defined features and prominent eyes

P Autoimmune disorder associated with increased circulating levels of T_3 and T_4

A Myxedema: round, swollen face with characteristic periorbital edema and dry, dull skin

P Associated with hypothyroidism

A Cachexia: sunken eyes and hollow cheeks (Figure 11-5)

P Profound state of wasting of the vital tissues associated with cancer, malnutrition, and dehydration

A Cushing's syndrome: rounded, "moon" face in conjunction with red cheeks and excess hair on the jaw and upper lip

P Increased production of adrenocorticotrophic hormone (ACTH)

A Dusky blue discoloration beneath the eyelids (allergic shiners)

P Chronic allergies

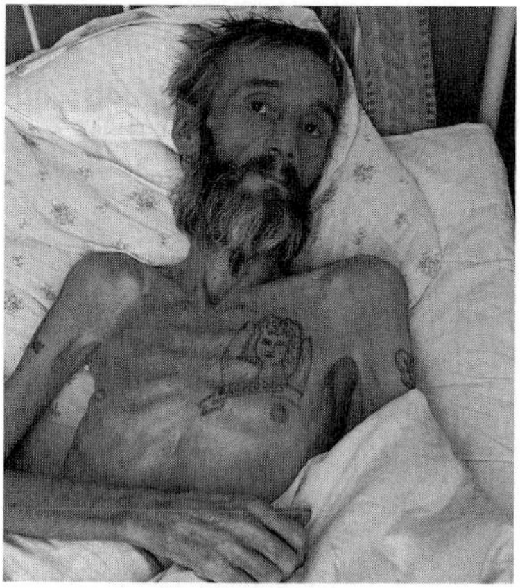

Figure 11-5 Cachectic Face in a 40-Year-Old Man with Tuberculosis. *Courtesy of WHO/STB/Colors Magazine/J. Mollison*

Palpation and Auscultation of the Mandible

E **1.** Use the fingertips of both index and both middle fingers to locate the temporomandibular joint anterior to the tragus of the ear on each side of the head.
2. Hold the fingertips firmly in place over the joints and ask the patient to open and close the mouth.
3. As the patient opens and closes the mouth, observe the relative smoothness of the movement and whether the patient notices any discomfort.
4. Remove the hands.
5. Hold the bell of the stethoscope over the joint.
6. Listen for any sound while the patient opens and closes the mouth.

N **The patient should experience no discomfort with movement. The temporomandibular joint should articulate smoothly and without clicking or crepitus.**

A Tenderness when the mouth is opened and closed

P Inflammation or arthritis

A Crepitus or clicking

P Osteoarthritis

A Mouth remains open and in a fixed position after either a wide yawn or trauma to the chin

P Temporomandibular joint dislocation; requires reduction

Inspection and Palpation of the Neck

Inspection of the Neck

E **1.** Have the patient sit facing you and with the head held in a central position.
2. Inspect for symmetry of the sternocleidomastoid muscles anteriorly and the trapezii posteriorly.

3. Have the patient touch the chin to the chest, to each side, and to each shoulder.
4. Assess for limitation of motion.
5. Note whether a stoma or tracheostomy or scar is present.

N **The muscles of the neck are symmetrical when the head is in a central position. The patient is able to move the head through a full range of motion without either complaint of discomfort or noticeable limitation. The patient may be breathing through a stoma or tracheostomy.**

A Pain upon flexion or rotation of the head

P Pain upon flexion: muscle spasm caused by meningeal irritation of meningitis (see Chapter 19); generalized discomfort: trauma, muscle spasm, inflammation, vertebral diseases

A Torticollis: slight or prominent lateral deviation of the neck (Figure 11-6); possible prominence of sternocleidomastoid muscles on the affected side

P **1.** Congenital: hematoma, partial sternocleidomastoid rupture occurring at birth and resulting in a shortened muscle
2. Ocular: head posture assumed to correct for ocular muscle palsy and resulting diplopia
3. Acute spasm: inflammation associated with viral myositis or trauma
4. Other: hysteria, phenothiazine therapy, Parkinson's disease

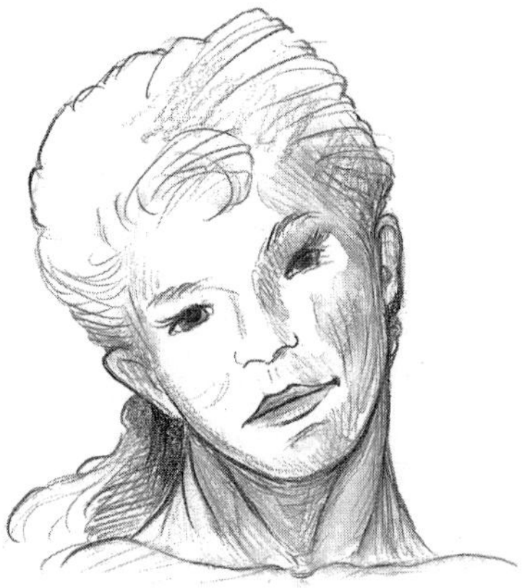

Figure 11-6 Torticollis

A Reduced range of motion of the neck, crepitus upon hyperextension of the neck

P Degenerative changes of osteoarthritis, usually painless unless nerve root irritation has occurred

Palpation of the Neck

E **1.** Stand in front of the patient.
2. Using your finger pads, palpate the sternocleidomastoids.
3. Note the presence of masses or tenderness.
4. Stand behind the patient.
5. Using your finger pads, palpate the trapezius.
6. Note the presence of masses or tenderness.

N **The muscles should be symmetrical and without palpable masses or spasm.**

A Palpable mass in the musculature

P Primary or metastatic tumor

A Palpable spasm in the musculature

P Infections, trauma, chronic inflammatory processes, neoplasms

Inspection of the Thyroid Gland

E **1.** Secure strong, tangential lighting and shine at an oblique angle on the patient's anterior neck.
2. Face the patient.
3. Ask the patient to look straight ahead and to slightly extend the head.
4. Have the patient drink a sip of water and swallow twice.
5. As the patient swallows, observe the front of the neck in the area of the thyroid and isthmus for masses and symmetrical movement.

N **Thyroid tissue moves up with swallowing, but the movement often is so small as to be invisible on inspection. In males, the thyroid cartilage, or "Adam's apple," is more prominent than in females.**

A Goiter (enlarged thyroid gland) or thyroid nodules

P Various thyroid diseases

Palpation of the Thyroid Gland

Posterior Approach (See Figure 11-7A)

E **1.** Have the patient sit comfortably. Stand behind the patient.

2. Have the patient lower the chin slightly in order to relax the neck muscles.

3. Place your thumbs on the back of the patient's neck and bring the other fingers around the neck anteriorly to rest their tips over the trachea on the lower portion of the neck.

4. Move the finger pads over the tracheal rings.

5. Instruct the patient to swallow. Palpate the isthmus for nodules or enlargement.

6. Have the patient incline the head slightly forward.

7. Press the fingers of your left hand against the left side of the thyroid cartilage to stabilize it while gently placing the fingers of your right hand against the right side of the cartilage.

8. Instruct the patient to swallow sips of water.

9. Note consistency, nodularity, or tenderness as the gland moves upward.

10. Repeat on the other side.

Anterior Approach (See Figure 11-7B)

E **1.** Stand in front of the patient.

2. Ask the patient to flex the head slightly forward.

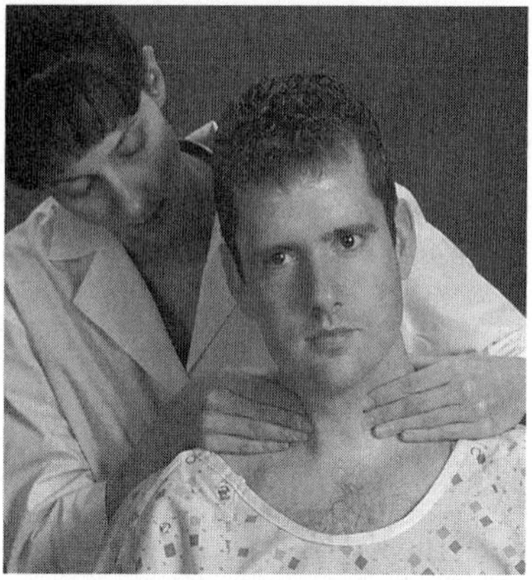

A. Posterior Approach

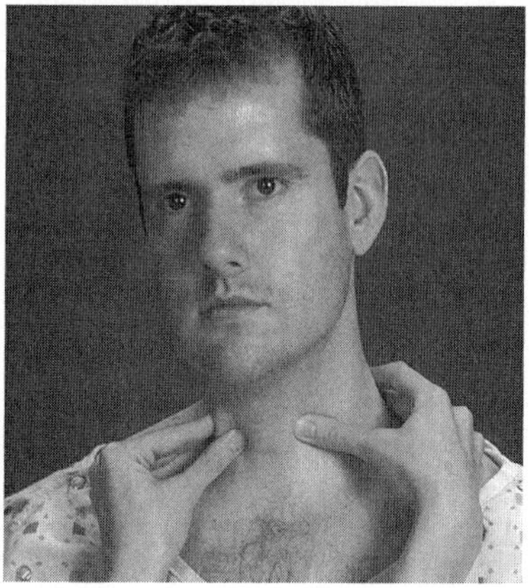

B. Anterior Approach

Figure 11-7 Examination of the Thyroid Gland

3. Place your right thumb on the thyroid cartilage and displace the cartilage to the patient's right.

4. Using the thumb and index and middle fingers of your left hand, grasp the elevated and displaced right lobe of the thyroid gland.

5. Palpate the surface of the gland for consistency, nodularity, and tenderness.

6. Have the patient swallow; palpate the surface again.

7. Repeat the procedure on the opposite side.

N **No enlargement, masses, or tenderness should be noted on palpation.**
A Physiological hyperplasia: smooth, soft gland slightly enlarged but to less than twice the size of normal
P Seen premenstrually, during pregnancy, or from puberty to young adulthood in the female; symmetric enlargement in iodine deficiency (nontoxic diffuse goiters or endemic goiters)
A Toxic hyperplasia: thyroid gland two to three times larger than normal size
P Graves' disease (hyperthyroidism)
A Thyroid adenomas: asymmetric enlargement with two or more nodules present on the gland
P Benign epithelial tumors usually occurring after the age of 30; a nontoxic diffuse goiter may become nodular as the patient ages
A Solitary nodule in the thyroid tissue
P Suggestive of carcinoma
A Lateral deviation of the trachea but no specific goiter
P Possible retrosternal goiter
A Tenderness of the thyroid
P Suggestive of thyroiditis

Auscultation of the Thyroid Gland

If the thyroid is enlarged, auscultation should be performed.

E **1.** Stand in front of the patient.
2. Place the bell of the stethoscope over the right thyroid lobe.
3. Auscultate for bruits.
4. Repeat on the left thyroid lobe.

N **Auscultation should not reveal bruits.**
A Bruit over an enlarged thyroid gland
P Increased vascularization due to diffuse toxic goiter

> **Nursing Alert**
>
> **Risk Factors for Thyroid Cancer**
>
> - Diets low in iodine
> - History of head or neck radiation, especially in childhood
> - Exposure to nuclear fallout
> - Genetics
> - Female gender

Inspection of the Lymph Nodes

E **1.** Stand in front of the patient.
2. Expose the head and neck areas to be assessed.
3. Inspect the nodal areas of the head and neck for any enlargement or inflammation.

N **Lymph nodes should not be visible or inflamed.**
A Enlargement and inflammation in specific nodes
P Localized or generalized infection

Palpation of the Lymph Nodes

E **1.** Have the patient sit comfortably.
2. Face the patient and conduct the assessment of both sides of the neck simultaneously.
3. Using gentle pressure, move the pads and tips of the middle three fingers of each hand in small circles.
4. Follow a systematic, routine sequence beginning with the preauricular, postauricular, occipital, submental, submandibular, and tonsillar nodes and moving down to the neck to the anterior cervical chain, posterior cervical chain, and supraclavicular nodes (Figure 11-8).
5. Note size, shape, delimitation (discrete or matted together), mobility, consistency, and tenderness.

N **Lymph nodes should not generally be palpable in the healthy adult patient; however, small, discrete, movable nodes are sometimes present, and are of no significance.**
A Palpable lymph nodes greater than 0.5 cm
P Acute bacterial infections, blood dyscrasias, AIDS, tuberculosis, surgical

procedures that traumatize the nodes, blood transfusions, chronic illness

A Enlarged, nontender, firm, immobile nodes

P Possible malignancy in the head and neck area, metastasis from the region the lymph node drains, malignant lymphomas such as Hodgkin's disease

A Enlarged, tender nodes

P Lymphadenitis, infectious mononucleosis

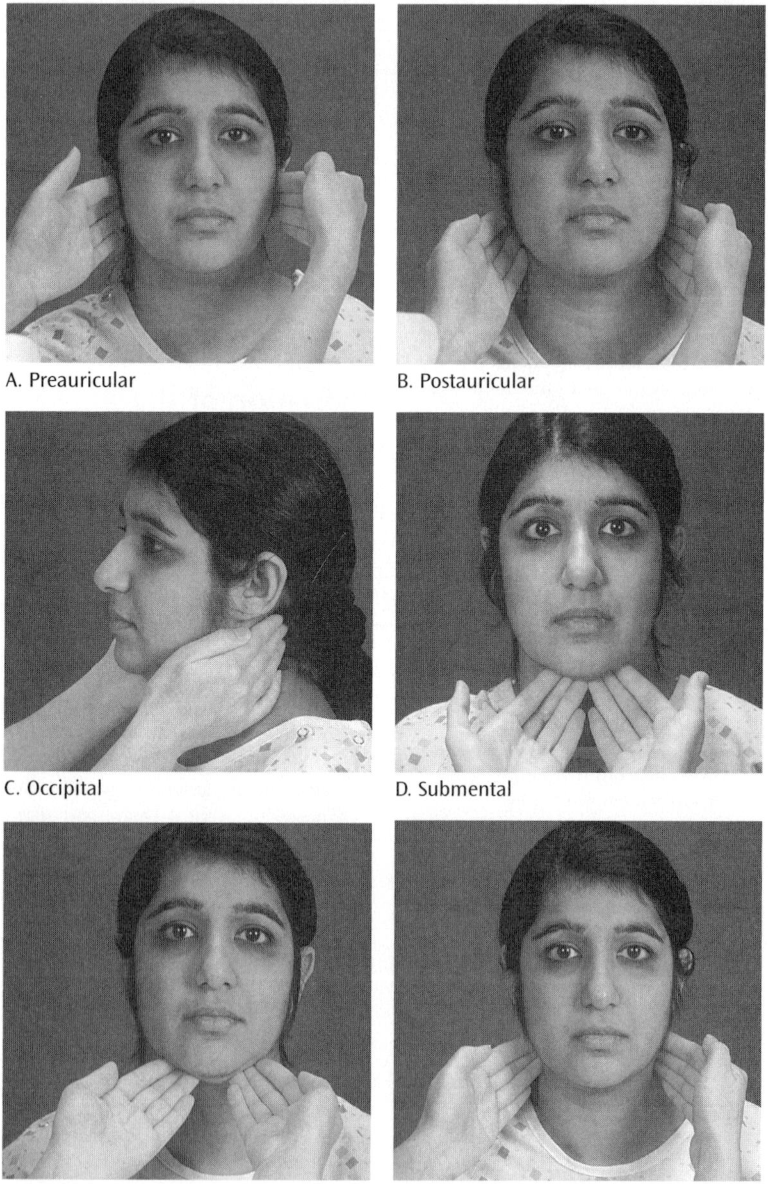

A. Preauricular

B. Postauricular

C. Occipital

D. Submental

E. Submandibular

F. Tonsillar

Figure 11-8 Palpation of Lymph Nodes

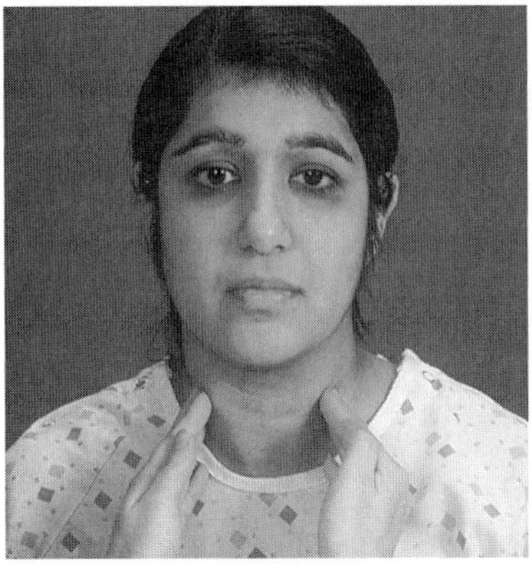

G. Anterior Cervical Chain

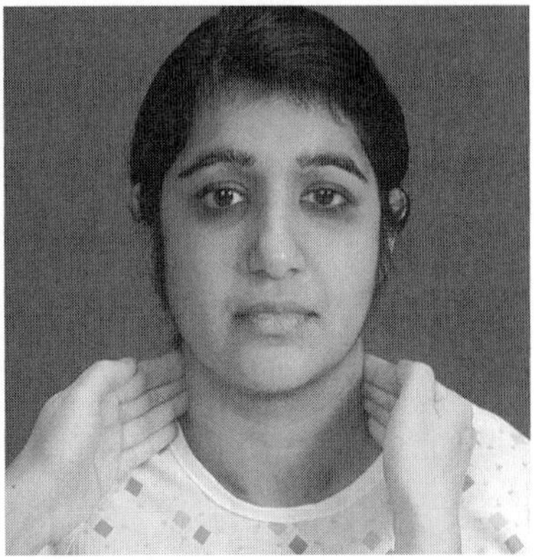

H. Posterior Cervical Chain

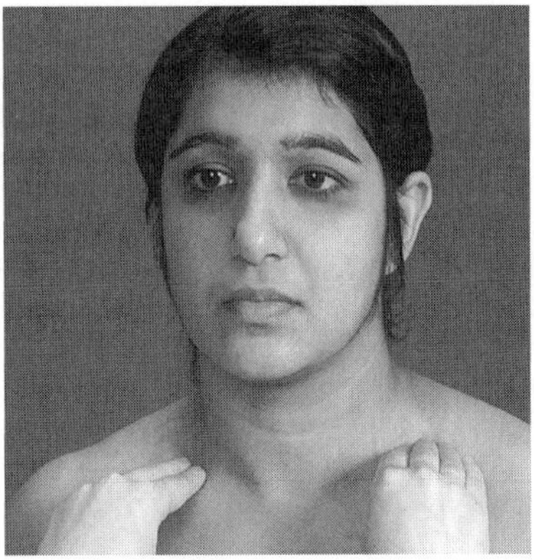

I. Supraclavicular

Figure 11-8 Palpation of Lymph Nodes *continued*

12

Eyes

Anatomy and Physiology

External Structures

The external structures of the eye are the eyelids (or palpebra), the conjunctiva, the lacrimal glands, and the extraocular muscles. The interior surface of the lid muscle is covered with a pink mucous membrane called the palpebral conjunctiva. Contiguous with the palpebral conjunctiva is the bulbar conjunctiva. The bulbar conjunctiva folds back over the anterior surface of the eyeball and merges with the cornea at the limbus, the junction of sclera and cornea (Figure 12-1). The conjunctiva contains blood vessels and pain receptors that respond quickly to outside insult. Eyelashes protect the eye by filtering particles of dirt and dust from the external environment.

The opening between the eyelids is called the palpebral fissure. The upper and lower eyelids meet at the inner canthus. Embedded just beneath the lid margins are the meibomian glands, which secrete a lubricating substance onto the surface of the eye.

The lacrimal glands, located above and to the temporal side of each eye, are responsible for the production of tears, which lubricate the eye.

Six extraocular muscles extend from the scleral surface of each eye and attach to the bony orbit. These muscles are the superior, inferior, medial, and lateral recti and the superior and inferior obliques.

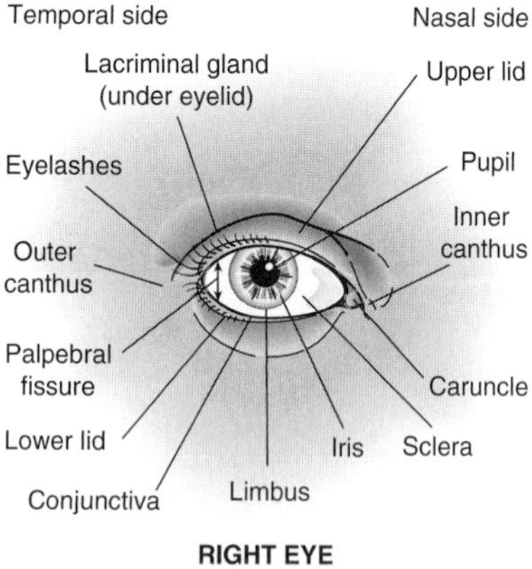

Figure 12-1 External View of the Eye

Internal Structures

The eye itself is approximately 1 inch in diameter and has three layers: a tough, outer, fibrous tunic (the sclera); a middle, vascular tunic; and the innermost layer, which contains the retina (Figure 12-2).

The innermost layer of the eyeball, or the retina, is an extension of the optic nerve, which lines the inside of the globe and receives light impulses to be transmitted to the occipital lobe of the brain.

The optic disc is a round or oval area that has distinct margins and is located on the nasal side of the retina.

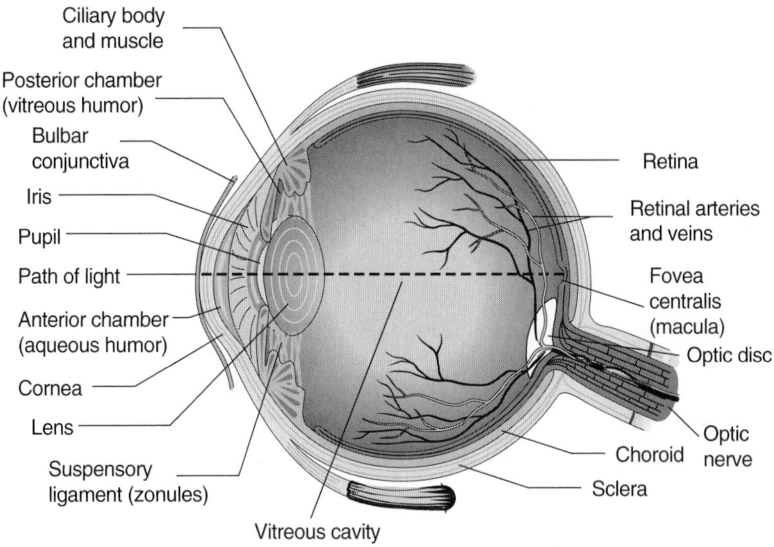

Figure 12-2 Lateral Cross Section of the Interior Eye

The physiologic cup (see Figure 12-10), a pale, central area in the optic disc, occupies one-third to one-fourth of the disc. In the temporal area of the retina, the tiny, darker macula, with the fovea centralis at its center, contains a high concentration of cones necessary for color vision, reading ability, and other tasks requiring fine visual discrimination. The fovea is the area of sharpest vision. Other portions of the retina contain a high concentration of rods, which provide dark and light discrimination and peripheral vision.

HEALTH HISTORY

Medical History

Glaucoma, conjunctivitis, cataracts, trachoma

Surgical History

Cataract extraction, lens implant, enucleation of eye, repair of detached retina, optic nerve decompression

Allergies

Pollen: watery or itchy eyes; insect stings: swelling around the eyes; animal dander: watery or itchy eyes

Special Needs

Legal blindness

Childhood Illnesses

Visual sequelae (blindness)

NURSING ◂CHECKLIST▸

General Approach to Eyes

1. Explain the assessment techniques that you will be using.
2. Ensure that the light in the room provides sufficient brightness to allow adequate observation of the patient.
3. Place the patient in an upright, sitting position on the examination table.
4. Always use a systematic approach and compare right and left eyes.

Equipment

- Ophthalmoscope
- Penlight
- Clean gloves
- Snellen chart, Snellen E chart, Rosenbaum near-vision pocket screening card
- Vision occluder
- Cotton-tipped applicator

Assessment of the Eye

Visual Acuity

The assessment of visual acuity (cranial nerve [CN] II) is performed using a Snellen chart and an occluder to cover the patient's eye.

Distance Vision

E 1. Ask the patient to stand or sit facing the Snellen chart at a distance of 20 feet.
2. If the patient normally wears glasses, ask that they be removed. If the glasses are used strictly for reading, do not have the patient wear the glasses for the examination. Contact lenses may be left in the eyes.
3. Instruct the patient to cover the left eye with the occluder and read as many lines on the chart as possible.
4. Note the number at the end of the last line the patient was able to read.
5. If the patient is unable to read the letters at the top of the chart, move the patient closer to the chart. Note the distance at which the patient is able to read the top line.
6. Repeat the test with the patient occluding the right eye.
7. If the patient normally wears glasses, the test should be repeated with the patient wearing the glasses and it should be so noted (corrected or uncorrected).

N **The patient who has a visual acuity of 20/20 is considered to have normal visual acuity.**

A Inability to read the chart with an uncorrected visual acuity of 20/30 in one eye; vision in both eyes is different by two lines or more; absent acuity

P Myopia (nearsightedness); corneal opacities that are either congenital, from lesions that have scarred the cornea (e.g., herpes simplex), from trauma, or from degeneration and dystrophies; opacities of the lens secondary to senile or traumatic cataracts; iritis; inflammation of the retina caused by infectious agents (toxoplasmosis) or hemorrhage; hypertension; diabetes mellitus; trauma

Near Vision

E 1. Use a pocket Snellen or Rosenbaum card or any printed material written at an appropriate reading level.
2. If using a pocket vision card, have the patient sit comfortably and hold the card 14 inches from the face without moving the card.
3. Ask the patient to read the smallest line possible. If printed material

other than a pocket card is used, you will be able to obtain only a general understanding of the patient's near vision.

N **Until the patient is in the late 30s to the late 40s, reading is generally possible at a distance of 14 inches.**

A Presbyopia (farsightedness)

P Nuclear sclerosis secondary to aging and resulting in decreased ability of the lens to change shape and to focus

Color Vision

E For routine testing of color vision, test the patient's ability to identify primary colors found on the Snellen chart or in the examination room. For more specific testing, ask the patient to view Ishihara plates and to identify the numerals on them.

N **The patient who is able to identify all six screening Ishihara plates correctly has normal color vision.**

A Color vision defect: designated as red/green, blue/yellow, or, if the patient sees only shades of gray, complete

P Diseases of the optic nerve, macular degeneration, pathology of the fovea centralis, nutritional deficiency, heredity

Visual Fields

The confrontation technique is used to test the visual field of each eye (CN II). The visual field of each eye is divided into quadrants, and a stimulus is presented in each quadrant.

E 1. Sit or stand approximately 2 to 3 feet opposite the patient and with your eyes at the same level as the patient's.

2. Have the patient cover the right eye with the right hand or an occluder. Cover your left eye in the same manner.

3. Have the patient look at your uncovered eye with his or her uncovered eye.

4. Hold your free hand at arm's length equidistant from you and the patient. Move your free hand or a held object such as a pen into your and the patient's field of vision from the nasal, temporal, superior, inferior, and oblique angles.

5. Ask the patient to say "now" when your hand is seen moving into the field of vision. Use your own visual fields as the control for comparison with the patient's.

6. Repeat the procedure for the other eye.

N **The patient is able to see the stimulus at approximately 90° temporally, 60° nasally, 50° superiorly, and 70° inferiorly.**

A Inability to identify movement perceived by the examiner

P Visual field defects: neurological diseases such as tumor and stroke, glaucoma, retinal detachment

External Eye and Lacrimal Apparatus

Eyelids

E 1. Ask the patient to sit facing you.

2. Observe the patient's eyelids for drooping, infection, tumors, or other abnormalities.

3. Note the distribution of the eyelashes and eyebrows.

4. Instruct the patient to focus on an object or a finger held approximately 10 to 12 inches away and slightly above eye level.

5. Move the object or finger slowly downward and observe for a white space of sclera between the upper lid and the limbus.

6. Observe the blinking of the eyes.

7. Ask the patient to elevate the eyelids.

N **The eyelids should appear symmetric and be without drooping, infection, and tumors. Eyelids of Asians normally slant upward. When the eyes are focused in a normal frontal**

gaze, the lids should cover the upper portion of the iris. The patient can raise both eyelids symmetrically (CN III). Slight ptosis, or drooping of the lid, can be normal. When the eye is closed, no portion of the cornea should be exposed. Normal lid margins are smooth, with the lashes evenly distributed and sweeping upward from the upper lids and downward from the lower lids. Eyebrows are present bilaterally, symmetric, and without lesions and scaling.

A Unilateral or bilateral, constant or intermittent ptosis of the lid (Figure 12-3)

P Congenital (failure of the levatator muscle to develop) or acquired and classified as one of the following:
1. *Mechanical:* heavy lids from lesions, adipose tissue, swelling, or edema
2. *Myogenic:* muscular diseases such as myasthenia gravis or multiple sclerosis
3. *Neurogenic:* paralysis from damage or interruption of the neural pathways

A Area of white sclera between the upper lid and the limbus and widening as the eye looks downward (lid lag)

P Thyrotoxicosis

A Lagophthalmos: incomplete lid closure (usually unilateral)

P Bell's palsy, stroke, trauma, ectropion (everted eyelid)

A Exophthalmos (proptosis): unilateral or bilateral disparity of the palpebral fissure with apparent lid retraction, indicating a protrusion of the globe

P Unilateral: orbital tumors, thyroid disease, trauma, inflammation; bilateral: thyroid disease

A Entropion: inversion of the lower lid

P Spasms or advancing age (associated with loss of muscle tone)

A Ectropion: eversion of the lower lid

P Normal aging process, Bell's palsy

A Excessive blinking (possibly with increased tearing and pain)

P Voluntary: irritation to the cornea or the conjunctiva, stress; involuntary: tonic spasms of the orbicularis oculi muscle that are called blepharospasms and are seen in the elderly, CN VII lesions, irritation of the eye, fatigue, or stress

A Lids that are black and blue, bluish, yellow, or red, depending on race and skin color

P 1. Generalized redness: nonspecific; redness in the nasal half of the lid: frontal sinusitis; redness adjacent to the lower lid: disease of the lacrimal sac or nasolacrimal duct, such as dacryocystitis; redness in the temporal portion of the lid: dacryoadenitis (inflammation of the lacrimal gland)
2. Bluish: orbital vein thrombosis, orbital tumors, aneurysms in the orbit
3. Black and blue: bleeding into the surrounding tissues following trauma (black eye)

A Swelling or edema in the eyelid

P Allergies, systemic diseases, or medications that contribute to swelling

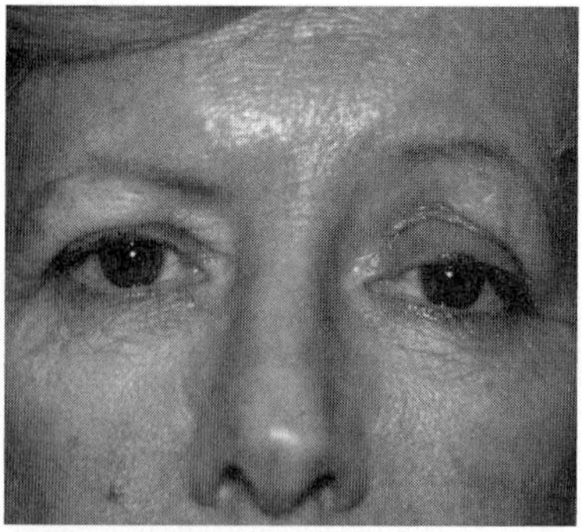

Figure 12-3 Mild Ptosis. *Courtesy of Salim I. Butrus, M.D., Senior Attending, Department of Ophthalmology, Washington Hospital Center, Washington, DC & Associate Clinical Professor, Georgetown University Medical Center, Washington, DC*

from fluid overload, trichinosis, early myxedema, thyrotoxicosis, contact dermatitis

A Hordeolum (sty): acute, localized inflammation, tenderness, redness, and pain

P Staphylococcus

A Chalazion: chronic inflammation of the meibomian gland in either the upper or lower lid and without tenderness and redness

P Unknown

A Blepharitis: bilaterally inflamed, red-rimmed lids with scales clinging to both the upper and lower lids, associated itching and burning along the lid margins, and possible loss of eyelashes

P Staphylococcal or seborrheic

A Xanthelasma: raised, yellow, nonpainful plaques on the upper and lower lids and near the inner canthus

P Hypercholesteremia

Lacrimal Apparatus

Inspection

E 1. Have the patient sit facing you.
2. Identify the area of the lacrimal gland. Note any swelling or enlargement of the gland or elevation of the eyelid. Note any enlargement, swelling, redness, increased tearing, or exudate in the area of the lacrimal sac at the inner canthus.
3. Compare with the other eye to determine whether any involvement is unilateral or bilateral.

N **There should be no enlargement, swelling, redness, or excessive exudate, and tearing should be minimal.**

A Dacryoadenitis: inflammation, swelling, and pain in the upper lateral aspect of one or both eyes

P Acute inflammation of the lacrimal gland secondary to trauma, measles, mumps, or mononucleosis

A Dacryocystitis: inflammation and painful swelling occurring beside the nose and near the inner canthus and possibly extending to the eyelid

P Inflammatory or neoplastic obstruction of lacrimal duct

Palpation

E 1. To assess the lacrimal sac for obstruction, don gloves.
2. Gently press the index finger near the inner canthus and just inside the rim of the bony orbit of the eye.
3. Note any discharge from the punctum.

N **There should not be excessive tearing or discharge from the punctum.**

A Mucopurulent discharge

P Obstruction anywhere along the lacrimal apparatus

A Epiphora: overflowing of tears from the eye

P Obstruction of the lacrimal duct

Extraocular Muscle Function

Six extraocular muscles control the movement of each eye in relation to three axes: vertical, horizontal, and oblique (Figure 12-4). Extraocular function is assessed by observing corneal light reflex or alignment, using the cover/uncover test, and testing the six cardinal fields of gaze (CN III, IV, and VI).

Corneal Light Reflex (Hirschberg Test)

E 1. Instruct the patient to look straight ahead.
2. Focus a penlight on the corneas from a distance of 12 to 15 inches away at the midline.
3. Observe the location of reflected light on the cornea.

N **The reflected light (light reflex) should be seen symmetrically and in the center of each cornea.**

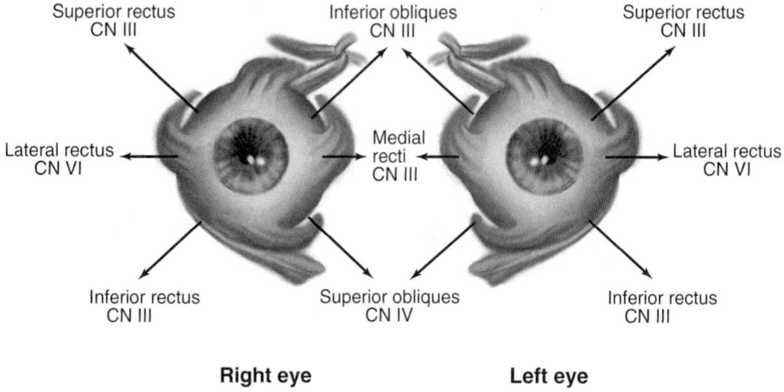

Figure 12-4 Direction of Movement of Extraocular Muscles

A Discrepancy in the location of one of the corneal light reflections (Figure 12-5):

1. Strabismus (tropia): one eye constantly deviated
2. Esotropia: inward turning of the eye
3. Exotropia: outward turning of the eye

P Extraocular muscle imbalance related to neurological conditions such as myasthenia gravis; multiple sclerosis; stroke; neuropathies of diabetes mellitus; uncorrected childhood strabismus (misalignment); trauma; or hypertension

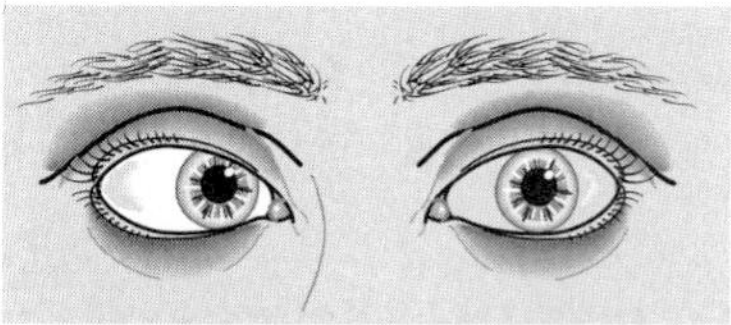

A. Right esotropia

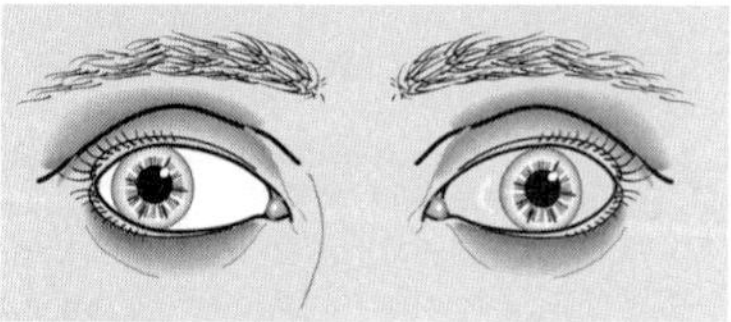

B. Right exotropia

Figure 12-5 Asymmetric Corneal Light Reflex

Cover/Uncover Test

E 1. Ask the patient to look straight ahead and to focus on an object in the distance.

2. Place an occluder over the patient's left eye for several seconds and observe for movement in the uncovered right eye.
3. As you remove the occluder, observe the covered eye for movement.
4. Repeat the procedure with the same eye, this time having the patient focus on an object held close to the eye.
5. Repeat on the other side.

N **The eyes are normally in alignment, as indicated by lack of movement of either eye.**

A Phoria: latent misalignment of an eye (the uncovered eye shifts position as the other eye is covered, or the covered eye shifts position as it is uncovered); esophoria: nasal, or inward, drift; exophoria: temporal, or outward, drift

P Mild muscle weakness

Cardinal Fields of Gaze (Extraocular Muscle Movements)

E 1. Have the patient sit facing you.
2. Place your nondominant hand just under the patient's chin or on top of the patient's head as a reminder to hold the head still.
3. Ask the patient to follow an object (finger, pencil, penlight) with the eyes.
4. Move the object through the six fields of gaze (Figure 12-6) in a smooth and steady manner, pausing in each extreme position to detect any nystagmus or involuntary movement and returning to the center after each field is tested.
5. Note the patient's ability to move the eyes in each direction.
6. Move the object forward to approximately 5 inches in front of the patient's nose at the midline.
7. Observe for convergence of gaze.

N **Both eyes should move smoothly and symmetrically in each of the six fields of gaze and converge on the held object as it moves toward the nose. A few beats of nystagmus with extreme lateral gaze can be normal.**

A Lack of symmetric eye movement in a particular direction

P Weakness in the muscle responsible for moving the eye in that direction

A Failure of an eye to move outward (CN VI), inability of an eye to move downward when deviated inward (CN IV), other defects in movement (CN III)

P Traumatic ophthalmoplegia secondary to fracture of the orbit near the foramen magnum and causing damage to the extraocular muscles or CN II, III, IV, or VI; basilar skull fracture; vitamin deficiency (especially of thiamine); herpes zoster; syphilis; scarlet fever; whooping cough; botulism

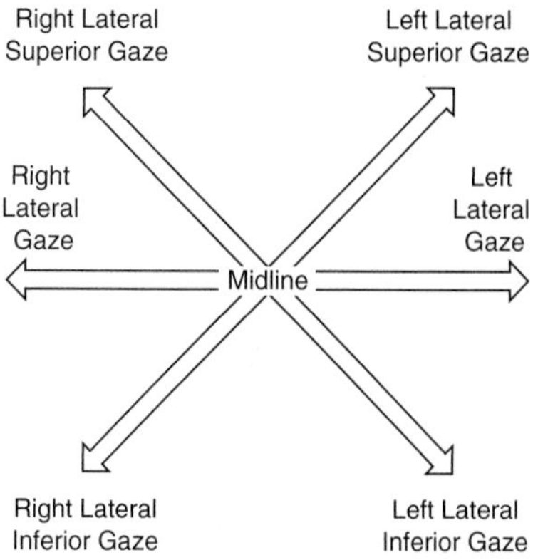

Figure 12-6 Cardinal Fields of Gaze

A Ophthalmoplegia: paralysis of one or more of the optic muscles

P Increased intracranial pressure, parasellar meningiomas or tumors in the sphenoid sinus

A Vertical gaze deviation

P Destruction of the midbrain-diencephalic junction or the medial longitudinal fasciculus, tumors of the pineal gland

A Horizontal gaze deviation

P Damage to the motor areas of the cerebral cortex (deviation tending toward the side of the lesion)

A Skew deviation: one eye deviates down, the other eye deviates up

P Lesion in the pons on the same side as the eye that deviates down, cerebellar disease

A Nystagmus: rhythmic, beating, involuntary oscillation of the eyes as an object is held at points away from the midline; usually lateral, vertical, or rotary

P Lesion in the brain stem, cerebellum, or vestibular system or along the visual pathways in the cerebral hemispheres

Anterior Segment Structures

Conjunctiva

E To assess the bulbar conjunctiva:

1. Use the fingers to separate the lid margins.
2. Have the patient look up, down, and to the right and left.
3. Inspect the surface of the bulbar conjunctiva for color, redness (injection), swelling, exudate, and foreign bodies.
4. Use the thumb to gently pull the lower lid toward the cheek; inspect the surface of the bulbar conjunctiva for color, inflammation, edema, lesions, and foreign bodies.

N **The bulbar conjunctiva is normally transparent and has small, visible blood vessels. It should appear white except for these few small blood vessels. No swelling, injection, exudate, foreign bodies, or lesions are present.**

E The palpebral conjunctiva is examined only when there is a concern about its condition. To examine the palpebral conjunctiva of the upper lid:

1. Explain the procedure to the patient to alleviate any fear of pain or damage to the eye.
2. Don gloves. Wash any glove powder off of gloves. Have the patient look down to relax the levator muscle.
3. Gently pull the eyelashes downward and place a sterile, cotton-tipped applicator approximately 1 cm above the lid margin.
4. Gently exert downward pressure on the applicator while pulling the eyelashes upward to evert the lid (Figure 12-7).
5. Inspect the palpebral conjunctiva for injection, swelling (chemosis), exudate, and foreign bodies.
6. Return the lid to its normal position by instructing the patient to look up and then pulling the eyelid outward and removing the cotton-tipped applicator. Ask the patient to blink.

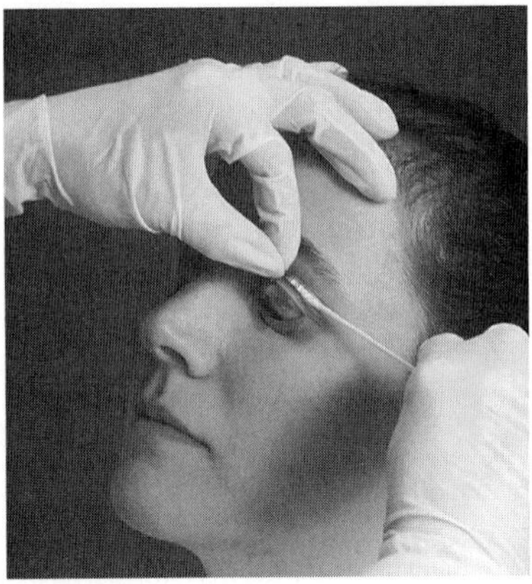

Figure 12-7 Assessing Palpebral Conjunctiva: Everting the Eyelid

N **The palpebral conjunctiva should appear pink and moist and be without swelling, lesions, injection, exudate, and foreign bodies.**

A Bilateral injected conjunctiva with purulent, sticky discharge and lid edema

P Bacterial conjunctivitis

A Unilateral injection with moderate pain and increased lacrimation but without purulent discharge

P Viral conjunctivitis (e.g., adenovirus or herpes simplex)

A Mild inflammation and injection and follicles of palpebral conjunctiva with scant discharge; associated itching and burning sensation with increased lacrimation

P Allergic conjunctivitis

A Pinguecula: usually painless yellow nodule on the nasal or temporal side of the bulbar conjunctiva and adjacent to the cornea

P Nodular degeneration of the conjunctiva resulting from exposure to ultraviolet light

A Pterygium: unilateral or bilateral, painless, triangular encroachment onto the nasal side of the conjunctiva (Figure 12-8)

P Excessive ultraviolet-light exposure

A Sudden onset of painless, bright-red appearance of the bulbar conjunctiva

P Subconjunctival hemorrhage resulting from pressure exerted during coughing, sneezing, or Valsalva maneuver; uncontrolled hypertension; anticoagulant medications

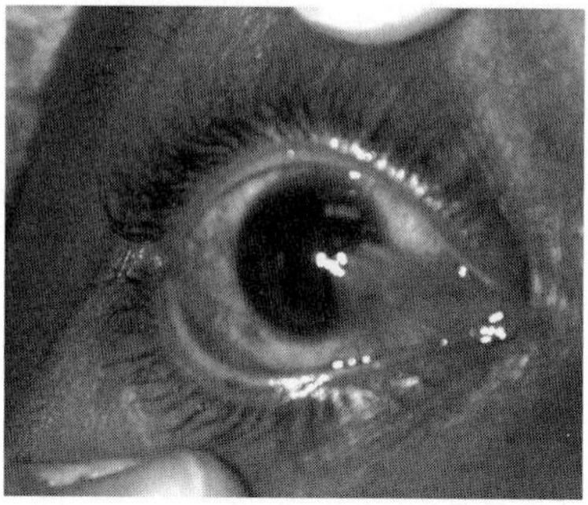

Figure 12-8 Pterygium. *Courtesy of Salim I. Butrus, M.D., Senior Attending, Department of Ophthalmology, Washington Hospital Center, Washington, DC & Associate Clinical Professor, Georgetown University Medical Center, Washington, DC*

Sclera

E While assessing the conjunctiva, inspect the sclera for color, exudates, lesions, and foreign bodies.

N **In light-skinned individuals, the sclera should be white with some small, superficial vessels and without exudate, lesions, and foreign bodies. In dark-skinned individuals, the sclera may have tiny brown patches of melanin or a grayish blue or "muddy" color.**

A Jaundice or scleral icterus: uniformly yellow sclera

P Coloring of the sclera by bilirubin (an early manifestation of systemic conditions such as hepatitis, sickle cell disease, gallstones, and physiological jaundice of the newborn)

A Blue sclera

P Osteogenesis imperfecta secondary to thinning of the sclera

Cornea

E 1. Stand in front of the patient.
2. Shine a penlight directly on the cornea.
3. Move the light laterally and view the cornea from that angle, noting color, discharge, and lesions.

N **The corneal surface should be moist and shiny and without discharge, cloudiness, opacity, and irregularity.**

A A grayish, well-circumscribed, ulcerated area on the cornea

P Corneal ulceration resulting from a bacterial invasion

A A treelike configuration on the corneal surface in conjunction with patient complaints of discomfort, photophobia, and, sometimes, blurred vision

P Ulceration caused by the herpes simplex virus

A Arcus senilis: a hazy gray ring approximately 2 mm in width and located just inside the limbus

P Bilateral benign degeneration of the peripheral cornea

A Glaucoma: steamy or cloudy corneal appearance with associated ocular pain

P Increased intraocular pressure

Iris

E With the penlight, inspect the iris for color, nodules, and vascularity.

N **The color is evenly distributed over the iris, although there can be a mosaic variant. The iris is normally smooth and without apparent vascularity.**

A Iris nevus: a heavily pigmented, slightly elevated area visible in the iris

P Benign iris nevus or malignant melanoma

A Hyphema: inferior portion of the iris obscured by blood

P Bleeding from vessels in the iris as a result of direct trauma to the globe; eye surgery

A Absent wedge portion of the iris

P Change in iris shape resulting from surgical removal of a cataract

Pupil

E **1.** Stand in front of the patient in a darkened room.
2. Note pupil shape and size (in millimeters).
3. Move a penlight from the side to the front of one eye without allowing the light to shine on the other eye.
4. Observe the pupillary reaction in that eye (the direct light reflex). Note the size of the pupil receiving the light stimulus and the speed of pupillary response to the light.
5. Repeat on the other eye.
6. Move the penlight in front of one eye and observe the other eye for pupillary constriction (the consensual light reflex).
7. Repeat on the other eye.
8. Instruct the patient to shift his or her gaze to a distant object for 30 seconds.
9. Instruct the patient to then look at your finger or an object held in your hand approximately 10 cm from the patient.
10. Note the reaction and size of the pupils. Accommodation occurs when pupils constrict and converge to focus on objects at close range.

N **The pupils should be deep black, round, and of equal diameter ranging from 2 to 6 mm. Pupils should constrict briskly to direct and consensual light and to accommodation (CN III). Small differences in pupil size (anisocoria) may be normal in some people.**

A Miotic: pupil constricted to less than 2 mm in diameter; mydriatic: pupil dilated to more than 6 mm in diameter

P Medications such as sympathomimetics or parasympathomimetics, iritis, CN-III paralysis resulting from carotid artery aneurysm (see Table 12-1 for further pathologies)

A Irregularly shaped pupil

P Surgical removal of cataract, iridectomy

A Hippus phenomenon: pupil constricts to light but then appears to rhythmically vacillate in size from a larger to a smaller diameter

P Lesion in the midbrain

A Marcus Gunn: pupil dilates to light (inappropriate consensual reaction)

P Optic nerve damage in the optic chiasm, such as in trauma

Lens

E **1.** Stand in front of the patient.
2. Shine a penlight directly on the pupil. The lens is behind the pupil.
3. Note lens color.

N **The lens is transparent.**

A Cataract: pearly gray appearance of one or both lenses

P Senile cataract; unilateral cataract: injury from a foreign body; bilateral cataracts: when found in infants or young children; most likely congenital but may result from maternal rubella in the first trimester of pregnancy

Posterior Segment Structures

The funduscopic assessment (CN II) requires the use of a direct ophthalmoscope to view the structures in the posterior segment of the eye.

Retinal Structures

E Ask the patient to remove eyeglasses; contact lenses may be left in place. In a darkened room:

TABLE 12-1 Pupil Abnormalities

A.

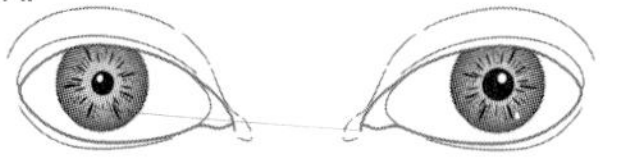

A: The size of pupils is unequal, but both pupils react to light and accommodation.
P: Inequality of pupillary size is called **anisocoria** and may be congenital or due to inflammation of ocular tissue or disturbances of neurophthalmic pathways.

B.

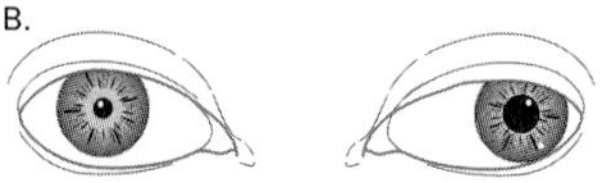

A: A fixed and dilated pupil is observed on one side. The abnormal pupil does not react to direct or consensual light stimulation and does not accommodate. Ptosis and lateral downward deviation may also be noted.
P: This abnormality is caused by **oculomotor nerve damage** due to head trauma and increased intracranial pressure. Atropine-like agents applied topically may cause an even more widely fixed and dilated pupil.

C.

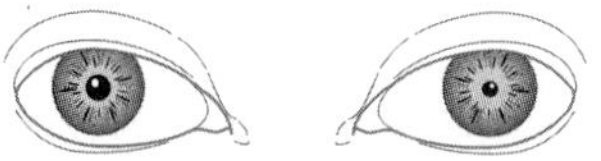

A: A unilateral, small, regularly shaped pupil is observed. Both pupils react directly and consensually and accommodate. Ptosis and diminished or absent sweating on the affected side may also be noted.
P: This finding is **Horner's syndrome,** which is caused by a lesion of the sympathetic nerve pathway.

D.

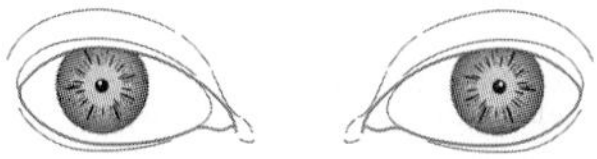

A: Pupils are bilaterally small and irregularly shaped. They react to accommodation but sluggishly or not at all to light.
P: These abnormalities are **Argyll Robertson** pupils and are usually caused by central lesions of neurosyphilis. Other causes include encephalitis, drugs, diabetes, brain tumors, and alcoholism.

E.

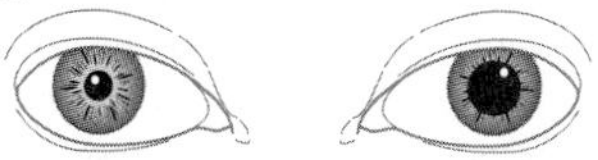

A: A unilateral, large, regularly shaped pupil is noted. The affected pupil's reaction to light and accommodation is sluggish or absent. The patient may report blurred vision because of the slow accommodation. You may observe diminished ankle and knee deep-tendon reflexes.
P: This abnormality, a tonic or **Adie's** pupil, is due to impaired sympathetic nerve supply.

F.

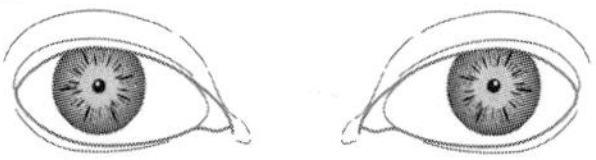

A: Both pupils are **small, fixed,** regularly shaped, and do not react to light or accommodation.
P: This abnormality may be caused by opiate ingestion, topical application of miotic drops, or lesions in the brain.

A: Pupils are small, equal, and reactive.
P: Diencephalic injury or metabolic coma may cause these findings.

G.

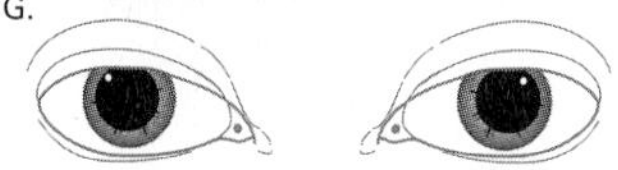

A: Both pupils are **dilated** and **fixed**, and do not react to light and do not accommodate.
P: Severe head trauma, brain stem infarction, cardiopulmonary arrest (after 4 to 6 min).

H.

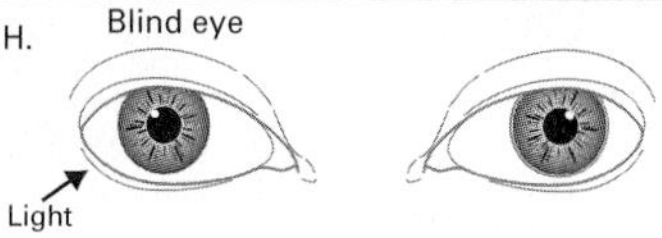

A: Light shone into a blind eye (**amaurotic pupil**) will cause no reaction (direct or consensual) in either pupil. If light is shone in the other eye, and CN III is intact, both pupils should constrict.
P: Due to a lesion in the retina or the optic nerve, the light stimulus shown in the amaurotic pupil is unable to pass along the sensory pathway; therefore, the oculomotor response in both eyes is absent.

1. Instruct the patient to look at a distant object across the room. (Looking at a distance helps dilate the pupils.)
2. Set the ophthalmoscope on the 0 lens and hold it in front of your right eye.
3. From a distance of 8 to 12 inches from the patient and approximately 15° to the lateral side, shine the light into the patient's right pupil to elicit a light reflection from the retina, called the red reflex.
4. While maintaining the red reflex in view, move closer to the patient and move the diopter wheel from 0 to the +, or black, numbers in order to focus on the anterior ocular structures.
5. For optimum visualization, keep the ophthalmoscope within 1 inch of the patient's eye (Figure 12-9).
6. Next, move the diopter wheel from the +, or black, numbers, through 0, and into the –, or red, numbers in order to focus on structures progressively more posterior.
7. Focus on the optic disc at the nasal side of the retina by following any retinal vessels centrally.
8. If the disc does not come into view, you may need to reverse direction along the vessel.
9. Observe the retina for color and lesions, the retinal vessels for configuration and characteristics of their crossing, and the optic disc for color, shape, size, margins, and comparison of cup-to-disc ratio.
10. Describe the size, position, and location of any abnormality. Use the diameter of the disc (DD) as a guide to describe the distance of the abnormality from the optic disc. Use the optic disc as a clock face to reference the location of the abnormality. Describe the size of the abnormality in relation to the size of the optic disc.
11. Repeat on the left eye.

N **Refer to Table 12-2. The red reflex is present. The optic disc is pinkish orange and has a yellow-white excavated center known as the physiologic cup (Figure 12-10). The ratio of the cup diameter to that of the entire disc is 1:3. The border of the disc may range from a sharp, round demarcation from the surrounding retina to a more blended demarcation but should be on the same plane as the retina. In general, there are four main vascular branches emanating from the disc; each branch consists of an arteriole and a venule. The venules are approximately**

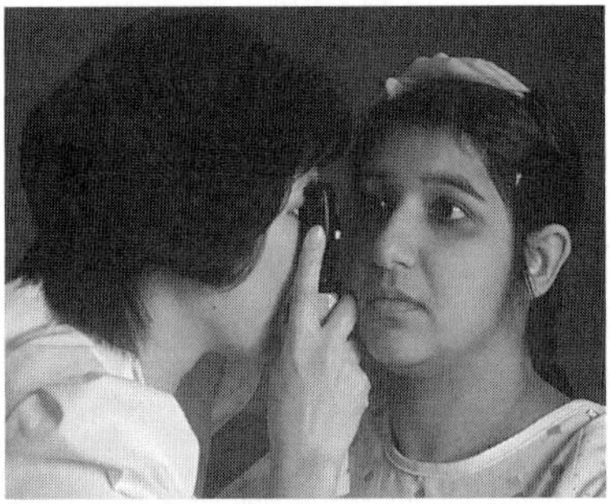

Figure 12-9 Examining Retinal Structures: Funduscopic Examination

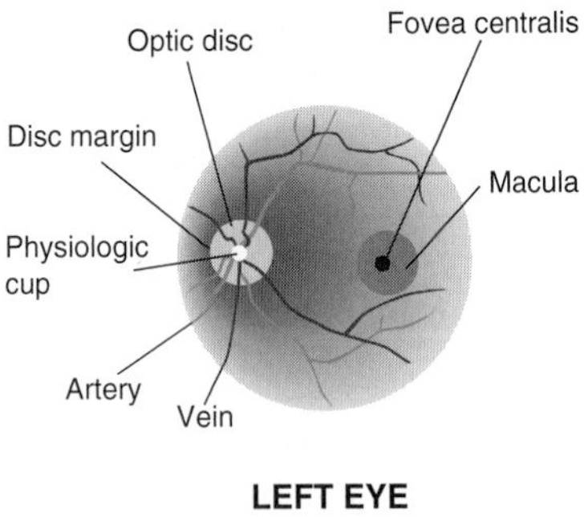

Figure 12-10 Retina

TABLE 12-2 Retinal Color Variations

SUBJECT	CHARACTERISTICS
Light-skinned individuals	Retina appears a light red-orange Tessellated appearance of the fundi (pigment does not obscure the choroid vessels)
Dark-skinned individuals	Fundi appear dark; grayish purple to brownish (from increased pigment in the choroid and retina) No tessellated appearance Choroidal vessels usually obscured
Aging individuals	Vessels are straighter and narrower than in younger subjects Choroidal vessels are easily visualized Retinal pigment epithelium atrophies and causes retina to become paler

four times the size of the accompanying arterioles and are darker. Light often produces a glistening "light reflex" from the arteriolar vessel. Normal arterial to venous ratio is 2:3 or 4:5.

A The red reflex is absent and the pupil appears white.

P Cataract, congenital cataract

A Pale optic disc

P Optic atrophy caused by increased intracranial pressure; congenital syphilis

A Papillitis: physiologic cup exceeds the normal 1:3 ratio; disc is edematous and hyperemic and has blurred margins and an elevated surface

P With loss of vision: optic neuritis; without loss of vision: choked disc, or papilledema, resulting from increased intracranial pressure obstructing return blood flow from the eye

A Roth spots: superficial, flame-shaped retinal hemorrhages or red hemorrhages with white centers, both found in the fundi

P Severe hypertension, occlusion of the central retinal vein, papilledema, infective endocarditis

A Deep retinal hemorrhages: small, red dots or irregular spots in the deep layer of the retina

P Diabetes mellitus

A Preretinal hemorrhages in the small space between the vitreous and the retina

P Sudden increase in intracranial pressure

A Microaneurysms: tiny, red dots seen in peripheral and macular areas of the retina

P Diabetic retinopathy

A Neovascularization: formation of new and extremely narrow and disorderly vessels

P Diabetic retinopathy

A Cotton wool spots: fluffy white areas on the retina

P Microscopic infarcts of the nerve fiber layer resulting from diabetic or hypertensive retinopathy

A Drusen: small white dots in the fundus that are arranged in an irregular pattern and may occur on the optic disc

P Normal aging process

A Detached retina: absent red reflex in area of detachment; area is pearly gray, elevated, and wrinkled

P Severe myopia, cataract surgery, trauma, diabetic retinopathy

Macula

E When the retinal structures and optic disc have been assessed:

1. Move the ophthalmoscope approximately 2 disc diameters temporally to view the macula, or ask the patient to look at the light. The red-free filter lens of the ophthalmoscope may also be helpful in assessing the macula. Because the macula is not clearly demarcated and is very light sensitive, you may have difficulty assessing it; the patient tends to turn away when the light strikes the fovea, making it difficult to assess details of the macular area.

2. Note the fovea centralis and observe for color, shape, and lesions.

3. Repeat on the other eye.

N **The macula is a darker, avascular area with a pinpoint, reflective center known as the fovea centralis.**

A Pale retina, macular region like a cherry-red spot

P Central retinal artery occlusion (indicative of Tay-Sachs disease)

A Microaneurysms: sharply defined, small, red spots in and around the macula

P Diabetes mellitus

A Blurred macular borders and a few spots of pigment near the macula; a hole may appear to be present in the center of the region

P Age-related macular degeneration

13

Ears, Nose, Mouth, and Throat

Anatomy and Physiology

Ear

External Ear

The external ear, which is also called the auricle or pinna, extends through the auditory canal to the tympanic membrane (Figure 13-1). The auricle receives sound waves and funnels them through the auditory canal to produce vibrations on the tympanic membrane.

The external auditory canal is lined with tiny hairs and modified sweat glands that secrete a thick, waxlike substance called cerumen. Cerumen ranges from a pale, honey color in light-skinned individuals to dark brown or black in dark-skinned individuals.

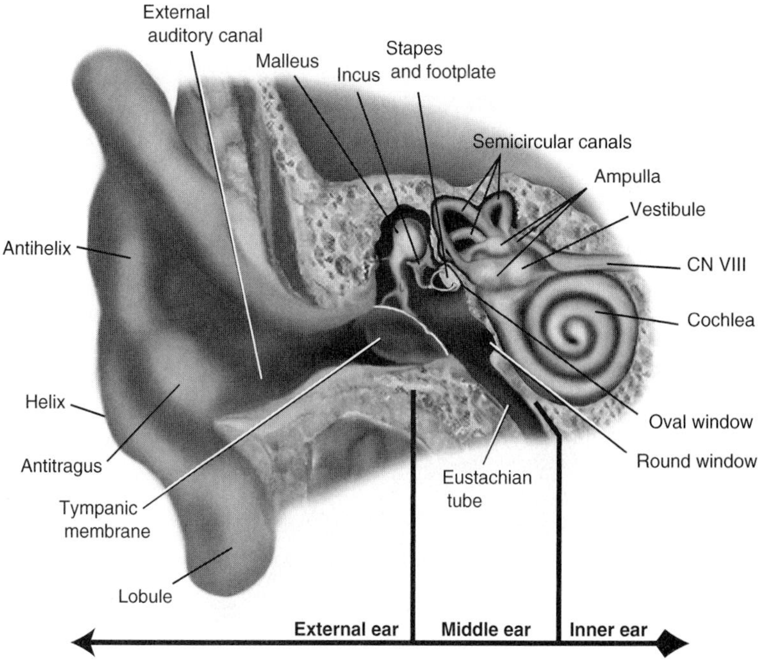

Figure 13-1 Cross Section of the Ear

Middle Ear

The middle ear is composed of the tympanic membrane, the ossicles, and the tympanic cavity. The cavity is an air-filled compartment that divides the external ear from the internal ear. The tympanic membrane is circular or oval and approximately 1 cm in diameter (Figure 13-2).

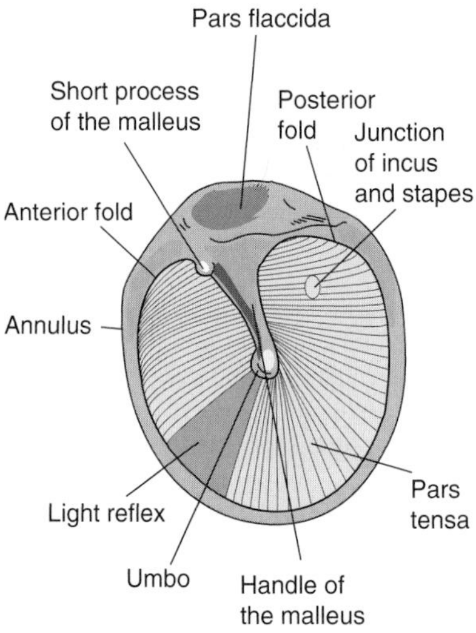

Figure 13-2 Landmarks of the Tympanic Membrane

Vibrations set up in the tympanic membrane by sound waves reaching it through the external auditory canal are transmitted to the inner ear via rapid movement of the ossicles.

The middle ear is connected to the nasopharynx via the auditory, or eustachian, tube.

Inner Ear

The inner ear is a complex, closed, fluid-filled system of interconnecting tubes called the labyrinth, which is essential for hearing and equilibrium. The inner ear is composed of the cochlea, the semicircular canals, and the vestibule. The human ear has a hearing frequency range of 20 to 20,000 Hz and 0 to 140 decibels.

Nose

The nose consists of the external, or outer, nose and the nasal fossae, or internal nose (Figure 13-3). The outer nose

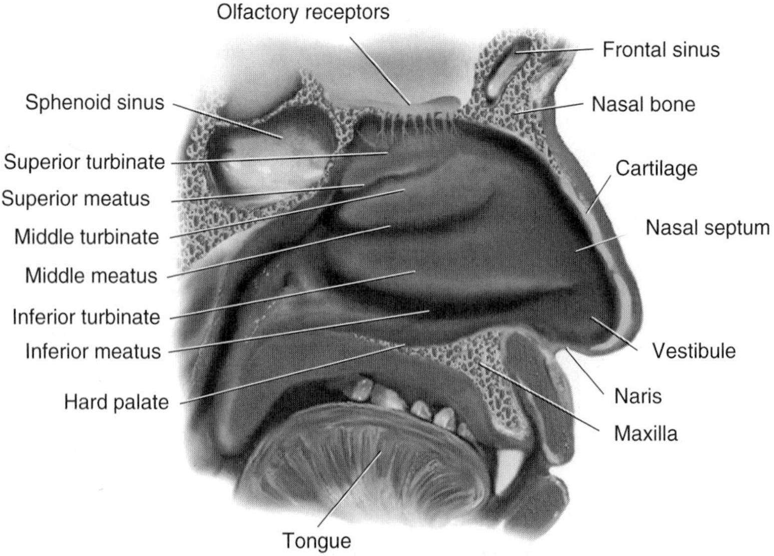

Figure 13-3 Lateral Cross Section of the Nose

is made up of bone and cartilage and is divided internally into two nasal fossae via the nasal septum. Anterior openings into the nasal fossae are nostrils, or nares.

Air enters the anterior nares, passes through the vestibule, and enters the fossa itself. The fossae clean, filter, humidify, and control the temperature of inspired air.

Olfactory receptor cells are located in the upper parts of the nasal cavity, in the superior nasal turbinate, and on parts of the nasal septum and are covered by hair-like cilia, which project into the cavity. Kiesselback's plexus is a vascular area on the nasal septum and a common site of epitaxia.

Sinuses

The frontal, maxillary, ethmoid, and sphenoid sinuses are air-filled cavities lined with mucous membranes and located in some of the cranial bones (Figure 13-4). Only the frontal and maxillary sinuses can be assessed in the physical exam.

Mouth and Throat

The lips are sensory structures found at the opening of the mouth (Figure 13-5). The area where the lips meet the facial skin is the vermillion border. The

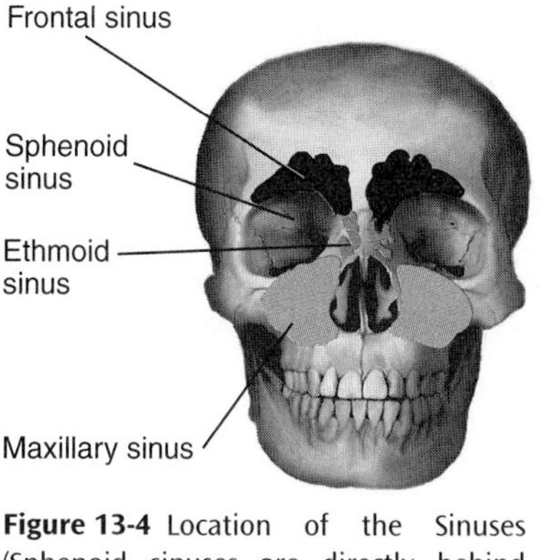

Figure 13-4 Location of the Sinuses (Sphenoid sinuses are directly behind ethmoid sinuses.)

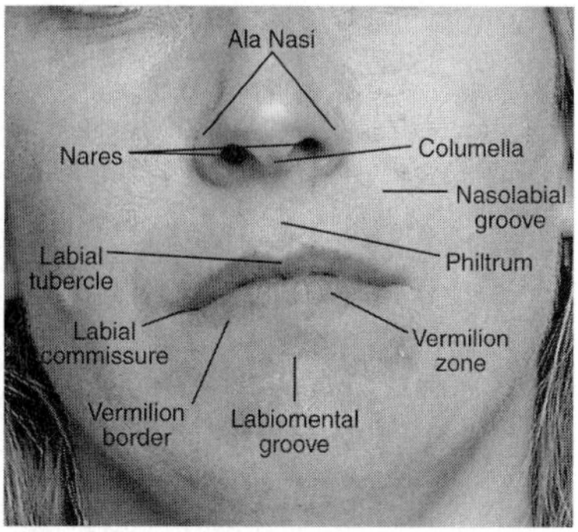

Figure 13-5 Landmarks of the Face

median groove superior to the upper lip is called the philtrum.

The roof of the mouth consists of the hard palate anteriorly and the soft palate posteriorly. The linear raphe is a linear ridge in the middle of the hard palate (Figure 13-6).

The tongue is a muscular organ connected to the hyoid bone posteriorly and to the floor of the mouth anteriorly via the frenulum. The tongue assists with mastication, swallowing, speech, and mechanical cleansing of the teeth.

Projections called papillae, which cover the upper surface of the tongue, assist in handling food and contain the taste buds. Four qualities of taste are found in taste buds: bitter is located at the base of the tongue, sour along the sides of the tongue, and salty and sweet near the tip of the tongue. The sulcus terminalis is the midline depression that separates the anterior two-thirds of the tongue from the posterior one-third.

Gums, or gingivae, hold the teeth in place.

Adults have 32 permanent teeth: four incisors, two canines, four premolars, and six molars in each half of the mouth (Figure 13-7). The three parts of the tooth are the top, or the crown, the root, which is embedded in the gum, and the neck, which connects the root and crown.

The uvula is a fingerlike projection of tissue that hangs down from the center of the soft palate.

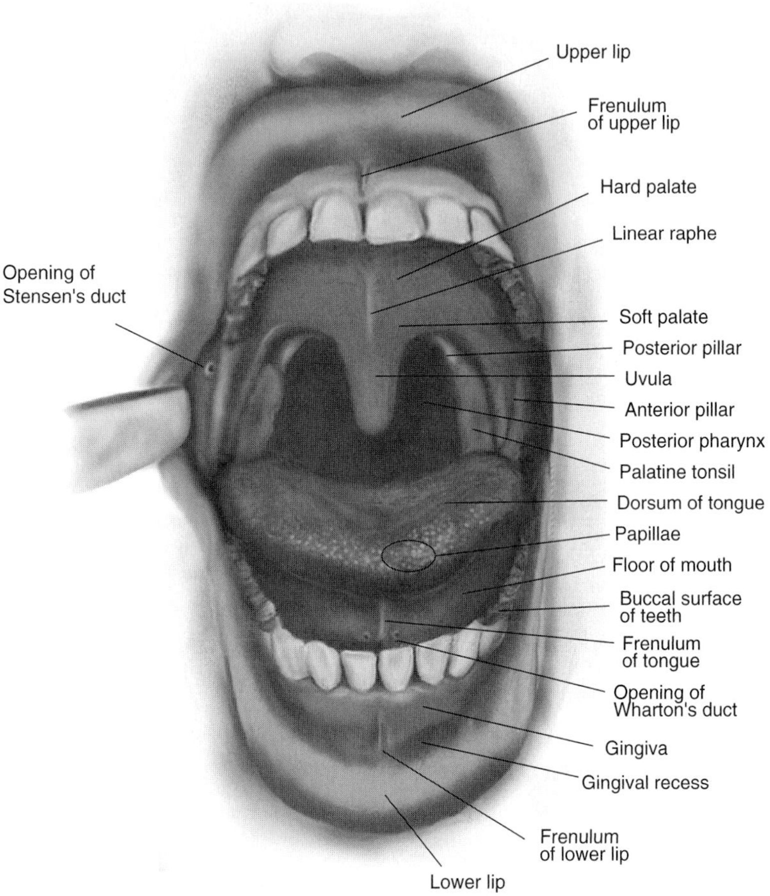

Figure 13-6 Structures of the Mouth

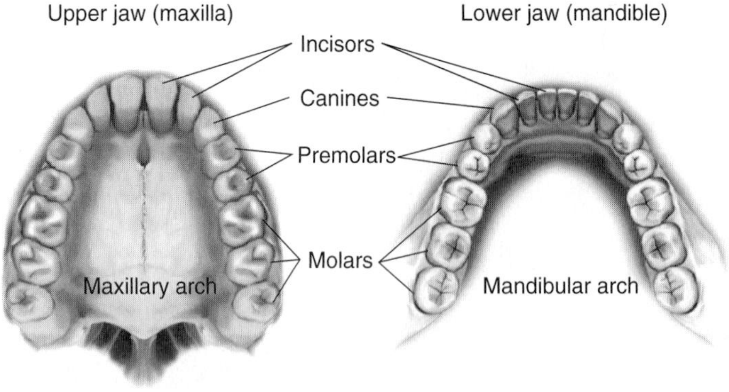

Figure 13-7 Permanent Teeth

HEALTH HISTORY

Medical History

Ear specific: Acute otitis media, serous otitis media, acute otitis externa, otorrhea, hearing changes, otalgia, tinnitus
Nose specific: Polyps, sinus infection, septal deviation, allergic rhinitis, rhinorrhea, congestion
Mouth and throat specific: Tonsillitis, herpes simplex virus, strep throat, tonsillar abscess, caries, candida infections, frequent URI, halitosis

Surgical History

Tonsillectomy, adenoidectomy, repair of septal deviation, tympanostomy tube placement, repair of detached retina, neurosurgery, tumor removal, cosmetic surgery of head or neck, oral surgery, foreign body removal

Allergies

Pollen: sneezing, nasal congestion, cough; insect stings: swelling of the throat; animal dander: sneezing, nasal congestion, cough

Special Needs

Deafness, speech disorders

Childhood Illnesses

Frequent ear infections, frequent tonsillitis, rubella

Social History

Tobacco use: snuff or chewing tobacco predisposes the patient to mouth, lip, and throat cancers; smoking pipes predisposes the patient to mouth, lip, and tongue cancers.
Drug use: snorting cocaine may cause perforation of the nasal septum.

Equipment

- Otoscope with ear pieces of different sizes and a pneumatic attachment
- Nasal speculum
- Penlight
- Tuning fork, 512 Hz
- Tongue blade
- Watch
- Gauze square
- Clean gloves
- Transilluminator
- Cotton-tipped applicator

NURSING CHECKLIST

General Approach to Ears, Nose, Mouth, and Throat Assessment

1. Explain the assessment techniques that you will be using.
2. Ensure that the light in the room provides sufficient brightness to allow adequate observation of the patient.
3. Place the patient in an upright, sitting position on the examination table.
4. For patients who cannot tolerate the sitting position, gain access to the patient's head so that it can be rotated from side to side for assessment.
5. Always use a systematic approach and compare right and left ears as well as right and left sides of the nose, sinuses, mouth, and throat.

Assessment of the Ear

Physical assessment of the ear consists of three parts:

1. Auditory screening (CN VIII)
2. Inspection and palpation of the external ear
3. Otoscopic assessment

Auditory Screening

Voice-Whisper Test

E 1. Instruct the patient to use a finger to occlude one ear.
2. Stand 2 feet behind the patient's other ear and whisper a two-syllable word or a phrase that is evenly accented.
3. Ask the patient to repeat the word or phrase.
4. Repeat the test on the other ear.

N **The patient should be able to repeat words whispered from a distance of 2 feet.**

A Inability to correctly repeat the words or to hear anything

P Hearing loss in the high-frequency range and associated with excessive exposure to loud noises

Tuning Fork Tests

Weber and Rinne tests help determine whether hearing loss is conductive or sensorineural. Air conduction refers to the transmission of sound through the ear canal, tympanic membrane, and ossicular chain to the cochlea and auditory nerve. Bone conduction refers to the transmission of sound through the bones of the skull to the cochlea and auditory nerve.

Weber Test

E 1. To activate the 513 Hz tuning fork, hold the handle and strike the tines on the ulnar border of the palm.
2. Firmly place the stem of the fork against the middle of the patient's forehead, on the top and at the midline of the patient's head, or on the patient's front teeth (Figure 13-8).
3. Ask the patient whether the sound is heard centrally or toward one side.

N **The patient should perceive the sound equally in both ears, or "in the middle." No lateralization of sound is known as a "negative" Weber test.**

A Unilateral conductive hearing loss: sound is conducted directly through the bone and lateralizes to the impaired ear.

P External or middle ear disorders such as impacted cerumen, perforation of the tympanic membrane, serum or pus in the middle ear, or fusion of the ossicles

A Sensorineural hearing loss: sound lateralizes to the unimpaired ear.

P Nerve damage in the impaired ear resulting from a disorder in the inner ear, the auditory nerve, or the brain (such as congenital defects, effects of ototoxic drugs, or repeated or prolonged exposure to loud noise)

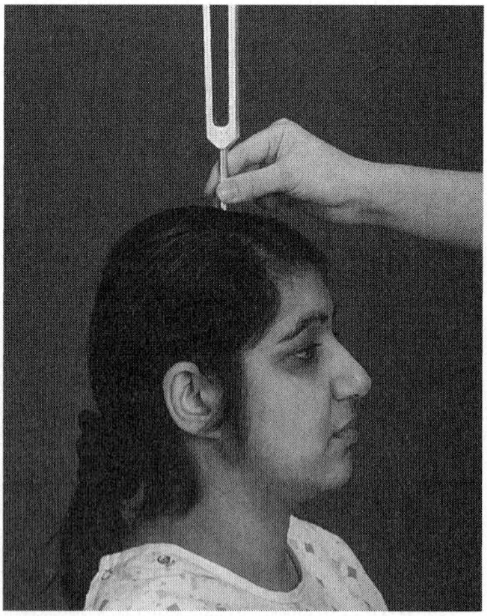

Figure 13-8 Weber Test

Rinne Test

E 1. Stand behind or to the side of the patient and strike the tuning fork.
2. To test bone conduction, place the stem of the tuning fork against the right mastoid process (Figure 13-9A).
3. Instruct the patient to indicate whether the sound is heard.
4. Ask the patient to tell you when the sound stops.
5. To test air conduction (Figure 13-9B), when the patient says that the sound has stopped, move the tuning fork (with the tines facing forward) in front of the right auditory meatus and ask the patient whether the sound is still heard. Note the length of time the patient hears the sound.
6. Repeat the test on the left ear.

N **Air-conducted sound (via the external auditory canal) is heard twice as long as is bone-conducted sound (via the mastoid process). This difference is denoted as AC>BC.**

A Sound is heard longer through bone conduction than through air conduction.

P Conductive hearing loss resulting from disease, obstruction, or damage to the outer or middle ear

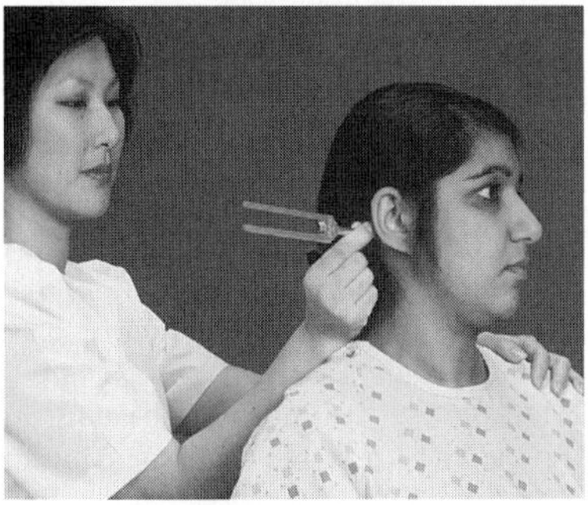

A. Assessing Bone Conduction

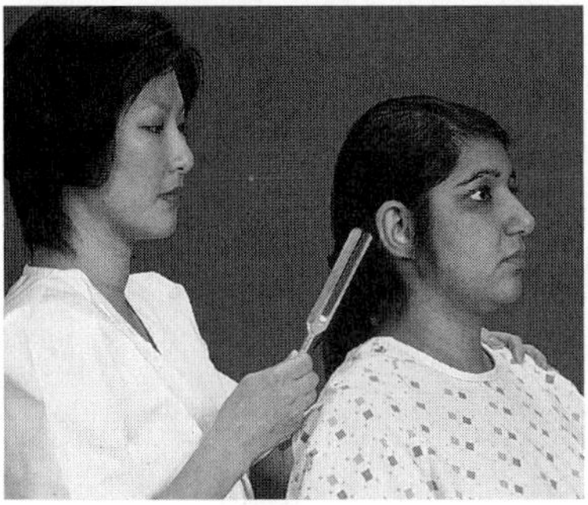

B. Assessing Air Conduction

Figure 13-9 Rinne Test

External Ear

Inspection

E 1. Inspect the ears, noting position, color, size, and shape.
2. Note any deformities, nodules, inflammation, and lesions.
3. Note color, consistency, and amount of cerumen.

N **The ear color should match the color of the rest of the patient's skin, and the ear should be positioned centrally and in proportion to the head. The top of the ear should cross an imaginary line drawn from the outer canthus of the eye to the occiput. Cerumen should be moist and should not obscure the tympanic membrane. There should be no foreign bodies, redness, drainage, deformities, nodules, or lesions.**

A Pale, red, or cyanotic ears

P Vasomotor disorders, fever, hypoxemia, cold weather

A Purulent drainage

P Infection

A Clear or bloody drainage

P Possible cerebrospinal spinal fluid leakage resulting from head trauma or surgery

A A hard, painless, irregularly shaped nodule on the pinna

P Tophi: uric acid nodules indicating gout; other nodules: possibly benign fibromas

Nursing Tip

Cerebrospinal Fluid Drainage from the Ear

If the patient is noted to have cerebrospinal fluid (clear liquid that tests positive for glucose on Dextrostix) leaking from the ear, use good handwashing technique and do not place any objects into the ear canal in order to prevent the development of meningitis. A patient with this finding needs immediate referral to a qualified specialist.

A Hematoma over mastoid bone
P Battle sign indicates head trauma
A Lymph nodes anterior to the tragus or overlying the mastoid
P Malignancy or infectious process
A Sebaceous cysts
P Blockage of the ducts to the sebaceous gland
A Abnormally large, small, or irregularly shaped ears
P Congenital or trauma

Palpation

E 1. Between your thumb and index finger, palpate the auricle; note any tenderness or lesions. If there is pain, assess the unaffected ear first.
2. Using the tips of the index and middle fingers, palpate the mastoid tip; note any tenderness.
3. Using the tips of the index and middle fingers, press inward on the tragus; note any tenderness.
4. Hold the auricle between the thumb and index finger and gently pull upward and downward; note any tenderness.

N **The patient should not complain of pain or tenderness during palpation.**
A Auricular pain
P Acute otitis externa
A Tenderness over the mastoid process
P Middle ear inflammation or mastoiditis
A Edematous or sensitive tragus
P Inflammation of the external or middle ear

Otoscopic Assessment

E 1. Ask the patient to tip the head away from the ear being assessed.
2. Select the largest speculum that will comfortably fit the patient.
3. In your dominant hand, securely hold the otoscope, with the head held downward and the handle held like a pencil between the thumb and forefinger (Figure 13-10.)
4. Rest the back of the dominant hand on the right side of the patient's head.
5. Use the ulnar aspect of your free hand to pull the right ear in a manner to straighten the canal. In adults and in children over 3 years old, pull the ear upward and backward. See Chapter 24 for the assessment of children.
6. If hair obstructs visualization, use water or a water-soluble lubricant to moisten the speculum.
7. If wax obstructs visualization, it should be removed by curettement (if

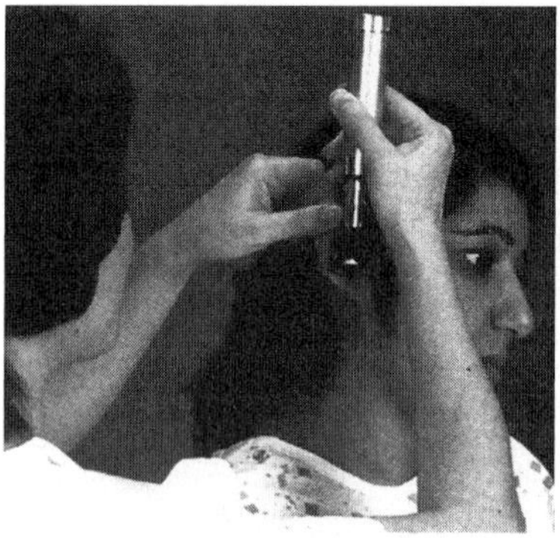

Figure 13-10 Position for Otoscope Examination

the cerumen is soft or the tympanic membrane is ruptured) or irrigation (if the cerumen is dry and hard and the tympanic membrane is intact).

8. Slowly insert the speculum into the canal, looking at the canal as the speculum passes.

9. Assess the canal for inflammation, exudates, lesions, and foreign bodies.

10. Continue to insert the speculum into the canal, following the path of the canal until the tympanic membrane is visualized.

11. If the tympanic membrane is not visible, gently pull the tragus slightly farther in order to straighten the canal to allow adequate visualization.

12. Identify color, light reflex, umbo, the short process, and the long handle of the malleus. Note the presence of perforations, lesions, bulging or retraction of the tympanic membrane, dilatation of blood vessels, and bubbles or fluid level.

13. Ask the patient to close the mouth, pinch the nose closed, and blow gently while you observe for movement of the tympanic membrane. If one is available, a pneumatic attachment may be used to create this movement.

14. Gently withdraw the speculum and repeat the process on the left ear.

N **The ear canal should have no redness, swelling, tenderness, lesions, drainage, foreign bodies, or scaly surface areas. Cerumen varies in amount, consistency, and color. The tympanic membrane should be pearly gray and have clearly defined landmarks and a distinct cone-shaped light reflex extending from the umbo toward the anterioinferior aspect of the membrane. This light reflex is seen at 5 o'clock in the right ear and at 7 o'clock in the left ear. Blood vessels should be visible only on the periphery, and the membrane should neither bulge nor retract and should have no evidence of fluid behind it. The tympanic membrane should move when the patient blows against resistance.**

A Otitis externa: redness, swelling, narrowing, and pain of the external ear; possible drainage

P Infectious organisms or allergic reactions (predisposing factors: excessive moisture in the ear and related to swimming; trauma from using a sharp instrument to cleanse the ears; allergies to substances such as hairspray)

A Hard, dry, very dark yellow-brown cerumen

P External canal impaction

A Otitis media (AOM): red tympanic membrane with decreased mobility and possible bulging

P Inflammation of the middle ear

A Otitis media with effusion (OME): amber-yellow fluid behind the tympanic membrane; possible fluid line or bubbles behind the membrane; possible bulging of the membrane; possible decreased mobility of the eardrum

P Allergies, infections, blocked eustachian tube

A Absent light reflex, redness of the eardrum in conjunction with hyperemic blood vessels and bulging

P Early stage of acute purulent otitis media

A Diffuse, displaced, or absent landmarks along with a bulging eardrum having decreased mobility

P Late stage of acute purulent otitis media

A Darkened area or hole in the tympanic membrane

P Perforated eardrum caused by increased pressure secondary to an untreated ear infection or by trauma

A Pearly gray tympanic membrane with plaques or patches

P Dense white plaques: calcification deposits of tympanic membrane scarring; dark patches: old perforations

See Table 13-1 for a comparison of AOM, OME, and otitis externa.

TABLE 13-1 Comparison of Acute Otitis Media (AOM), Otitis Media with Effusion (OME), and Otitis Externa

	AOM	OME	OTITIS EXTERNA
Tympanic membrane (TM) color	Diffuse red, dilated peripheral vessels	Yellowish	Within normal limits (WNL)
TM appearance	Bulging	Bubbles, fluid line	WNL
TM landmarks	Decreased	Retracted with prominent malleus	WNL
Movement of tragus	Painless	Painless	Painful
Hearing	WNL/decreased	WNL/decreased	WNL
External auditory canal (EAC)	WNL	WNL	Erythematous, edematous

Nursing Alert

Hearing Loss Risk Factors

- Noise exposure
- Smoking
- Ototoxic drugs
- Congenital or heredity
- Cardiovascular disease
- Aging
- Tumors
- Trauma
- Chronic Infection
- Systemic disease
- Tympanic membrane perforation
- Ménière's disease
- Barotrauma

Assessment of the Nose

External Inspection

E Inspect the nose, noting any trauma, bleeding, lesions, masses, swelling, and asymmetry.

N **The shape of the external nose can vary greatly among individuals. Normally, it is located symmetrically in the midline of the face and is without swelling, bleeding, lesions, and masses.**

A Misshapen, broken, or swollen nose

P Genetics, trauma, cosmetic surgery

Patency

E **1.** Have the patient use a finger to occlude one nostril.
2. Ask the patient to breathe in and out through the nose as you observe and listen for air movement into and out of the nostril.
3. Repeat on the other side.

N **Each nostril is patent.**

A No or limited air movement through the nostril(s)

P Deviated septum, foreign body, upper respiratory infection, allergies, nasal polyps

Internal Inspection

E 1. Position the patient so that the head is in an extended position.
2. Place your nondominant hand firmly on top of the patient's head.
3. Using the thumb of the same hand, lift the tip of the patient's nose.
4. Gently insert a nasal speculum or an otoscope with a short, wide, nasal speculum. If using a nasal speculum, use the light of a penlight to view the nostrils.
5. Assess each nostril separately.
6. Inspect the mucous membranes for color and discharge.
7. Inspect the middle and inferior turbinates and the middle meatus for color, swelling, drainage, lesions, and polyps.
8. Observe the nasal septum for deviation, perforation, lesions, and bleeding.

N **The nasal mucosa is pink or dull red and without swelling and polyps. The septum is at the midline and without perforation, lesions, and bleeding. A small amount of clear, watery discharge is normal.**

A Rhinitis: red, swollen nasal mucosa with copious, clear, watery discharge

P Common cold (coryza); possible purulent discharge if a secondary bacterial infection develops

A Pale, edematous nasal mucosa: with clear, watery discharge

P Allergic rhinitis

A Following head trauma, clear, watery, nasal discharge in conjunction with normal-appearing mucosa

P Cerebrospinal fluid secondary to head injury, surgery

A Red, swollen nasal mucosa with purulent nasal discharge

P Bacterial sinusitis

A Unilateral purulent discharge with nasal mucosa on the unaffected side appearing normal

P Local infection commonly associated with the presence of a foreign body

A Inflamed, friable nasal mucosa with possible septal perforation but no infection

P Cocaine or amphetamine use, overuse of nasal spray

Assessment of the Sinuses

Inspection

E Observe the patient's face for any swelling around the nose and eyes.

N **There is no evidence of swelling around the nose and eyes.**

A Swelling above or below the eyes

P Acute sinusitis

Palpation and Percussion

E To palpate and percuss the frontal sinuses:
1. Stand facing the patient.
2. Gently press the thumbs under the bony ridges of the upper orbits (Figure 13-11A). Avoid applying pressure to the globes themselves.
3. Observe for the presence of pain.
4. Using the middle or index finger of the dominant hand, percuss the areas (immediate percussion).
5. Note the sound.

E To palpate and percuss the maxillary sinuses:
1. Stand in front of the patient.
2. Using the thumbs or middle fingers, apply gentle pressure in the areas under the infraorbital ridges (Figure 13-11B).
3. Observe for the presence of pain.
4. Using the dominant middle or index finger, percuss the areas.
5. Note the sound.

N **The patient should experience no discomfort during palpation or percussion. The sinuses should be air filled and, therefore, resonant to percussion.**

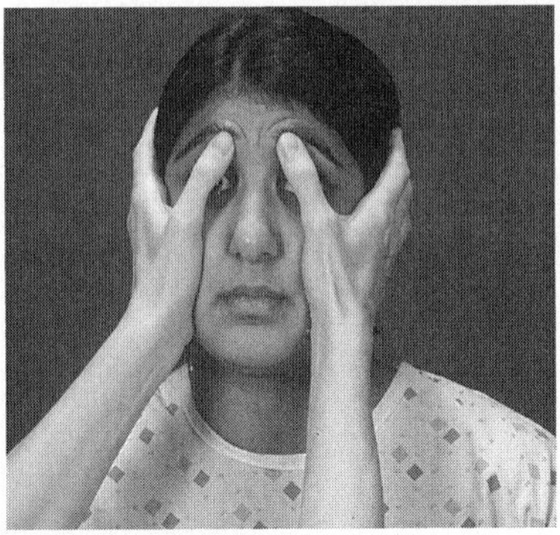

A. Palpation of Frontal Sinuses

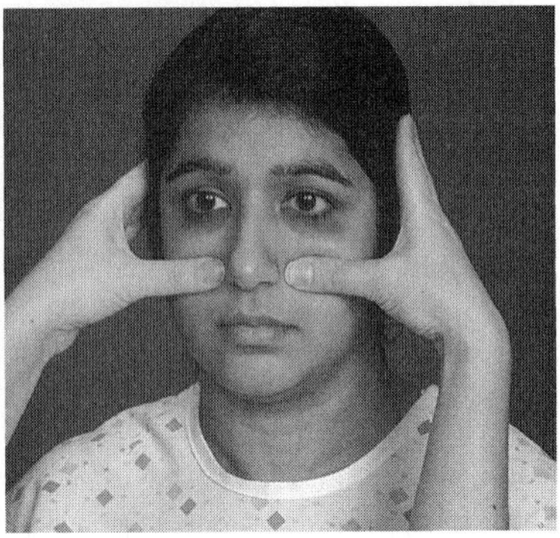

B. Palpation of Maxillary Sinuses

Figure 13-11 Palpation of Sinuses

A Pain or tenderness at the site of palpation or percussion
P Sinusitis: viral, bacterial, or allergic processes

A Sinuses percuss dull
P Fluid or cells in sinus secondary to infection, allergic process, or congenital absence of sinus

Advanced Technique

Transillumination of the Sinuses

If palpation and percussion of the sinuses suggest sinusitis, transillumination of the frontal and maxillary sinuses should be performed.

To evaluate the frontal sinuses:

E
1. Place the patient in a sitting position facing you in a dark room.
2. Place a strong light source such as a transilluminator, penlight, or tip of an otoscope with the speculum under the bony ridge of the upper orbits (Figure 13-12A).
3. Observe the red glow over the sinuses and compare the symmetry of the two sides.

To evaluate the maxillary sinuses:

E
1. Place the patient in a sitting position facing you in a dark room.
2. Place the light source firmly under each eye and just above the infraorbital ridge (Figure 13-12B).
3. Ask the patient to open the mouth; observe the red glow on the hard palate.
4. Compare the two sides.

N **The glow on the two sides is equal, indicating air-filled frontal and maxillary sinuses.**
A Absence of glow is abnormal.
P Absence of glow suggests sinus congestion or the congenital absence of a sinus.

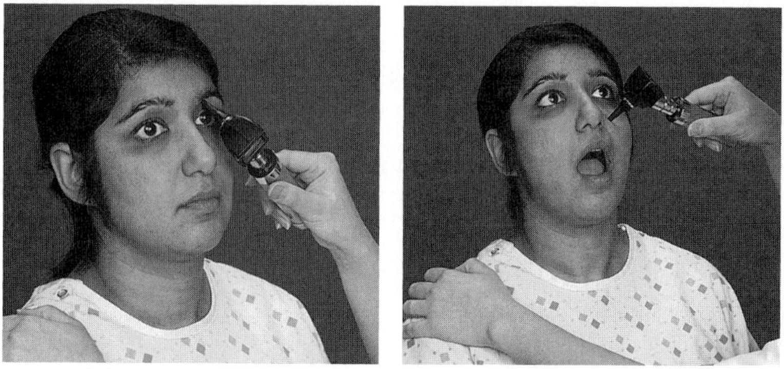

A. Frontal Sinuses B. Maxillary Sinuses

Figure 13-12 Transillumination of Sinuses

NURSING CHECKLIST

Preparing for the Assessment of the Mouth and Throat

- If the patient is wearing dentures or removable orthodontia, ask that they be removed before the assessment begins.
- Use gloves and a good light source, such as a penlight, for optimum visualization of the oral cavity and pharynx.

Assessment of the Mouth and Throat

Assessment of the Mouth

Breath

E 1. Stand facing the patient and approximately 12 inches away.
2. Smell the patient's breath.

N **The breath should smell fresh.**

A Halitosis: foul-smelling breath

P Tooth decay; poor oral hygiene; diseases of the gums, tonsils, or sinuses

A Breath smells of acetone (fruity)

P Malnourishment, diabetic ketoacidosis

A Breath smells of ammonia

P End-stage renal failure (uremia)

Lips

Inspection

E 1. Observe the lips for color, moisture, and swelling, lesions, and other signs of inflammation.
2. Instruct the patient to open the mouth.
3. Use a tongue blade to inspect the membranes that connect the upper and lower lips to the gums for color, inflammation, lesions, and hydration.

N **The lips and membranes should be pink and moist and show no evidence of lesions or inflammation.**

A/P Pale or cyanotic lips: refer to Chapter 16

A Swelling of the lips

P Allergic reaction

A Angular cheilosis: skin at the outer corners of the mouth is atrophic, irritated, and cracked

P Nutritional deficiencies (such as of riboflavin), poorly fitting dentures, immune system deficiencies

A Herpes simplex lesions (cold sores or fever blisters): vesicles on erythematous bases, with serous fluid, and found either singly or in clusters on the lips, gums, or hard palate

P Common viral infection precipitated by febrile illness, sunlight, stress, or allergy

A Chancre: round, painless lesion with central ulceration

P Syphilis

A A plaque, wart, nodule, or ulcer on the lower lip

P Possible squamous cell carcinoma (the most common form of oral cancer); basal cell carcinoma lesions: pearly borders, crusting, and central ulcerations

A Leukoplakia: persistent, painless, white, painted-looking patches on the lips

P Premalignant lesions often occurring at sites of chronic irritation from dentures, tobacco, or excessive alcohol intake

Palpation

E 1. Don clean gloves.
2. Gently pull down the patient's lower lip using the thumb and index finger of one hand and pull up the patient's upper lip using the thumb and index finger of the other hand.
3. Note the tone of the lips as they are manipulated.
4. If lesions are present, palpate them for consistency and tenderness.

N **Lips should not be flaccid, and no lesions should be present.**

A/P See inspection of the lips for pathologies.

Tongue

E 1. Ask the patient to stick out the tongue (CN XII).
2. Observe the dorsal surface for color, hydration, texture, symmetry, fasciculations, atrophy, position in the mouth, and the presence of lesions.
3. Ask the patient to move the tongue from side to side and up and down.
4. With the patient's tongue back in the mouth, ask the patient to press it against the cheek. Use your finger pads held on the outside of the cheek to apply resistance. Note the strength of the tongue and compare bilaterally.
5. Ask the patient to touch the tip of the tongue to the roof of the mouth. You may also grasp the tip of the tongue in a gauze square held between the thumb and index finger of a gloved hand.
6. Inspect the ventral surface of the tongue, the frenulum, and Wharton's ducts for color, hydration, lesions, inflammation, and vasculature.
7. Using the gauze square, pull the tongue to the left and inspect; use the finger pads to palpate the tongue.
8. Repeat with the tongue held to the right side.

N **The tongue is in the midline of the mouth. The dorsum of the tongue is pink, moist, rough, and without lesions. The tongue is symmetric and moves freely. The strength of the tongue is symmetric and strong. The ventral surface of the tongue has prominent blood vessels and is moist and without lesions. Wharton's ducts are patent and without inflammation or lesions. The lateral aspects of the tongue are pink, smooth, and lesion free.**

A Enlarged tongue

P Myxedema, acromegaly, Down syndrome, amyloidosis; transient enlargement: glossitis, stomatitis, cellulitis of the neck, angioneurotic edema, hematoma, abscess

A Glossitis: red, smooth tongue without papillae

P Secondary to vitamin B_{12}, iron, or to niacin deficiency or chemotherapy

A Candidiasis (thrush): thick, white, curdlike coating on the tongue

P Changes in the normal oral flora resulting from chemotherapy, radiation therapy, disorders of the immune system (such as AIDS), antibiotic therapy, or excessive use of alcohol, tobacco, or cocaine

A Aphthous ulcer (canker sore): painful, small, round, white, ulcerated lesion with erythematous border

P Stress, extreme fatigue, food allergies, oral trauma

A Hairy leukoplakia: tongue hairy in appearance and yellow, black, or brown in color

P Benign condition resulting from antibiotic therapy (hairy appearance is elongated papillae)

A Lesions on the ventral surface of the tongue

P Malignancies, especially in patients who drink alcohol and smoke or use smokeless tobacco

A Indurations or ulcerations on the lateral surfaces of the tongue

Nursing Alert

Oral Cancer Risk Factors

- Male gender
- African American
- Age >40 years
- Tobacco use (snuff, chewing tobacco, pipes, cigars, cigarettes)
- Excessive alcohol use
- Sun exposure (lips)
- History of leukoplakia
- History of erythroplakia

(American Cancer Society, 2003; National Cancer Institute, 2003)

P Lingual cancers

A Engorged blood vessels in the tongue

P Hemangioma of the tongue: benign overgrowth of vascular tissue

A Tongue deviated toward one side, atrophied, and asymmetric in shape

P Unilateral paralysis of the tongue muscles that causes the tongue to deviate toward the affected side and that is secondary to hypoglossal nucleus damage

Buccal Mucosa

E **1.** Ask the patient to open the mouth as wide as possible.
2. Use a tongue depressor and a penlight to assess the inner cheeks and the openings of Stensen's ducts.
3. Observe for color, inflammation, hydration, and lesions.

N **The color of the oral mucosa on the inside of the cheek may vary according to race. African Americans have bluish mucosa; Caucasians have pink, wrinkled mucosa. Freckle-like macules may appear on the inside of the buccal mucosa. The buccal mucosa should be moist, smooth, and free of lesions.**

A Cyanotic mucosa

A/P Leukoplakia, aphthous ulcers; see *Tongue*

A Pale mucosa

P Vasoconstriction secondary to shock

A Xerostomia (excessively dry mucosa)

P Diminished salivary gland activity, hypovolemia, mouth breathing, Sjögren syndrome, or salivary gland obstruction

P Systemic hypoxemia: refer to Chapters 10 and 16

A Erythematous mucosa

P Stomatitis

A Lichen planus: flat-topped papules with thin, bluish-white, spider-web lines resembling leukoplakia

P Inflammatory and pruritic disease of the skin and mucous membranes with uncertain etiology

Gums

E 1. Instruct the patient to open the mouth.
2. Observe dentures or orthodontics for fit.
3. Remove any dentures or removable orthodontia.
4. Shine the penlight in the mouth.
5. Use the tongue depressor to move the tongue to visualize the gums.
6. Observe for redness, swelling, bleeding, retraction from the teeth, and discoloration.

N **In light-skinned individuals, the gums have a pale-red, stippled surface. Patchy, brown pigmentation may be present in dark-skinned individuals. The gum margins are well defined and without pockets between the gums and teeth, and without swelling, and bleeding.**

A Gingivitis: red, tender, swollen gingivae that bleed easily

P Poor dental hygiene, improperly fitted dentures, scurvy, stomatitis

A Periodontitis: red gingival borders with associated infection of the pockets formed between receding gums and teeth

P Chronic gingivitis

A Blue lines approximately 1 mm from the gingival margin

P Chronic exposure to lead or bismuth

A Brownish coloration of the gums

P Addison's disease

A Gingival hyperplasia: hypertrophy of gum tissue

P Pregnancy, medications such as phenytoin, in wearers of orthodontia braces, caused by dental plaque

Teeth

E 1. Instruct the patient to open the mouth.
2. Count the upper and lower teeth.
3. Observe the teeth for discoloration, loose or missing teeth, caries, malocclusion, and malformation.

N **The adult normally has 32 teeth, which should be white with smooth edges, in proper alignment, and without caries.**

A Absent teeth

P Trauma, loss, malnourishment, developmental failure

A Dental caries: white or black patches on the surface of a tooth

P Bacteria and poor oral hygiene

A Teeth worn at an angle

P Bruxism: grinding of the teeth

Palate

E 1. Instruct the patient to tilt the head back and to open the mouth as wide as possible.
2. Shine the penlight in the patient's mouth.
3. Observe both the hard and soft palates.
4. Note their shape and color and the presence of any lesions or malformations.

N **The hard and soft palates are concave and pink. The hard palate has many ridges; the soft palate is smooth. No lesions or malformations are noted.**

A Palates are red, swollen, and tender or have lesions.

P Infection

A Fibroma: fibrous, encapsulated tissue growth

P Idiopathic or neoplastic in origin; chronic trauma

A Lesion that becomes eroded on the palate

P Cancerous lesion in the epithelium of the hard palate

A Highly arched palate

P Turner's syndrome, Marfan's syndrome

A Palatine perforation: hole in the hard palate

P Syphilis, radiation therapy

Inspection of the Throat

E 1. Instruct the patient to tilt the head back and to open the mouth widely. The patient can either stick the tongue out or leave it resting on the floor of the mouth.

2. With your right hand, place the tongue blade on the middle third of the tongue.

3. With your left hand, shine a light at the back of the patient's throat.

4. Ask the patient to say "ah."

5. Observe the position, size, color, and general appearance of the tonsils and uvula.

6. Touch the tongue depressor to the posterior third of the tongue.

7. Note the movement of the palate and the presence of the gag reflex.

8. Assess the color of the oropharynx. Note the presence of swelling, exudate, and lesions.

N **When the patient says "ah," the soft palate and the uvula should rise symmetrically (CN IX and X). The uvula is midline. The throat is normally pink, vascular, and without swelling, exudate, and lesions. The gag reflex should be present but is congenitally absent in some patients (CN IX and X).**

A Uvular deviation, induration and swelling of the tonsils, gray membrane, absence of gag reflex, asymmetry of the oropharynx

P Infection; tumor; gray membrane: acute tonsillitis, infectious mononucleosis, or diphtheria.

A Red posterior pharynx, enlarged and reddened uvula, enlarged tonsils

P Bacterial or viral tonsillitis or pharyngitis

REFERENCES

American Cancer Society & Silverman, S. (2003). *Oral cancer* (5th ed.). Hamilton, Ontario: B. C. Decker.

National Cancer Institute. (2003). Risk Factors for Oral Cancer. www.cancer.gov

14

Breasts and Regional Nodes

Anatomy and Physiology

Breasts

The female breasts are a pair of mammary glands located on the anterior chest wall, each extending vertically from the second to the sixth rib and laterally from the sternal border to the axilla. Anatomically, the breast can be divided into four quadrants: the upper inner quadrant, the lower inner quadrant, the upper outer quadrant, and the lower outer quadrant (Figure 14-1). The upper outer quadrant, which extends into the axilla, is known as the tail of Spence. The breasts are supported by a bed of muscles: the pectoralis major and minor, latissimus dorsi, serratus anterior, rectus abdominus, and external oblique muscles, which extend vertically from the deep fascia (Figure 14-2). Cooper's ligaments, which extend vertically from the deep fascia and through the breast to the inner layer of the skin, provide support for the breast tissue.

In the center of each breast is the nipple, a round, hairless, pigmented protrusion of erectile tissue approximately

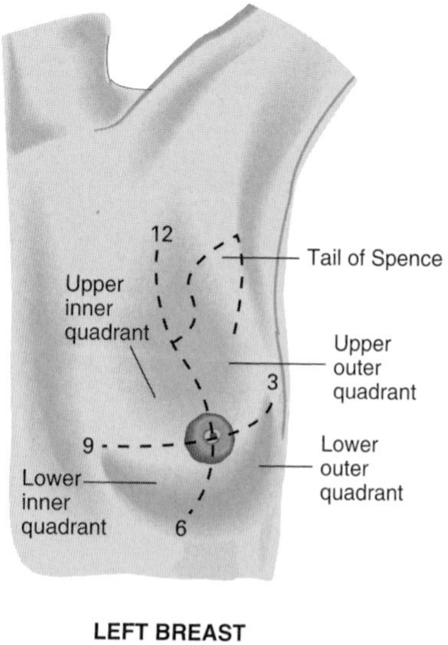

Figure 14-1 Quadrants of the Left Breast

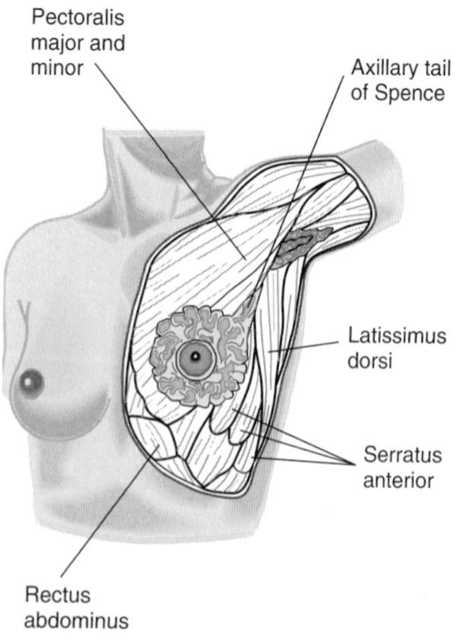

Figure 14-2 Muscles Supporting the Breast

0.5 to 1.5 cm in diameter. There are 12 to 20 minute openings on the surface of the nipple. These are openings of the lactiferous ducts through which milk and colostrum are excreted.

Surrounding the nipple is the areola, a pigmented area approximately 2.5 to 10.0 cm in diameter. Several sebaceous glands (Montgomery's tubercles) are present on the surface of the areola. These glands lubricate the nipple, helping to keep it supple during lactation. Hair follicles punctuate the border of the areola.

The breast is composed of glandular, connective (Cooper's ligaments), and adipose tissue. The glandular tissue is arranged radially in the form of 12 to 20 lobes. This disbursement resembles the structure of a bicycle wheel. Each lobe is composed of 20 to 40 lobules that contain milk-producing glands called alveoli, or acini. The lobules are clustered around several ducts; these ducts gradually form one main lactiferous (excretory) duct per lobe (Figure 14-3). Each lactiferous duct widens to form a sinus that acts as a reservoir for milk during lactation. The duct opens onto the surface of the nipple. The lobes are lodged in tissue composed of subcutaneous and retromammary adipose tissue, and this tissue composes the bulk of the breast.

The functions of the female breast are to produce milk for the nourishment and protection of neonates and infants, to provide sensual pleasure during sexual foreplay, and to provide some protection to the anterior thoracic chest wall.

The male breast is composed of a well-developed areola and small nipple with immature tissue underneath. Gynecomastia, the enlargement of male breast tissue, may occur normally in adolescent and elderly males.

Regional Nodes

Lymphatic drainage (of the yellow, alkaline drainage composed primarily of lymphocytes) of the breast occurs via a complex network of lymph vessels and nodes. The axillary nodes are composed of four groups: brachial nodes (lateral), central axillary nodes (midaxillary), pectoral nodes (anterior), and subscapular nodes (posterior), and lateral nodes (Figure 14-4). The axillary nodes are easily accessible to palpation because of their superficial location. The internal mammary nodes are very deep in the chest wall and are inaccessible to palpation.

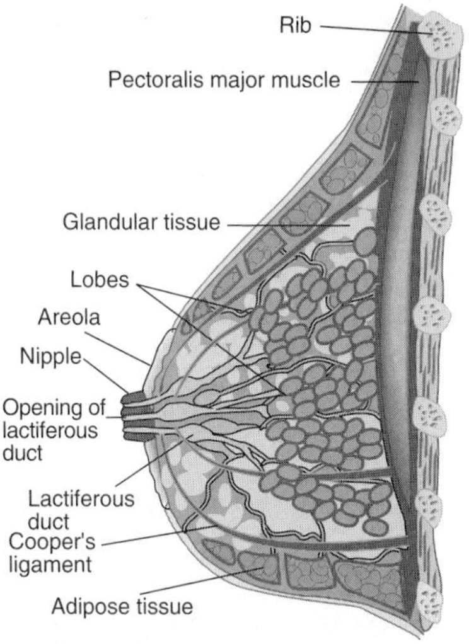

Figure 14-3 Glandular Tissue of the Right Breast

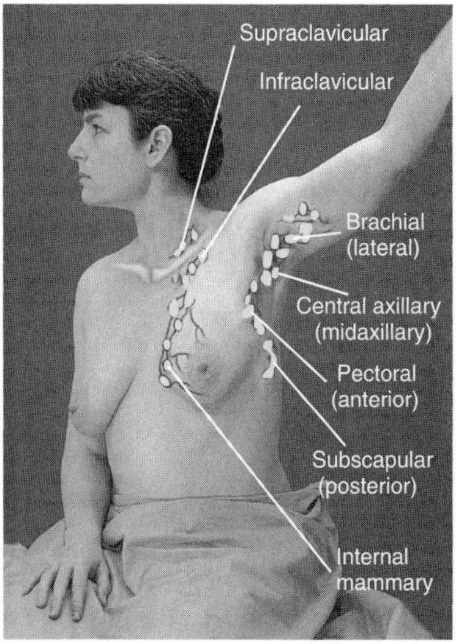

Figure 14-4 Regional Lymphatics and Drainage Patterns of the Left Breast

HEALTH HISTORY

Medical History

Benign breast disease, cysts, fibroadenomas, intraductal papillomas, mammary duct ectasia, mastitis, areas of greater density, breast cancer, masses, breast abscess, Paget's disease

Surgical History

Breast biopsy, lumpectomy, quadrantectomy, partial mastectomy, radical mastectomy, breast reduction or augmentation

Medications

Oral contraceptives, chlorpromazine, alpha-methyldopa, diuretics, digitalis, steroids, and tricyclics may precipitate nipple discharge. Hormone replacement therapy has been linked with increased relative risk of breast cancer.

Family Health History

8% to 20% of breast cancers are thought to have a familial link (*BRCA 1* or *BRCA 2* gene mutation) via a primary relative (e.g., mother, sister, or grandmother).

Equipment

- Towel
- Drape
- Centimeter ruler
- Teaching aid for breast self-examination

Assessment of the Female Breasts and Regional Nodes

Inspection of the Breasts

E **1.** Ask the patient to uncover to the waist. Position the patient so that she is seated at the edge of the examination table and facing you.
2. Instruct the patient to let her arms relax by her sides (Figure 14-5).
3. Inspect the breasts, axillae, areolar areas, and nipples for color, vascularity, thickening, edema, size, symmetry, contour, lesions, masses, and exudate.

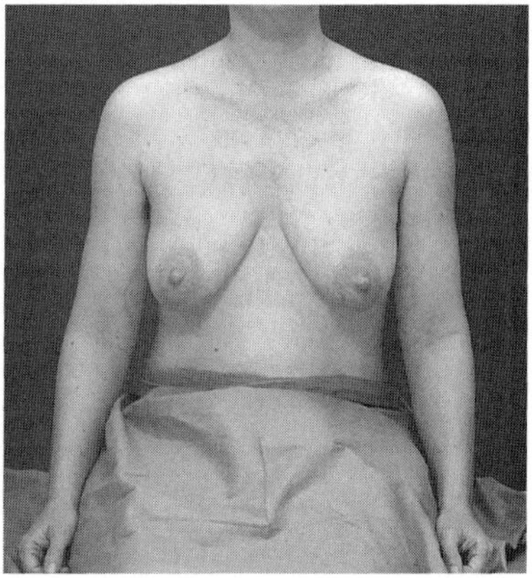

Figure 14-5 Position of Patient for Breast Inspection: Arms at Side

4. Repeat the previous inspection sequence, this time with the patient's arms raised over her head (Figure 14-6). This position will accentuate any retraction (drawing back of tissue) if present.

NURSING CHECKLIST

General Approach to Breast Assessment

1. When possible, instruct the patient neither to use creams, lotions, or powders nor to shave her underarms 24 to 48 hours before the scheduled examination. Application of toiletry products may mask or alter the nature of the surface integument of the breasts, and shaving the underarms may cause folliculitis, which may result in pain upon palpation.
2. Encourage the patient to express any anxieties and concerns about the physical examination. Acknowledge anxieties and validate concerns. Many women avoid having their breasts assessed because they fear abnormal findings. Assure the patient that she has taken a positive step in her own health care by having her breasts assessed.
3. Inform the patient that the examination should not be painful but may be uncomfortable at times. This is especially true if the patient is currently experiencing menses, ovulation, or pregnancy.
4. Be aware of the impact of culture on breast assessment and breast self-examination. In Asian cultures, for example, breast self-examination may be considered a form of masturbation, and in some Middle Eastern cultures, baring the breasts to a male is taboo, even if the male is a health care provider.
5. Instruct the patient to remove any jewelry that may interfere with the assessment.
6. Ensure that the room is warm enough to prevent chilling, and provide additional draping material as necessary.
7. Always compare right and left breasts.
8. Wear gloves if the patient has any discharge from the breast.
9. Assess whether the patient needs assistance in dressing.

5. Repeat the inspection sequence, this time with the patient pressing her hands into her hips to contract the pectoral muscles (Figure 14-7). Once again, if retraction is present, it will be more pronounced with this maneuver.

6. Have the patient lean forward to

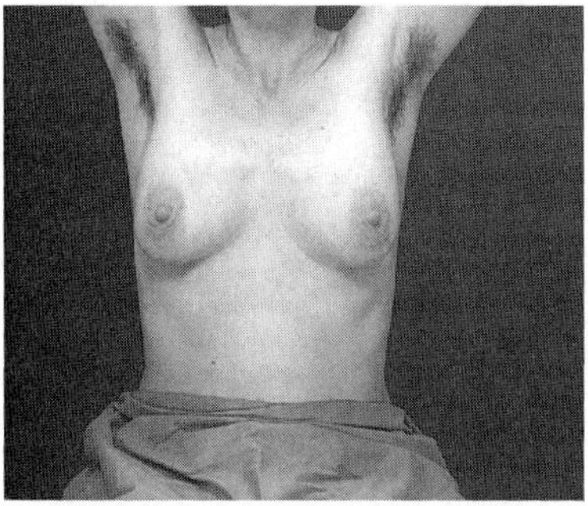

Figure 14-6 Position of Patient for Breast Inspection: Arms Overhead

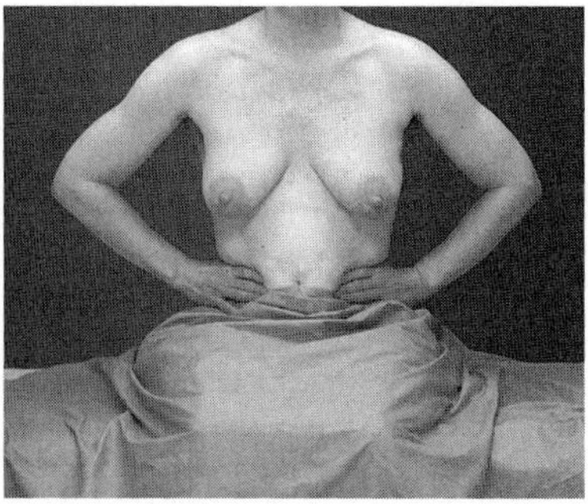

Figure 14-7 Position of Patient for Breast Inspection: Hands Pressed against Hips

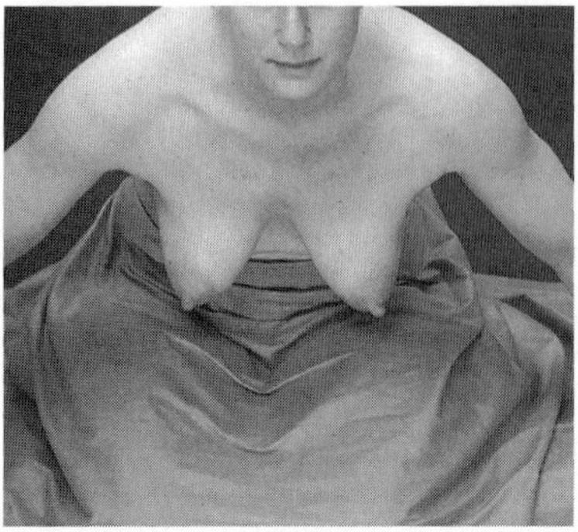

Figure 14-8 Position of Patient for Breast Inspection: Leaning Forward

allow the breasts to hang freely away from the chest wall (Figure 14-8); repeat the inspection sequence. Provide support to the patient as necessary.

Color

E Inspect the breasts, areolar areas, nipples, and axillae for coloration.

N **The breasts and axillae are normally flesh colored, and the areolar areas and nipples are normally darker in pigmentation. This pigmentation typically is enhanced during pregnancy. Moles and nevi are normal variants, and terminal hair may be present on the areolar areas.**

A Reddened areas of the breasts, nipples, or axillae

P Inflammation, an infection such as mastitis, inflammatory carcinoma

A Striae: streaks over the breasts or axillae (In light-skinned individuals, new striae are red and with age become silver to white in coloration; in dark-skinned individuals, new striae are a ruddy, dark-brown color and with age become lighter than the skin color.)

P Rapid stretching of the skin, as seen in pregnancy and obesity and which damages the elastic fibers found in the dermis

Vascularity

E Observe the entire surface of each breast for superficial vascular patterns.

N **Normal superficial vascular patterns are diffuse and symmetric.**

A Abnormal patterns of vascularity (focal or unilateral)

P Increased blood supply possibly secondary to tumor formation

Thickening or Edema

E Observe the breasts, axillae, and nipples for thickening and edema.

N **Thickening and edema are not normally found in the breasts, axillae, and nipples.**

A Enlarged skin pores that give the appearance of an orange rind (peau d'orange) and are more prevalent in the dependent, or inferior, portions of the breast

P Obstructed lymphatic drainage due to a tumor

Size and Symmetry

E Observe the breasts, axillae, areolar areas, and nipples for size and symmetry.

N **There is usually some difference in the size of the breasts and areolar areas, with the breast on the side of the dominant arm being larger. Nipple inversion, which is present from puberty, is a normal variant. Nipples should point upward and laterally or may point outward and downward. Supernumerary nipples are a variant of normal.**

A Significant differences in the size or symmetry of the breasts, axillae, areolar areas, or nipples

P Tumor formation

A Recent inversion, flattening, or depression of a nipple

P Nipple retraction, which is suggestive of an underlying cancer

A Nipples that have been inverted

since puberty and become broader or thicker

P Tumor formation

A Lack of breast tissue unilaterally

P Trauma, mastectomy, breast reduction

Contour

E 1. Assess the breasts for contour.
2. Compare the breasts with each other.

N **The breast is normally convex and without flattening, retractions, or dimpling.**

A Dimpling, retractions, flattening, or other changes in breast contour

P Suggestive of cancer, fat necrosis, and mammary duct ectasia

Lesions or Masses

E Inspect the breasts, axillae, areolar areas, and nipples for lesions and masses.

N **The breasts, axillae, areolar areas, and nipples are normally free of masses, tumors, and primary and secondary lesions.**

A Breast masses, tumors, nodules, or cysts

P See Table 14-1 for common pathologies of breast masses.

TABLE 14-1 Characteristics of Common Breast Masses

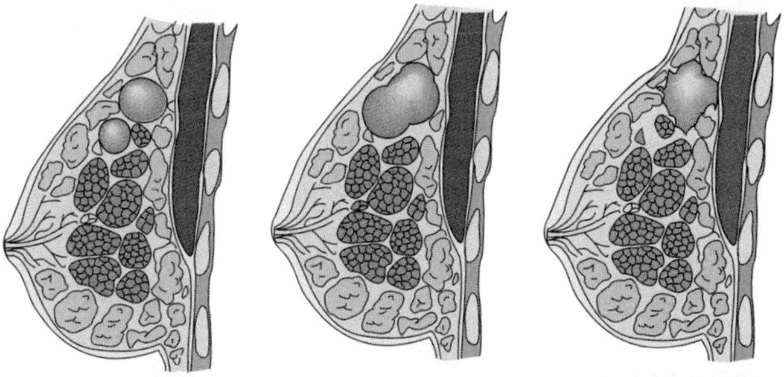

	Gross Cyst	Fibroadenoma	Carcinoma
Age	30–50; diminishes after menopause	puberty to menopause peaks between ages 20–30	most common after 50 years
Shape	round	round, lobular, or ovoid	irregular, stellate, or crab-like
Consistency	soft to firm	usually firm	firm to hard
Discreteness	well defined	well defined	not clearly defined
Number	single or grouped	most often single	usually single
Mobility	mobile	very mobile	may be mobile or fixed to skin, underlying tissue, or chest wall
Tenderness	tender	nontender	usually nontender
Erythema	no erythema	no erythema	may be present
Retraction/dimpling	not present	not present	often present

Nursing Tip

Ductal Lavage

There is now a procedure known as FirstCyte Ductal Lavage that is done in the provider's office. This procedure involves rinsing the inside of the milk ducts to collect cells. The procedure takes approximately 30 minutes. The nipple is anesthetized and a small tube is inserted into the milk ducts on the nipple. The duct is rinsed and cells are sent for evaluation to see if they are atypical. It is recommended for women who have had breast cancer in the past, have a close relative with breast cancer, have a 5-year GAIL risk of 1.7% or greater, or have a *BRCA 1* or *BRCA 2* gene mutation. The GAIL model consists of a set of calculations that evaluate the relative risk of breast cancer based on age at menarche, number of breast biopsies, age at first live birth, number of first-degree relatives with breast cancer, and a woman's age. It is named after Dr. Mitchell H. Gail, who developed the model. The risk of breast cancer can be calculated by entering data into special calculators that are available now.

A A scaly, eczema-like erosion of the nipple, or persistent dermatitis of the areola and nipple

P Suggestive of Paget's disease, a malignant, usually unilateral neoplasm

Discharge

E Observe for spontaneous discharge from the nipples or other areas of the breast.

N **In the nonpregnant, nonlactating female, there should be no discharge. During pregnancy and up through the first week after birth, there may be a yellow discharge known as colostrum. During lactation, there is a white discharge of breast milk.**

A Nipple discharge in the nonpregnant, nonlactating woman

P Possible causes: tranquilizer and/or oral contraceptive use, manual stimulation, infection, pituitary tumor, malignant or benign breast disease

Nursing Alert

Examining Nipple Discharge

If a patient is found to have abnormal nipple discharge:

1. Don gloves before proceeding with the assessment.
2. Note the following: color, consistency, amount of discharge, unilateral or bilateral involvement, spontaneous or provoked occurrence.
3. With a sterile, cotton-tipped swab, obtain a sample of the discharge so that a culture and sensitivity as well as a gram stain can be performed.
4. Consider checking the sample for occult blood.
5. Follow your institution's guidelines for sample preparation.

Palpation

Palpation is performed in a sequential manner:

1. Supraclavicular and infraclavicular lymph node areas
2. Breasts, with the patient in sitting position
   a. arms at side
   b. arms raised over head
3. Axillary lymph node regions
4. Breasts, with the patient in supine position

Supraclavicular and Infraclavicular Lymph Nodes

E **1.** The patient should remain uncovered to the waist and be seated with her arms at her sides.

2. Encourage the patient to relax the muscles of the head and neck, because relaxing these muscles pulls the clavicles down and allows a thorough exploration of the supraclavicular area.

3. Flex the patient's head to relax the sternocleidomastoid muscle.

4. Standing in front of the patient, in a bilateral and simultaneous motion, place your finger pads over the patient's clavicles, lateral to the tendinous portion of the sternocleidomastoid muscles.

5. Using a rotary motion of the palmar surfaces of the fingers, probe deeply into the scalene triangles in order to palpate the supraclavicular lymph nodes (Figure 14-9).

6. Using the same rotary motion of the palmar surfaces of the fingers, palpate the infraclavicular nodes (Figure 14-10).

N **Palpable lymph nodes less than 1 cm in diameter are usually considered normal and clinically nonsignificant, provided that there are no additional enlarged lymph nodes found in other regions such as the axilla. Palpation should not elicit pain.**

A Fixed, firm, immobile, irregular lymph nodes more than 1 cm in diameter

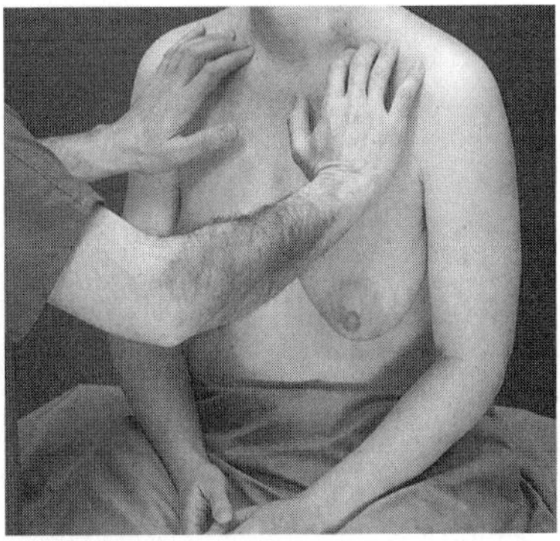

Figure 14-9 Palpation of Supraclavicular Nodes

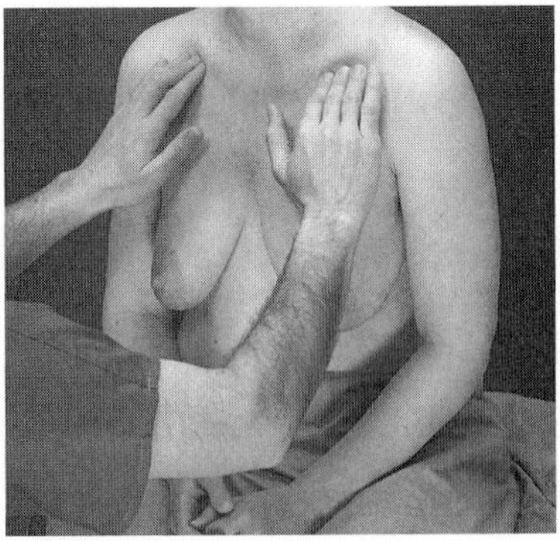

Figure 14-10 Palpation of Infraclavicular Nodes

Nursing Alert

Risk Factors for Breast Cancer

- Over 50 years of age; risk increases with age
- Personal history of breast cancer
- Mother, grandmother, or sister with breast cancer
- Menarche at an early age, menopause at an advanced age
- Obesity after menopause
- Alcohol intake of greater than three servings per day
- American or European descent
- Urban dweller
- Estrogen replacement therapy, hormone replacement therapy
- Nulliparous
- First birth after age 30
- Higher education and socioeconomic status
- Atypical hyperplasia
- Significant mammographic breast density
- *BRCA 1* or *BRCA 2* gene mutation

P Suggestive of metastasis from a variety of sources or of primary lymphoma

A Enlarged, painful, or tender nodes that are matted together

P Systemic infection or carcinoma

Breasts: Patient in Sitting Position

E 1. Place the patient in a sitting position with the arms at the sides.
2. Stand to the patient's right side and facing the patient.
3. Using the palmar surfaces of the fingers of the dominant hand, begin the palpation at the outer quadrant of the patient's right breast.
4. Use the nondominant hand to provide support to the inferior aspect of the breast.
5. If the breasts are small, you can use your dominant hand to palpate the tissue against the chest wall; if the breasts are pendulous, use a bimanual technique of palpation (Figure 14-11).
6. Palpate in a downward fashion, sweeping from the outer quadrants to the sternal border of each breast.
7. Repeat this sequence on the other breast.
8. Repeat the entire assessment, this time with the patient's arms raised over her head to enhance any potential retraction.

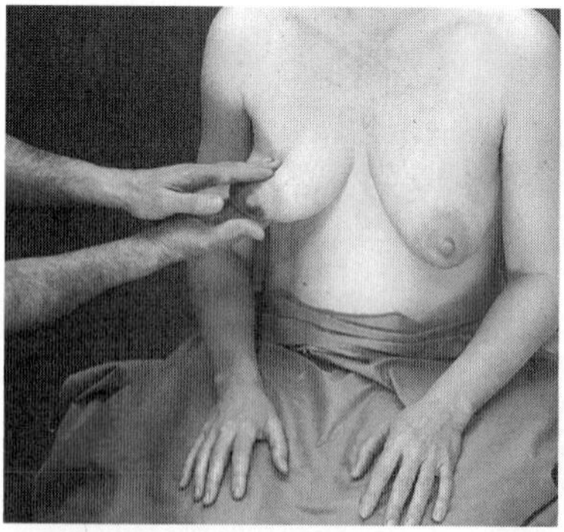

Figure 14-11 Bimanual Palpation of the Breasts while Patient Is Sitting

N **Normal consistency of the breasts varies widely and depends on age, time in menstrual cycle, and proportion of adipose tissue. The breasts may have a nodular or granular consistency that may be enhanced before the onset of menses. The inferior aspect of the breast is somewhat firmer because of a transverse inframammary ridge. Palpation should not elicit significant tenderness, although the breasts and, especially, the nipples may become full and slightly tender premenstrually. Breasts that feel fluid filled or firm throughout and with accompanying inferior suture line scars are indicative of breast augmentation.**

A Any lump, mass, thickening, or unilateral granulation that is noticeably different from the rest of the breast tissue

P See Table 14-2 for a description of breast masses and their pathologies.

A Significant breast tenderness

P Possible mammary duct ectasia: benign condition characterized by inflamed lactiferous ducts

A Erythema, swelling

P Mastitis caused by *Staphylococcus aureus*

Nursing Alert

Risk Factors for Benign Breast Disease

The following risk factors enhance a woman's potential for benign breast disease:

- Caffeine use
- Imbalance between estrogen and progesterone
- Estrogen excess
- Hyperprolactinemia
- Age 20–50 years

TABLE 14-2 Evaluation of Breast Mass Characteristics

If a mass is noted during palpation, the following information should be obtained regarding the mass. Always note if one or both breasts are involved.

LOCATION
Identify the quadrant involved or visualize the breast with the face of a clock superimposed upon it. The nipple represents the center of the clock. Note where the mass lies in relation to the nipple (e.g., 3 cm from the nipple in the 3 o'clock position).

SIZE
Determine size in centimeters in all three planes (height, width, and depth).

SHAPE
Masses may be round, ovoid, matted, or irregular.

NUMBER
Note if lesions are singular or multiple. Note if one or both breasts are involved.

CONSISTENCY
Masses may be firm, hard, soft, fluid, or cystic.

DEFINITION
Note if the mass borders are discrete or irregular.

MOBILITY
Determine if the mass is fixed or freely movable in relation to the chest wall.

TENDERNESS
Note if palpation elicits pain.

ERYTHEMA
Note any redness over involved area.

DIMPLING OR RETRACTION
Observe for dimpling or retraction as the patient raises arms overhead and presses her hands into her hips.

LYMPH ADENOPATHY
Note if the mass involves any of the regional lymph nodes, and indicate whether there is associated lymph adenopathy.

Axillary Lymph Node Region

E **1.** Stand to the patient's right side and facing the patient.

2. Tell the patient to take a deep breath and to relax the shoulders and arms. (This relaxes the areas to be palpated.)

3. Using your left hand, adduct the patient's right arm so that it is close to the chest wall. (This maneuver relaxes the muscles.)

4. Support the patient's right arm with your left hand.

5. Using the palmar surfaces of the fingers of your right hand, place your fingers into the apex of the axilla. Your fingers will be positioned behind the pectoral muscles.

6. Gently roll the tissue against the chest wall and axillary muscles as you work downward.

7. Locate and palpate the four axillary lymph node groups:

a. Brachial (lateral) at the inner aspect of the upper part of the humerus and close to the axillary vein

b. Central axillary (midaxillary) at the thoracic wall of the axilla

c. Pectoral (anterior) behind the lateral edge of the pectoralis major muscle

d. Subscapular (posterior) at the anterior edge of the latissimus dorsi muscle

8. With the patient's arm abducted (i.e., with the patient's upper arm and elbow lifted away from the body), repeat this sequence of palpation. Support the patient's abducted arm on your right shoulder (Figure 14-12).

9. Using the same technique, palpate the patient's left axilla.

N **Palpable lymph nodes less than 1 cm in diameter are usually considered normal and clinically nonsignificant, provided there are no additional enlarged lymph nodes found in other regions. Palpation should not elicit pain.**

A Fixed, firm, immobile, irregular lymph nodes more than 1 cm in diameter

P Suggestive of metastasis from a variety of sources or of primary lymphoma

A Enlarged, painful, or tender nodes that are matted together

P Systemic infection or carcinoma

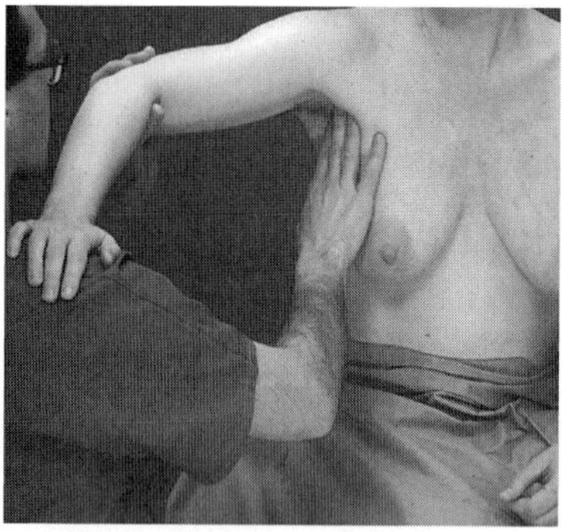

Figure 14-12 Palpation of Axillary Nodes

Breasts: Patient in Supine Position

E **1.** The patient should remain uncovered to the waist.

2. Instruct the patient to assume a supine position. This position spreads the breast tissue thinly and evenly over the chest wall. Palpation is most accurate when there is the least amount of breast tissue between the skin and the chest wall.

3. If the breasts are pendulous, place a small towel or folded sheet under the patient's right shoulder to help further flatten the breast.

4. Stand to the patient's right side. Palpation can be performed with the patient's arms at her sides or with her right arm above her head.

5. Using the palmar surfaces of the fingers, palpate the right breast by compressing the mammary tissues gently against the chest wall. Do not press too hard. You may mistake a rib for a hard breast mass. If the patient has a known breast mass, start with the unaffected breast. Palpation should be performed from the periphery to the nipple, in either concentric circles or wedge sections (Figure 14-13A).

6. Palpation must include the tail of Spence, periphery, and areola (Figure 14-13B).

7. Don gloves and compress the nipple to express any discharge (Figure 14-13C). If discharge is noted, palpate the breast along the wedge radii to distinguish from which lobe the discharge is originating.

8. Repeat the procedure on the left breast.

N **See previous section on normal breast tissue findings upon palpation. The nipple should be elastic and should readily return to its previous shape. No discharge should be expressed in the nonpregnant, nonlactating patient.**

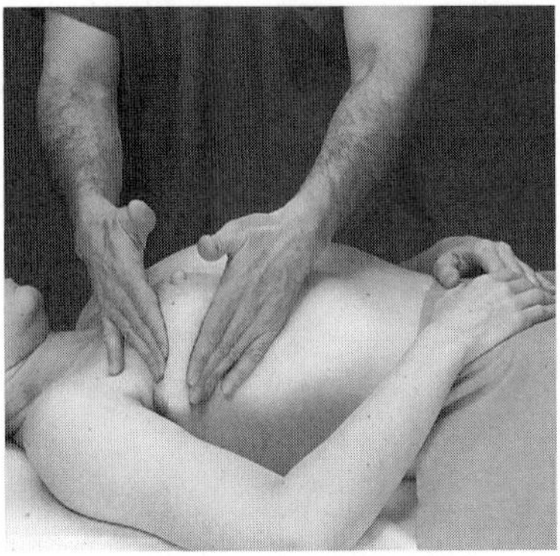

A. Palpation of the Glandular Area

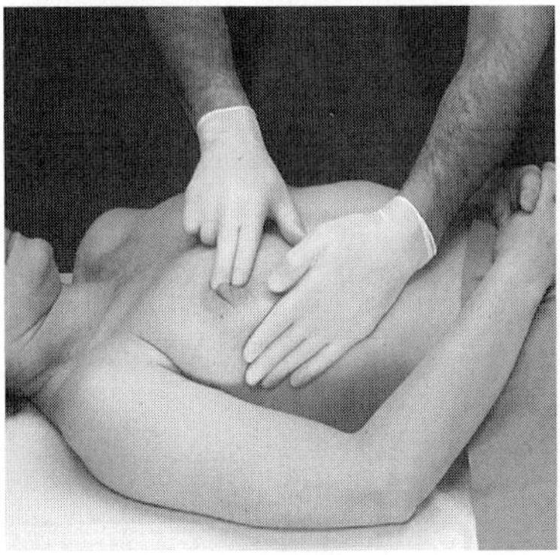

B. Palpation of the Areola

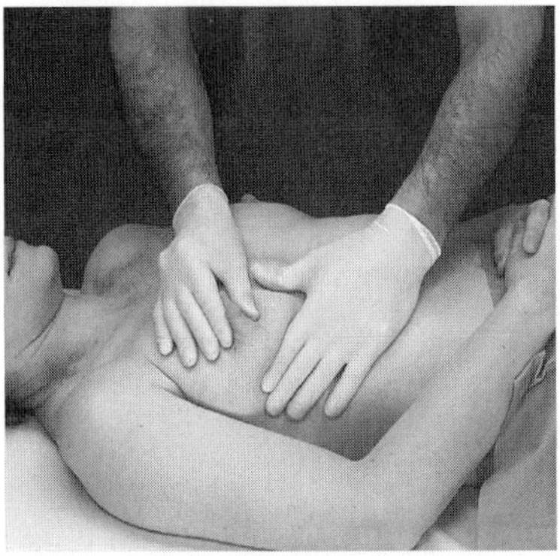

C. Compression of the Nipple

Figure 14-13 Palpation of the Breasts while Patient Is Supine

Nursing Tip

The Mastectomy Patient

There are four types of mastectomy (excision of the breast) procedure. In a simple mastectomy, only the breast is removed. In a modified radical procedure, the breast and lymph nodes from the axilla are removed. In a radical mastectomy, the breast, lymph nodes from the axilla, and pectoral muscles are removed. In a subcutaneous mastectomy, the skin and nipple are left intact, but the underlying breast tissue and lymph nodes are removed. The patient who has undergone a simple or modified radical mastectomy has the breast amputated from the chest wall.

Assessment of the mastectomy patient will be guided by the type of mastectomy and the presence or absence of reconstructive surgery. Follow the standard assessment procedures and modify your technique to suit the amount of breast tissue and the presence, if any, of a nipple. Always begin the assessment on the unaffected breast. Mastectomy patients should continue to perform monthly breast self-examinations to determine whether masses have returned to the excised area. Annual clinical evaluations and mammography are also recommended.

Refer to Table 14-1 for a description of breast masses and to Table 14-2 for a list of breast mass characteristics used to evaluate abnormal findings.

A Nipple thickening or lack of nipple elasticity

P Tumor formation

Nursing Tip

Breast Self-Examination (BSE)

Teaching BSE can be quick and simple.

1. Breast self-examination should be performed once a month, 8 days after menses or on any given fixed date. Advise the patient to avoid the time when her breasts might be tender because of menstruation or ovulation. Encourage her to put the BSE on her calendar and to include her significant other in the process.
2. *B (bed):* Show the patient how to use the palmar surfaces of her fingers to palpate her breast while lying supine in bed. She should start by placing her right arm over her head and palpating her right breast with her left hand, moving in concentric circles from the periphery inward and including the periphery, tail of Spence, and areola (Figure 14-14A). Finally, instruct her to squeeze the nipple to check for discharge. Using the reverse procedure, she should examine the other breast.
3. *S (standing):* Instruct the patient to repeat the above palpation method while standing (Figures 14-14B and 14-14C).
4. *E (examination in front of a mirror):* The patient should stand in front of a mirror, first with her arms at her sides, then with her arms raised over her head, and finally with her hands pressed into her hips (Figures 14-14D, 14-14E, and 14-14F). She should examine her breasts for symmetry, retraction, dimpling, inverted nipples, and nipple deviation.

See Table 14-3 for recommended breast cancer screening for asymptomatic women.

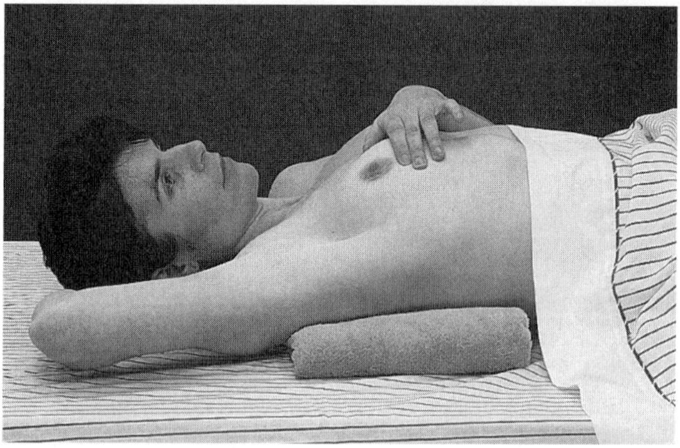

A. In Bed

Figure 14-14 Breast Self-Examination *continues*

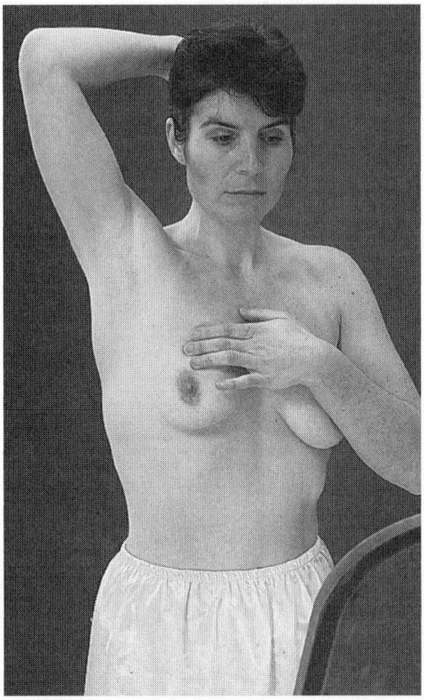

B. Standing

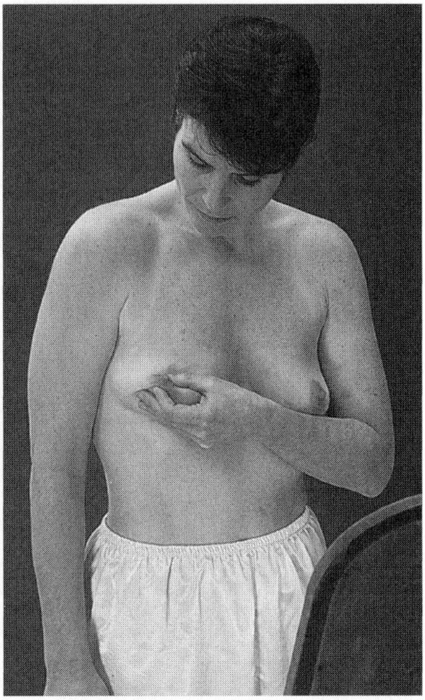

C. Compression of the Nipple

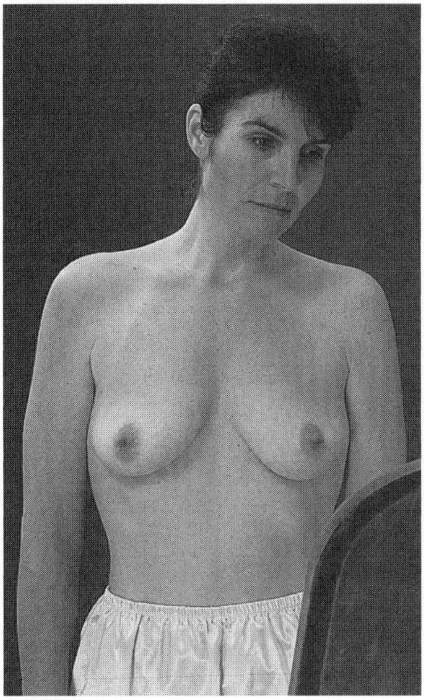

D. Before a Mirror: Arms at Side

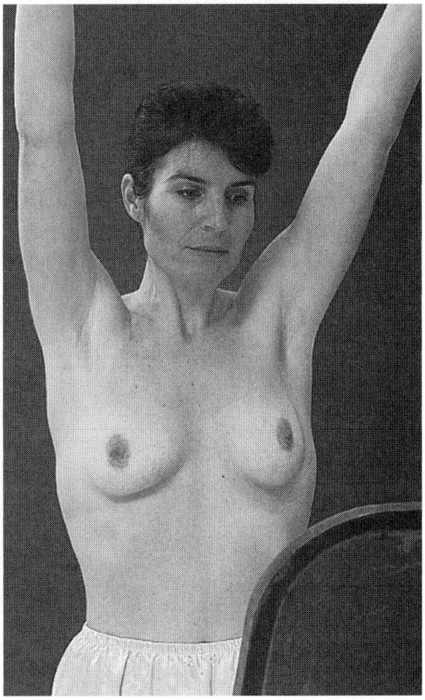

E. Before a Mirror: Arms Overhead

Figure 14-14 Breast Self-Examination *continues*

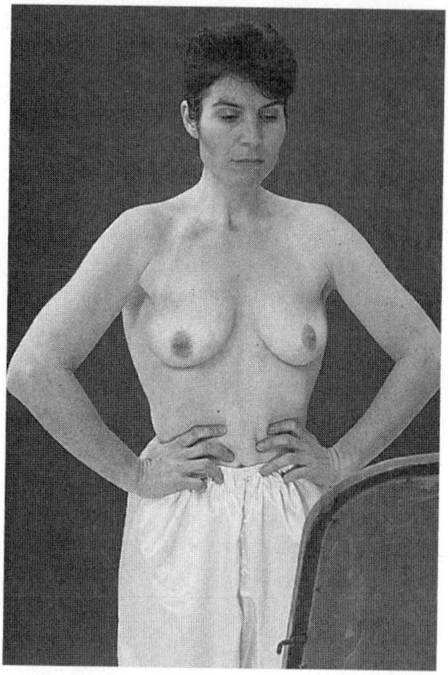

F. Before a Mirror: Hands Pressed into Hips

Figure 14-14 Breast Self-Examination *continued*

TABLE 14-3

Recommended Breast Cancer Screening for Asymptomatic Women

AGE	RECOMMENDATION
20–39	Monthly breast self-exam, clinical breast exam every 3 years
40 and over	Monthly breast self-exam, annual clinical breast exam, baseline mammography at 40 followed by annual mammography

Note. *From* Cancer Facts and Figures *[Online], by the American Cancer Society, 2005. Retrieved 4/1/05 from www.cancer.org.*

A Milky-white discharge in a nonpregnant, nonlactating patient
P Possible nonpuerperal galactorrhea (drug induced or hormonally induced by lesions of the anterior pituitary)
A Nonmilky discharge from the nipple
P Benign or malignant breast disease such as intraductal papilloma
A Bleeding from nipple
P Intraductal papilloma

Inspection and Palpation of the Male Breasts

Modify the technique used for a smaller breast with less tissue bulk. Males should perform breast self-examinations every month and should have clinical examinations of the breast every 1 to 3 years because 1% of all breast cancer is found in men.

REFERENCE

American Cancer Society.

15

Thorax and Lungs

Anatomy

The respiratory system extends from the nose to the alveoli (Figure 15-1). The normal air pathway is nose, pharynx, larynx, trachea, mainstem bronchus, right and left main bronchi, lobar/secondary bronchi, tertiary/segmental bronchi, terminal bronchioles, respiratory bronchioles, alveolar ducts, alveolar sacs, and alveoli.

The respiratory system is divided into the upper and lower tracts. The nose, pharynx, larynx, and upper trachea constitute the upper respiratory tract. These are discussed in Chapter 13. The lower respiratory tract is composed of the

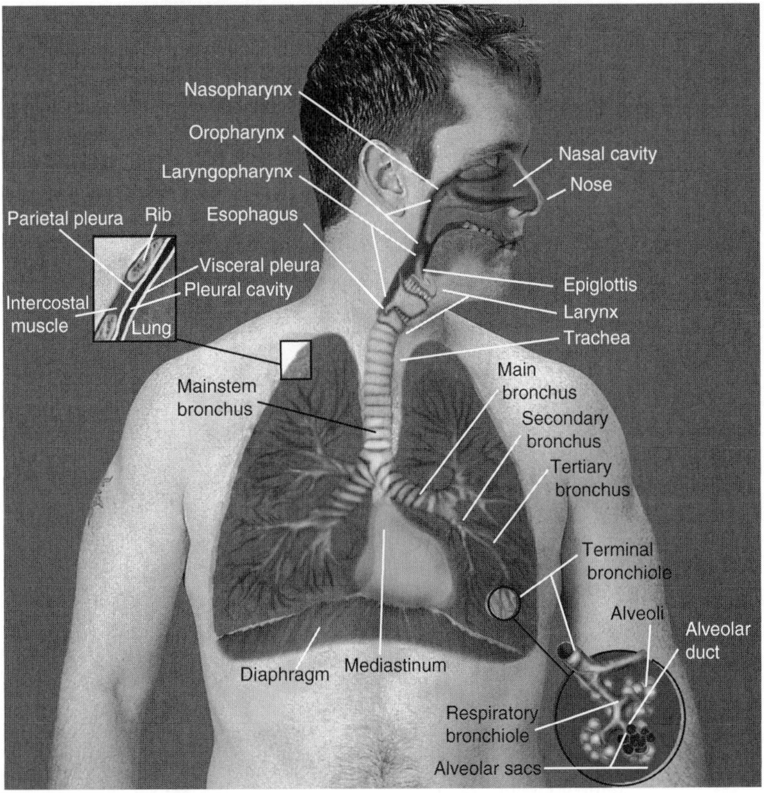

Figure 15-1 The Respiratory Tract

lower trachea to the lungs. This chapter deals only with those components of the respiratory system that are located in the thorax.

Thorax

The thorax is a cone-shaped structure (narrower ar the top and wider at the bottom) that consists of bones, cartilage, and muscles. On the anterior thorax, these bones are the 12 pairs of ribs and the sternum. Posteriorly, there are the 12 thoracic vertebrae and the spinal column.

Sternum

The sternum, or breastbone, is a flat, narrow bone approximately 15 cm in length. It is located at the median line of the anterior chest wall and is divided into three sections: the manubrium, the body, and the xiphoid process.

Ribs

The first seven pairs of ribs are articulated to the sternum via the costal cartilages and are called the vertebrosternal, or true, ribs. The false ribs, or rib pairs 8–10, articulate with the costal cartilages just above them. The remaining two pairs of ribs (ribs 11 and 12) are termed floating ribs and do not articulate at their anterior ends. All ribs articulate posteriorly to the vertebral column. When a rib is palpated, the costal cartilage cannot be distinguished from the rib itself (Figure 15-2).

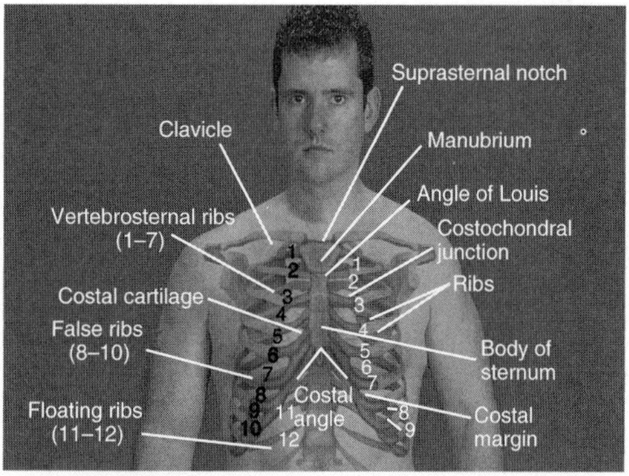

A. Anterior View

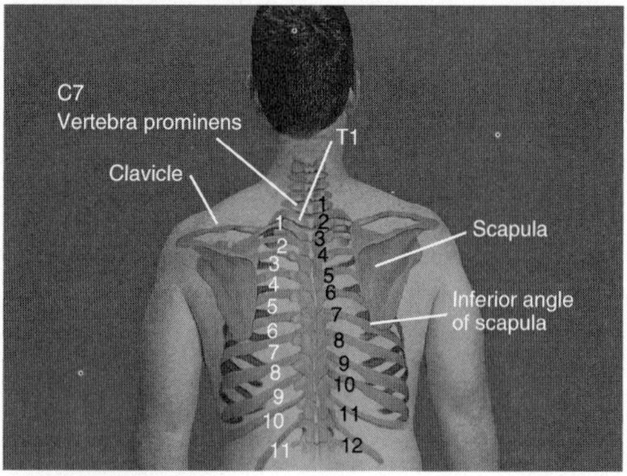

B. Posterior View

Figure 15-2 Thorax: Rib number is shown on the patient's right; intercostal space number is shown on the patient's left.

Intercostal Spaces

Each area between the ribs is called an intercostal space (ICS). There are 11 ICSs. Each ICS is named for the rib directly above it.

Lungs

The lungs are cone-shaped organs that fill the lateral chamber of the thoracic cavity. The right lung is broader than the left lung because of the position of the heart. The right lung consists of three lobes (upper, middle, and lower), whereas the left lung consists of two lobes (upper and lower) (Figure 15-3A, B).

The lobes of the right and left lungs are divided by grooves called fissures. It is important to know the location of the fissures when describing clinical findings. Figures 15-3C and 15-3D illustrate the right oblique (or diagonal) fissure, the right horizontal fissure, and the left oblique (or diagonal) fissure.

When one is assessing the thorax, it is helpful to envision it as a rectangular box, with the four sides being the anterior,

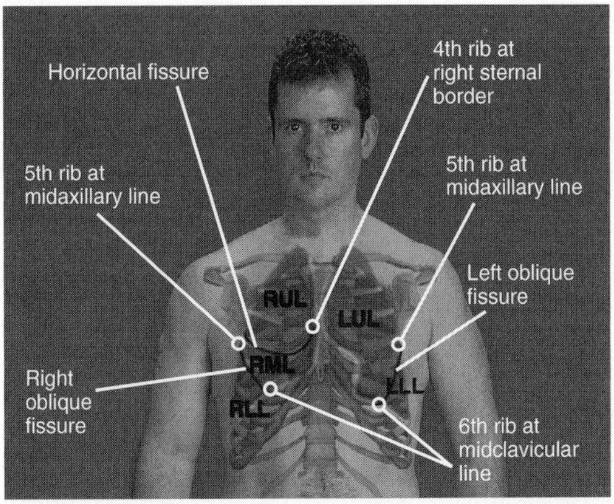

A. Anterior View

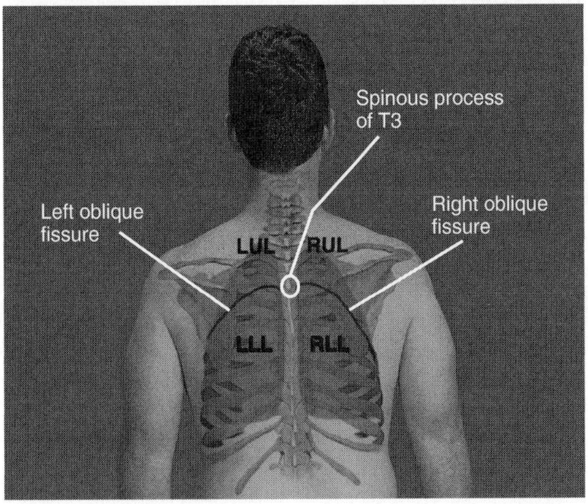

B. Posterior View

Figure 15-3 Lung Fissures

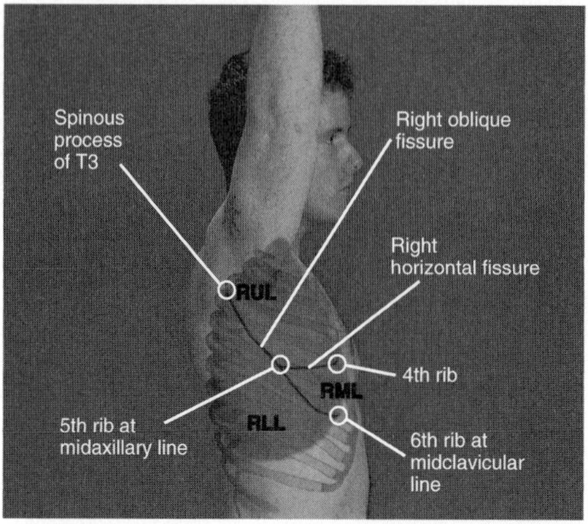

C. Right Lateral View

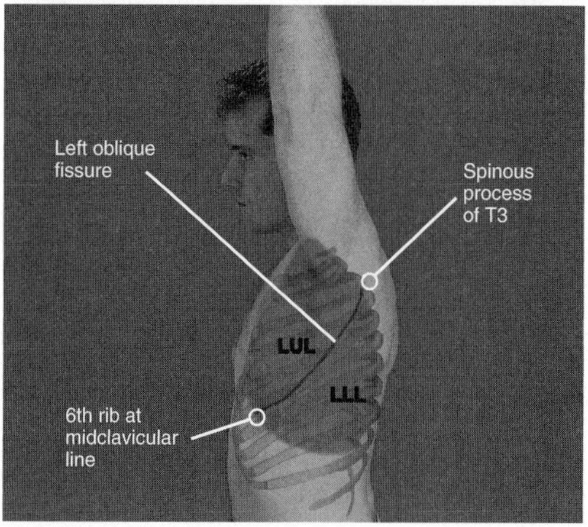

D. Left Lateral View

Figure 15-3 Lung Fissures *continued*

posterior, right lateral, and left lateral thoraces. Figure 15-4 illustrates the imaginary thoracic lines on each of the four sides. These landmarks are helpful when describing clinical findings.

Pleura

Each lung is encased in a serous sac, or pleura. The parietal pleura lines the chest wall and the superior surface of the diaphragm. The visceral pleura lines the external surface of the lung.

Mediastinum

The mediastinum, or interpleural space, is the area between the right and left lungs. It extends from the sternum to the spinal column and contains the heart, great vessels, trachea, esophagus, and lymph vessels.

Bronchi

The trachea bifurcates into the left and right mainstem bronchi at the level of the

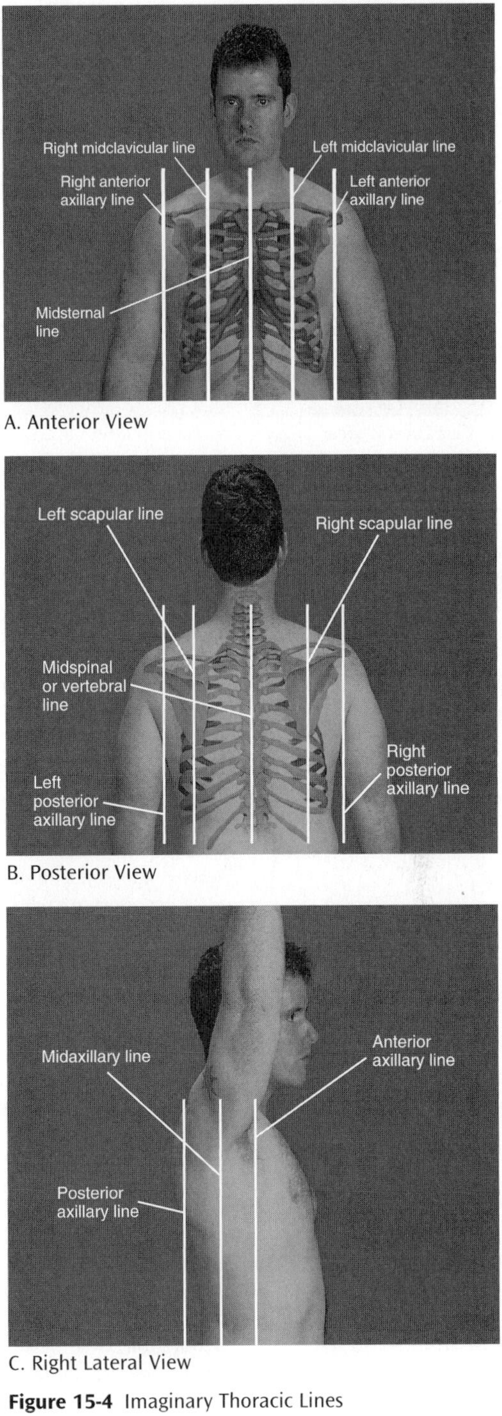

Figure 15-4 Imaginary Thoracic Lines

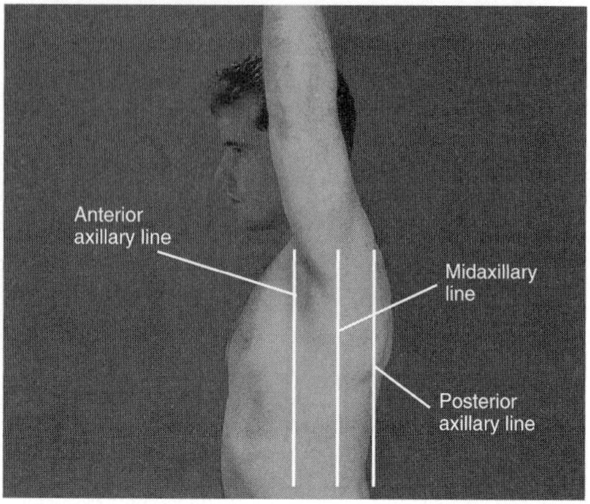

D. Left Lateral View

Figure 15-4 Imaginary Thoracic Lines *continued*

fourth or fifth vertebral process posteriorly and the sternal angle anteriorly. The mainstem bronchi further divide into lobar, or secondary, bronchi. The bronchi transport gases as well as trap foreign particles in their mucus. Cilia aid in sweeping the foreign particles upward in the respiratory tract for possible elimination. Culmination of the tracheobronchial tree is in the alveoli.

Alveoli

The alveoli are the smallest functional units of the respiratory system. It is here that gas exchange occurs.

Diaphragm

The diaphragm, which is innervated by the phrenic nerve, is a dome-shaped muscle that forms the inferior border of the thorax. The diaphragm is the principal muscle of respiration. Contraction of the diaphragm leads to an increase in volume in the thoracic cavity.

External Intercostal Muscles

The external intercostal muscles are located in the ICS. During inspiration, the external intercostal muscles elevate the ribs, thus increasing the size of the thoracic cavity. The internal intercostal muscles draw adjacent ribs together, thereby decreasing the size of the thoracic cavity in expiration.

Accessory Muscles

Accessory respiratory muscles are used to accommodate increased oxygen demand. Exercise and some diseases lead to the use of accessory muscles. The accessory muscles are the scalene, sternocleidomastoid, trapezius, and abdominal rectus.

Physiology

The primary functions of the respiratory system are to deliver oxygen to the lungs and to remove carbon dioxide from the lungs. The breathing process is composed of inspiratory and expiratory phases. During inspiration, atmospheric air is pulled into the respiratory tract until intraalveolar pressure equals atmospheric pressure. Lung size increases as air is taken in.

Expiration is a passive process and occurs more rapidly than inspiration. In expiration, the intrapulmonic volume decreases and the intrapulmonic pressure increases above the atmospheric pressure. The lungs possess elastic recoil capabilities that allow air to be expelled until intrapulmonic pressure equals atmospheric pressure.

External Respiration

External respiration is the process by which gases are exchanged between the lungs and the pulmonary vasculature. Oxygen diffuses from the alveoli into the blood, and carbon dioxide diffuses from the blood to the alveoli. Diffusion is a passive process in which gases move across a membrane from an area of higher concentration to an area of lower concentration. In the lungs, the membrane is the alveolar-capillary network.

Internal Respiration

Internal respiration is the process by which gases are exchanged between the pulmonary vasculature and the body's tissues. Oxygen from the lungs diffuses from the blood into body tissue. Carbon dioxide diffuses from the tissue into the blood. This blood is then carried back to the right side of the heart for reoxygenation.

Control of Breathing

Control of breathing is influenced by neural and chemical factors. The pons and medulla are the central nervous system structures primarily responsible for involuntary respiration. The stimulus for breathing is an increased carbon dioxide level, a decreased oxygen level, or an increased blood pH level.

HEALTH HISTORY

Medical History

Asthma, bronchitis, croup, cystic fibrosis, emphysema, pneumonia, pneumothorax, pulmonary edema, COPD, lung cancer, TB, plural effusion, frequent coryza, epiglottitis, pleurisy, pulmonary embolus

Surgical History

Lobectomy, pneumonectomy, tracheostomy, chest tube, intubation, wedge resection, bronchoscopy

Social

Tobacco use: Cigarette smoking is the primary risk factor for chronic bronchitis, emphysema, and lung cancer, among other disorders.

Work environment: Repeated exposure to materials in the workplace can create respiratory complications ranging from minor problems to life-threatening events. These diseases are listed along with the industries and agents related to them.

- Silicosis: glass making, tunneling, stone cutting, mineral mining, insulation work, quarrying, cement work, ceramics, foundry work, semiconductor manufacturing
- Asbestosis: mining, shipbuilding, construction
- Coal worker's pneumoconiosis: coal mining
- Pneumoconioses: tin and aluminum production, welding, insecticide manufacturing, rubber industry, fertilizer industry, ceramics, cosmetics industry
- Occupational asthma: electroplating, grain working, woodworking, photography, printing, baking, painting

continues

continued

- Chronic bronchitis: coal mining, welding, firefighting
- Byssinosis: cotton mill dust, flax
- Extrinsic allergic alveolitis (hypersensitivity pneumonia): animal hair, contamination of air conditioning or heating systems, moldy hay, moldy grains, moldy dust, sugar cane
- Toxic gases and fumes: welding, cigarette smoke, auto exhaust, chemical industries, firefighting, hair spray
- Pulmonary neoplasms: radon gas, mustard gas, printing ink, asbestos
- Pneumonitis: furniture polish: gasoline, or kerosene ingestion; mineral oil, olive oil, or milk aspiration

Home environment: air pollution, cigarette smoke, wood-burning stoves, gas stoves or heaters, kerosene heaters, radon gas, pet hair or dander

Hobbies and leisure activities: Birds (bird breeder's lung), mushroom grower's lungs, scuba diving (lung rupture, oxygen toxicity, decompression sickness)

Equipment

- Stethoscope
- Centimeter ruler or tape measure
- Washable marker
- Watch with second hand

NURSING CHECKLIST

General Approach to Thorax and Lung Assessment

1. Ensure that the examination room is well lit, quiet, and at a warm, comfortable temperature to prevent patient chilling and shivering.
2. Instruct the patient to remove all street clothes from the waist up and to don an examination gown.
3. Place the patient in an upright sitting position on the examination table or, for the patient who cannot tolerate the sitting position, rotate the supine patient from side to side to gain access to the thorax.
4. Expose the entire area being assessed. For women, provide a drape to cover the breasts (if desired) when the posterior thorax is being assessed.
5. When palpating, percussing, or auscultating the anterior thorax of female or obese patients, ask them to displace the breast tissue. Assessing directly over breast tissue does not yield accurate findings with regard to underlying structures.
6. Visualize the underlying respiratory structures in order to accurately describe the location of any pathology.
7. Always compare the right and left sides of the anterior thorax and the posterior thorax with one another, as well as the right lateral thorax and the left lateral thorax.
8. Use a systematic approach every time the assessment is performed. Proceed from the lung apices to the bases, right to left to lateral.

Assessment of the Thorax and Lungs

Inspection

Shape of Thorax

E 1. Stand in front of the patient.

2. Estimate visually the transverse diameter of the thorax.

3. Move to either side of the patient.

4. Estimate visually the anteroposterior (AP) diameter of the thorax.

5. Compare the estimates of these two visualizations.

N **In the normal adult, the ratio of the AP diameter to the transverse diameter is approximately 1:2 to 5:7. In other words, the normal adult is wider from side to side than from front to back. The normal thorax is slightly elliptical. A barrel chest is normal in infants and sometimes in the older adult. Figure 15-5 illustrates the normal and abnormal configurations of the thorax.**

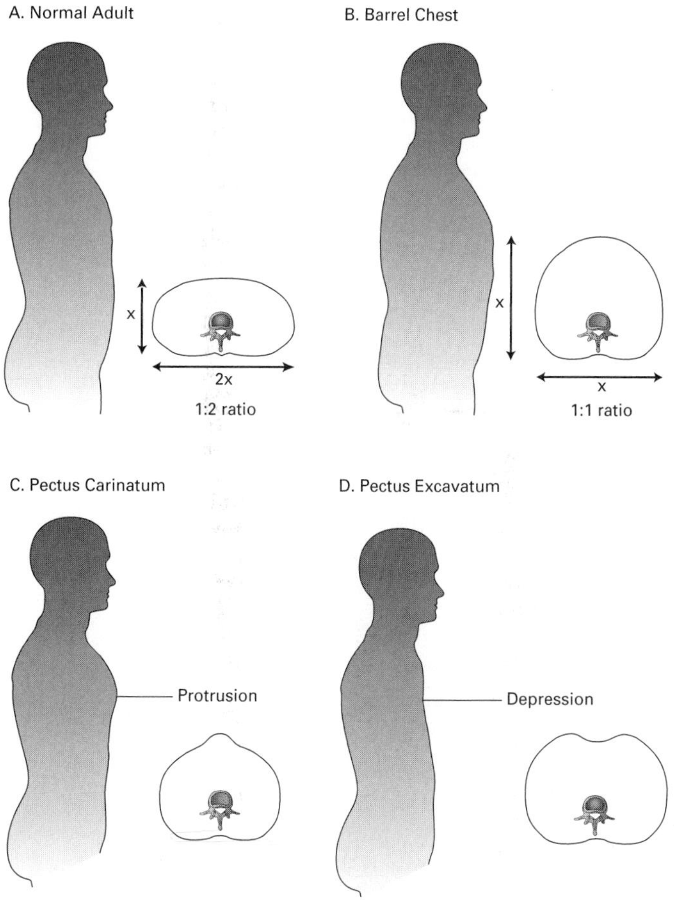

Figure 15-5 Chest Configurations

A Barrel chest: ratio of the AP diameter to the transverse diameter approximately 1:1; circular or barrel-shaped chest

P Chronic obstructive pulmonary disease (COPD): barrel chest results from air trapping in the alveoli and subsequent lung hyperinflation.

A Pectus carinatum, or pigeon chest: marked protrusion of the sternum

P Congenital anomaly (severe pectus carinatum may cause respiratory difficulty); rickets: vitamin D deficiency causing demineralization and weakness in bones so that the intercostal muscles pull the ribs and sternum forward

A Pectus excavatum, or funnel chest: depression in the lower body of the sternum (possibly leading to myocardial and respiratory disturbances and decreased AP diameter of chest)

P Congenital anomaly

A Kyphosis, or humpback: excessive concavity of the thoracic vertebrae (and associated respiratory compromise, if severe)

P Idiopathic, osteoporosis

A Scoliosis: lateral curvature of the thorax or lumbar vertebrae (and, possibly, associated hindered respiratory function, if severe): refer to Chapter 18

P Idiopathic, neuromuscular diseases, connective tissue diseases, and osteoporosis

> **Nursing Alert**
>
> **Risk Factors for Lung Cancer**
>
> - Smoking tobacco
> - Secondhand tobacco exposure
> - Smokers with COPD
> - Hereditary predisposition for some smokers
> - Occupational or environmental exposure to known carcinogens (e.g., asbestos, radon, heavy metals)

Symmetry of Chest Wall

E **1.** Inspect the right and left anterior thoraces.
2. Note shoulder height. Observe any differences between the two sides of the chest wall, such as the presence of masses.
3. Move behind the patient.
4. Inspect the right and left posterior thoraces comparing right and left sides.
5. Note the position of the scapula.

N **The shoulders should be at the same height. Likewise, the scapulae should be the same height bilaterally. There should be no masses.**

A One shoulder or scapula higher than the other

P Scoliosis

A Visible mass in chest wall

P Mediastinal tumors or cysts

Presence of Superficial Veins

E Inspect the anterior thorax for the presence of dilated superficial veins.

N **In the normal adult, dilated superficial veins are not seen.**

A Dilated superficial veins on the anterior chest wall

P Superior vena cava obstruction

Costal Angle

E **1.** In a patient whose thoracic skeleton is easily viewed, visually locate the costal margins (medial borders created by the articulation of the false ribs and floating ribs).
2. Estimate the angle formed by the costal margins during exhalation, or rest. This is the costal angle.
3. In a heavy or obese patient, place your fingertips on the lower anterior borders of the thoracic skeleton.
4. Gently move your fingertips medially to the xiphoid process.
5. As your hands approach the midline, feel the ribs where they meet at the apex of the costal margins. Visualize the line that is created by your fingers as you move them up the floating ribs toward the sternum.

This is the costal angle. Approximate this angle.

N **The costal angle is less than 90° during exhalation. The costal angle widens slightly during inhalation because the thorax expands.**

A Costal angle greater than 90°

P Hyperinflation of the lungs (emphysema) or dilation of bronchi (bronchiectasis)

Angle of the Ribs

E **1.** In a patient whose thoracic skeleton is easily viewed, visually locate the midsternal area.
2. Estimate the angle at which the ribs articulate with the sternum.
3. In a heavy or obese patient, place your fingertips on the midsternal area.
4. Move your fingertips along a rib laterally to the anterior axillary line. Visualize the line that is created by your hand as it traces the rib. Approximate this angle.

N **The ribs articulate at a 45° angle with the sternum.**

A Angle greater than 45°

P Hyperinflation of the lungs or dilation of the bronchi caused by emphysema, bronchiectasis, or cystic fibrosis

Intercostal Spaces

E **1.** Inspect the ICS throughout the respiratory cycle.
2. Note any bulging or retractions of the ICS.

N **There should be neither bulging nor retractions of the ICS.**

A Bulging and retractions of the ICS (bulging typically on expiration, retractions typically on inspiration)

P Bulging: emphysema, asthma, enlarged heart, aortic aneurysm, massive pleural effusion, tension pneumothorax, tumor

P Retractions: emphysema, asthma, tracheal or laryngeal obstruction, foreign body or tumor that compresses the respiratory tract; tension pneumothorax

Muscles of Respiration

E **1.** Observe the patient's breathing for several respiratory cycles, paying close attention to the anterior thorax and the neck.
2. Note all of the muscles that are being used by the patient.

N **No accessory muscles are used in normal breathing.**

A Use of the accessory muscles

P Hypoxemia or hypermetabolism as caused by hypermetabolic states such as exercise, fever, or infection or by hypoxic states such as COPD, pneumonia, pneumothorax, pulmonary edema, or pulmonary embolus

Respirations

Rate

E **1.** Observe the patient's breathing without stating that you are doing so.
2. Count the number of respiratory cycles in 1 minute. A respiratory cycle consists of one inhaled breath and one exhaled breath.

N **In the resting adult, the normal respiratory rate is 12 to 20 breaths per minute. This type of breathing is termed eupnea, or normal breathing.**

A Tachypnea: respiratory rate greater than 20 breaths per minute

P Hypermetabolic and hypoxic states (during which the body tries to supply additional oxygen to meet the body's demands): pneumonia, bronchitis, asthma, pneumothorax; stress (resulting in the release of catecholamines, which elevate the respiratory rate to supply sufficient oxygen)

A Bradypnea: respiratory rate less than 12 breaths per minute

P Injury to the brain, drug overdose (barbiturates, alcohol, opiates), lowered metabolic state of the body during non-REM sleep

A Apnea: lack of spontaneous respirations for 10 or more seconds

P Traumatic brain injury: herniation of the brain stem

P Central or obstructive sleep apnea

Nursing Alert

Respiratory Rate Emergencies

Extreme tachypnea (greater than 30 breaths per minute in an adult), bradypnea, and apnea are emergency conditions. Immediate intervention is necessary to prevent complications.

Pattern (Figure 15-6)

E While counting the respiratory rate, note the breathing rhythm, or pattern, for regularity or irregularity.

N **Normal respirations are regular and even in rhythm.**

A Cheyne-Stokes respirations: crescendo and decrescendo patterns interspersed between periods of apnea lasting 15 to 30 seconds (a normal finding in elderly and young children)

P Central-cerebral or high brain-stem lesions; sleep

A Biot's respirations, or ataxic breathing: irregularly irregular respiratory pattern (i.e., lack of identifiable pattern) without crescendo and decrescendo patterns and with deep and shallow breaths occurring at random intervals and intertwined with short

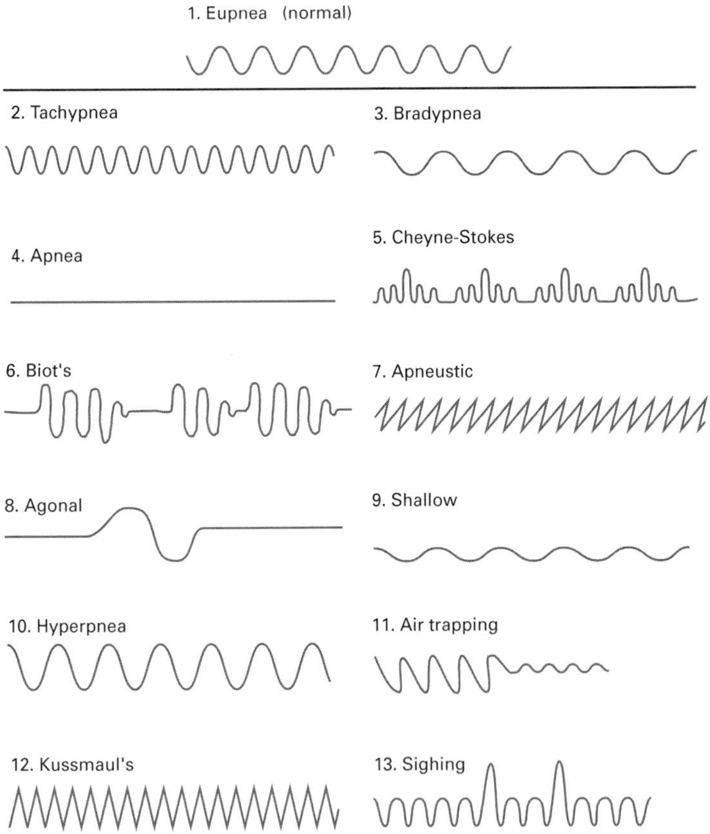

Figure 15-6 Respiratory Patterns

and long, sometimes frequent periods of apnea

P Damage to the medulla

A Apneustic respirations: prolonged gasping on inspiration followed by a very short, inefficient expiration (pauses between respiratory cycles can last 30 to 60 seconds)

P Injury to the upper portion of the pons

A Agonal respirations: irregularly irregular respirations of varying depth and pattern

P Hypoxia, compression of the respiratory center

Depth

E Observe the relative depth with which the patient draws a breath on inspiration.

N **The normal depth of inspiration is nonexaggerated and effortless.**

A Hypoventilation, or shallow respirations; minimal movement of chest wall during inspiration and expiration (small tidal volume inspired)

P Obesity (due to the sheer weight of the chest wall), pain or recent abdominal or thoracic incision (due to discomfort of moving the rib cage, the integument, and the respiratory muscles with each breath), pulmonary embolus, pneumonia, pneumothorax

A Hyperpnea: breath greater in volume than the resting tidal volume (normal respiratory rate and pattern)

P Warm-up and cool-down periods of exercise, highly emotional states, high altitudes (decreased partial pressure of oxygen)

A Air trapping: rapid, shallow respirations with forced expirations

P COPD, acute asthmatic attacks

A Kussmaul's respirations: regular respirations characterized by extreme increased depth and rate and active inspiratory and expiratory processes

P Diabetic ketoacidosis, metabolic acidosis

A Sighing: normal respirations interrupted by a deep respiration followed by a deep expiration and accompanied by an audible sigh (pathological if frequent)

P Central nervous system lesions

Symmetry

E Observe the symmetry with which the chest rises and falls during the respiratory cycle.

N **The healthy adult's thorax symmetrically rises and falls in unison with the respiratory cycle. There is no paradoxical movement.**

A Unilateral expansion of either side of the thorax

P Conditions in which the lung is absent or collapsed (pneumonectomy, pneumothorax), pulmonary fibrosis (thickening and decreased elasticity of the lung), acute pleurisy with massive atelectasis

A Paradoxical, or seemingly contradictory, chest wall movement

P Flail chest, broken ribs from trauma to the chest wall

Audibility

E Listen for the audibility of the respirations.

N **A patient's respirations can normally be heard by the unaided ear within several centimeters of the patient's nose or mouth.**

A Breathing audible from a distance of several feet

P Any condition in which air hunger exists (exercise, COPD, pneumonia, pneumothorax)

Patient Position

E **1.** Ask the patient to sit upright for the respiratory assessment.

2. View the patient either before or after the assessment and note the assumed position for breathing. Ask whether the assumed position is required for respiratory comfort.

3. Note whether the patient can breathe normally when in a supine position.

4. Note whether pillows are used to prop the patient upright to facilitate breathing.

N **The healthy adult breathes comfortably in a supine, prone, or upright position.**

A Orthopnea: difficulty breathing in positions other than upright

P COPD, congestive heart failure, pulmonary edema

Mode of Breathing

E 1. Note whether the patient is using the nose, mouth, or both, to breathe.
2. Note for which part of the respiratory cycle each is used.

N **Normal findings vary among individuals, but most patients inhale and exhale through the nose.**

A Continuous mouth breathing

P Any type of nasal or sinus obstruction

A Pursed-lip breathing (prolongs the expiration phase of the respiratory cycle)

P COPD

Sputum

E 1. Ask the patient to expectorate a sputum sample.
2. If the patient is unable to expectorate, ask the patient for a recent sputum sample from a handkerchief or tissue.
3. Note the color, odor, amount, and consistency of the sputum.

N **A small amount of sputum is normal. The color is light yellow or clear. Normal sputum is odorless. Depending on the hydration status of the patient, the sputum can be thick or thin.**

A Abnormal colors of sputum

P Table 15-1 lists the pathologies associated with different colors of sputum.

A Foul-smelling sputum

P Anaerobic infections

A Copious amounts of sputum

P Chronic bronchitis, infectious process (pneumonia), pulmonary edema (fluid leaked from pulmonary capillary membranes into large airways)

A Very thick sputum

P Dehydration

A Significantly thin sputum

P Overhydration

A Thin, pink, frothy sputum

P Pulmonary edema

Palpation

General Palpation

E To perform anterior palpation:
1. Stand in front of the patient.
2. Place the finger pads of the dominant hand on the apex of the right lung (above the clavicle).
3. Using light palpation, assess the integument of the thorax in that area.

TABLE 15-1 Pathologies Associated with Different Colors of Sputum

SPUTUM COLOR	PATHOLOGY
Mucoid	Tracheobronchitis, asthma
Yellow or green	Bacterial infection
Rust or blood tinged	Pneumococcal pneumonia, pulmonary infarction, tuberculosis, lung cancer
Black	Black lung disease
Pink	Pulmonary edema

E Examination **N** Normal Findings **A** Abnormal Findings **P** Pathophysiology

4. Move the finger pads down to the clavicle and palpate.
5. Proceed with the palpation, moving down to each rib and ICS of the right anterior thorax. Palpate any area(s) of tenderness last.
6. Repeat the procedure on the left anterior thorax.

E To perform posterior palpation:
1. Stand behind the patient.
2. Place the finger pads of the dominant hand on the apex of the right lung (approximately at the level of T1).
3. Using light palpation, assess the integument of the thorax in that area.
4. Move the finger pads down to the first thoracic vertebra and palpate.
5. Proceed with the palpation, moving down to each thoracic vertebra and ICS of the right posterior thorax.
6. Repeat the procedure on the left posterior thorax.

E To perform lateral palpation:
1. Stand to the patient's right side.
2. Have the patient lift the arms overhead.
3. Place the finger pads of the dominant hand beneath the right axillary fold.
4. Using light palpation, assess the integument of the thorax in that area.
5. Move the finger pads down to the first rib beneath the axillary fold.
6. Proceed with the palpation, moving down to each rib and ICS of the right lateral thorax.
7. Move to the patient's left side.
8. Repeat the procedure on the left lateral thorax.

Pulsations

N **No pulsations should be present.**

A Thoracic pulsations

P Thoracic aortic aneurysm

Masses

N **No masses should be present.**

A Thoracic mass

P Thoracic tumor or cyst

Thoracic Tenderness

N **No thoracic tenderness should be present.**

A Thoracic tenderness

P Fractured ribs from blunt chest trauma, infection, contusion from trauma

Crepitus

N **Crepitus should not be present.**

A Crepitus: fine beads of air escape the lung and are trapped in the subcutaneous tissue, yielding a crackling sound on palpation.

P Any condition that interrupts the integrity of the pleura and the lungs (pneumothorax, chest trauma, thoracic surgery, mediastinal emphysema, alveolar rupture, tearing of pleural adhesions)

Thoracic Expansion

E To perform anterior thoracic expansion: (Figure 15-7A)
1. Stand directly in front of the patient. Place the thumbs of both hands on the costal margins and pointing toward the xiphoid process. Gather a small fold of skin between the thumbs to assist with the visualization of the results of this technique.
2. Lay your outstretched palms on the anterolateral thorax.
3. Instruct the patient to take a deep breath.
4. Observe the movement of the thumbs, both in direction and in distance.
5. Ask the patient to exhale.
6. Observe the movement of the thumbs as they return to the midline.

E To perform posterior thoracic expansion: (Figure 15-7B)
1. Stand directly behind the patient. Place the thumbs of both hands at

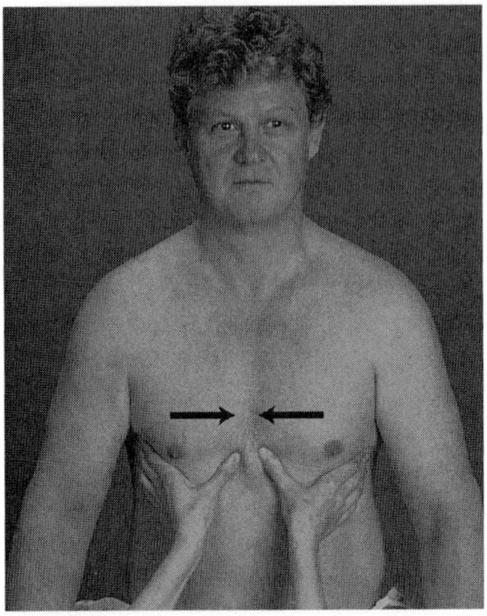

A. Anterior

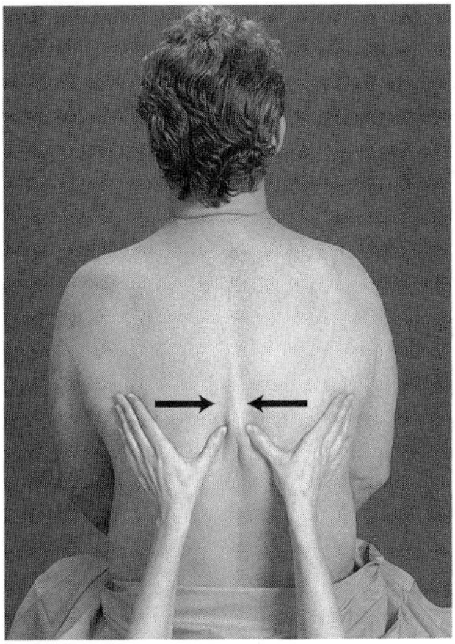

B. Posterior

Figure 15-7 Thoracic Expansion

the level of the 10th spinal vertebra, equidistant from the spinal column and approximately 1 to 3 inches apart. Gather a small amount of skin between the thumbs.

2. Place your outstretched palms on the posterolateral thorax.

3. Instruct the patient to take a deep breath.

4. Observe the movement of the thumbs, both in direction and in distance.

5. Ask the patient to exhale.

6. Observe the movement of the thumbs as they return to the midline.

N **The thumbs separate an equal amount from the xiphoid process (distance) or spinal column and remain in the same plane or costal margin (direction) as the 10th spinous vertebra. The normal distance for the thumbs to separate during thoracic expansion is 3 to 5 cm.**

A Unilateral decreased thoracic expansion

P Absent or incomplete expansion of alveoli on the affected side secondary to pathology inside or external to the lung (pneumothorax, pneumonia, atelectasis, lower-lobe lobectomy, pleural effusion, bronchiectasis)

A Bilateral decreased thoracic expansion

P Bilateral disease external or internal to the lungs (hypoventilation, emphysema, pulmonary fibrosis, pleurisy)

A Displacement of thumbs from the 10th spinal vertebral region (thumbs do not meet in the midline when the patient exhales)

P Scoliosis with lateral deviation to a particular side

Tactile Fremitus

Tactile, or vocal, fremitus is the palpable chest wall vibration produced by the spoken word.

E **1.** Firmly place the ulnar aspect of an open hand (the palmar bases of the fingers or the ulnar aspect of a closed fist) on the patient's right anterior apex (above the clavicle).

2. Instruct the patient to say the words "99" or "1, 2, 3" with the same intensity every time you place your hand on the thorax.

3. Feel any vibration as the patient phonates. If no fremitus is palpated, you may have to instruct the patient to speak more deeply and loudly.
4. Move your hand to the same location on the left anterior thorax.
5. Repeat steps 2 and 3.
6. Compare the vibrations palpated on the right and left apices.
7. Move the hand down 2 to 3 inches and repeat the process on the right and then the left. Ensure that your hand is in the ICS in order to avoid the bony structures.
8. Continue this process down the anterior thorax to the base of the lungs.
9. Repeat this procedure on the lateral chest wall and compare symmetry. Either do the entire right thorax and then the entire left thorax or alternate right and left at each ICS.
10. Repeat this procedure on the posterior chest wall. Figure 15-8 illustrates the progression of the assessment.

N **Normal fremitus is felt as a buzzing. The fremitus is more pronounced near the major bronchi (second ICS anteriorly, and T1 and T2 posteriorly) and the trachea, and is less palpable in the periphery of the lung.**

A Increased tactile fremitus

P Diseases involving consolidation (pneumonia, atelectasis, bronchitis), because solids conduct sound better than does air

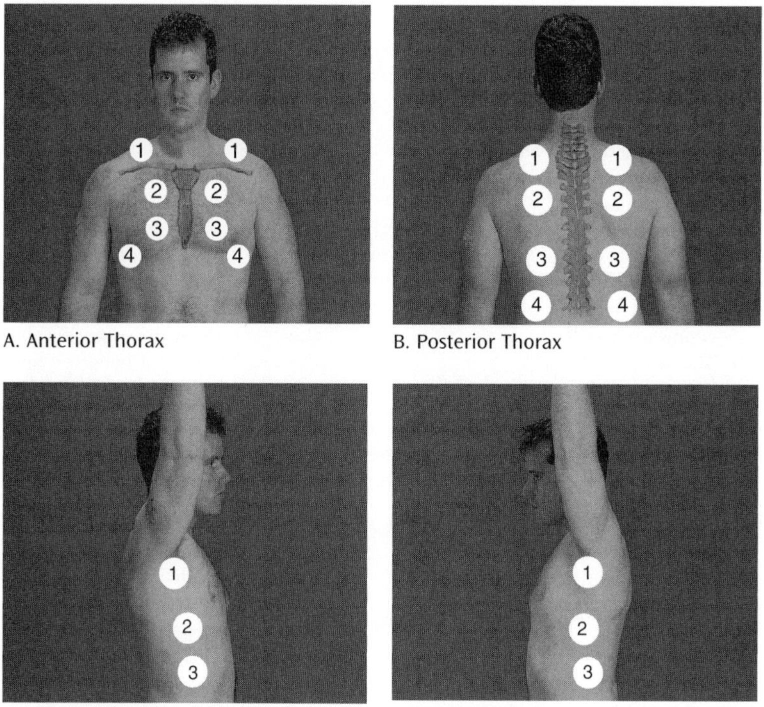

A. Anterior Thorax

B. Posterior Thorax

C. Right Lateral Thorax

D. Left Lateral Thorax

Figure 15-8 Pattern for Tactile Fremitus

A Decreased or absent tactile fremitus

P Pneumothorax, emphysema, asthma (because porous materials conduct vibrations less effectively than do fluids and solids); pleural effusion (exudate external to the alveoli serves to block the transmission of sound waves); large chest wall; obesity

A Pleural friction fremitus: palpable grating sensation that feels more pronounced on inspiration

P Inflammatory process between the visceral and parietal pleuras

A Tussive fremitus; palpable vibration

P Coughing

A Rhonchial fremitus: coarse, palpable vibration

P Passage of air through thick exudate in large bronchi or the trachea

Tracheal Position

E To assess the position of the trachea:
1. Place the finger pad of your index finger on the patient's trachea in the suprasternal notch.
2. Move the finger pad laterally to the right and gently move the trachea in the space created by the border of the inner aspect of the sternocleidomastoid and the clavicle.
3. Move the finger pad laterally to the left and repeat the procedure.

N **The trachea is midline in the suprasternal notch.**

A Tracheal deviation

P Deviation to the affected side: atelectasis and pneumonia (alveoli are closed to some degree or filled with exudate, and the trachea is slightly pushed by the healthy lung to the affected side, which contains less air); deviation to the unaffected side: tension pneumothorax, pleural effusion, tumor, enlarged thyroid

Percussion

Indirect or mediate percussion is used to further assess the underlying structures of the thorax. Remember that percussion reverberates a sound that is generated from structures approximately 5 cm below the chest wall. Deep pathological conditions will not be revealed during the percussion process.

General Percussion

E To perform anterior thoracic percussion: (Figure 15-9A)
1. Place the patient in an upright sitting position with the shoulders back.
2. Percuss two or three strikes along the right lung apex.
3. Repeat this process along the left lung apex.
4. Note the sound produced from each percussion strike and compare the sound from each. If different sounds are produced or the sounds are not resonant, pathology is suspected.
5. Move down approximately 5 cm, or every other ICS, and percuss in that area.
6. Percuss in the same position on the contralateral side.
7. Continue to move down until the entire lung has been percussed.

E To perform posterior percussion: (Figure 15-9B)
1. Place the patient in an upright sitting position with a slight forward tilt. Have the patient bend the head down and fold the arms in front at the waist. These actions move the scapula laterally and maximize the lung area that can be percussed.
2. Percuss the right lung apex, located along the top of the shoulder. Approximately three percussion strikes should be made along this area.
3. Repeat the process along the left lung apex.
4. Note the sound produced from each percussion strike and compare the sound from each. If different

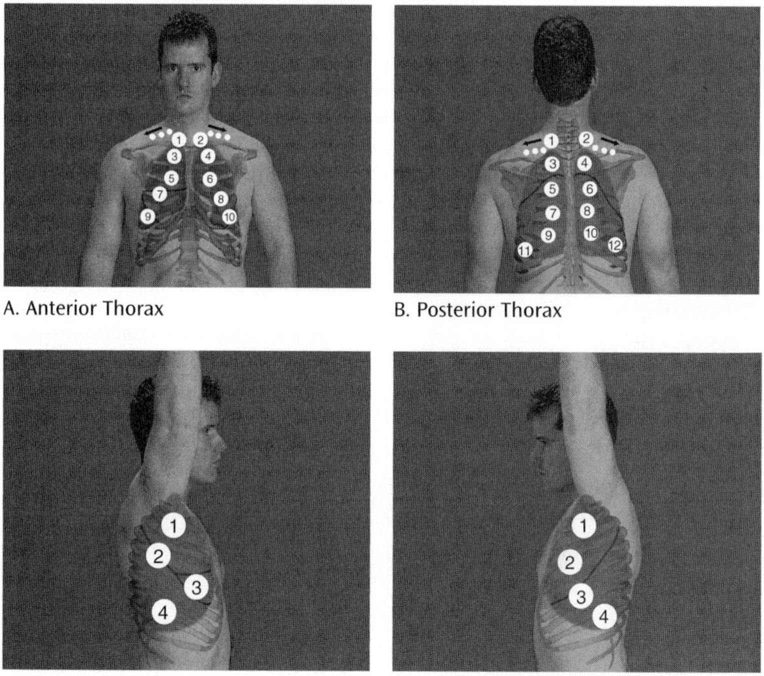

A. Anterior Thorax B. Posterior Thorax

C. Right Lateral Thorax D. Left Lateral Thorax

Figure 15-9 Percussion Patterns

sounds are produced or the sounds are not resonant, pathology is suspected.

5. Move down approximately 5 cm, or every other ICS, and percuss in that area.

6. Percuss in the same position on the contralateral side.

7. Continue to move down the thorax until the entire posterior lung field has been percussed.

E To perform lateral thorax percussion: (Figures 15-9C and 15-9D)

1. Place the patient in an upright sitting position and with the arms raised directly overhead. This position affords the greatest exposure of the thorax.

2. Either percuss the entire right lateral thorax and then the entire left lateral thorax or alternate right and left sides. Start to percuss in the ICS directly below the axilla.

3. Note the sound produced from that strike.

4. Move down approximately 5 cm, or every other ICS, and percuss in that area.

5. Percuss down to the base of the lung.

N **Normal lung tissue produces a resonant sound. The diaphragm and the cardiac silhouette emit dull percussion. Rib sounds are flat. Hyperresonance is normal in thin adults and in patients with decreased musculature.**

A Hyperresonance

P Air-filled spaces such as occur in conjunction with pneumothorax, emphysema, asthma, and emphysematous bullae

A Dullness

P Solid or fluid-filled structures such as occur in conjunction with pneumonia, atelectasis, pulmonary edema, pleural effusion, pulmonary fibrosis, hemothorax, emphysema, and tumor

Diaphragmatic Excursion

Diaphragmatic excursion provides information on the patient's depth of ventilation. Diaphragmatic excursion is the distance the diaphragm moves on inspiration and expiration.

E To evaluate diaphragmatic excursion:

1. Position the patient as for posterior thorax percussion.

2. With the patient breathing normally, percuss the right lung from the apex (resonant in healthy adults) to below the diaphragm (dull). To orient your assessment to the patient's percussion sounds, note the level at which the percussion sound changes quality. If full posterior thorax percussion has already been performed, this step can be eliminated.

3. Instruct the patient to inhale as deeply as possible and to hold that breath.

4. With the patient holding the breath, percuss the right lung in the scapular line from below the scapula to the location where resonance changes to dullness.

5. Mark this location and tell the patient to exhale and to breathe normally.

6. When the patient has recovered, instruct the patient to inhale as deeply as possible, exhale fully, and hold this exhaled breath.

7. Repercuss the right lung below the scapula in the scapular line in a caudal direction. Mark the spot where resonance changes to dullness.

8. Measure the distance between the two marks.

9. Repeat the procedure on the left posterior thorax.

N **Normal diaphragmatic excursion is 3 to 5 cm. The level of the diaphragm is T12 on inspiration and T10 on expiration. The right side of the diaphragm is usually slightly higher than the left.**

A A diaphragmatic excursion less than 3 cm

P Hypoventilation secondary to pain, obesity, lung congestion, emphysema, asthma, or pleurisy

A A high diaphragm level

P Lower lobe lobectomy, pneumonectomy (paralyzed diaphragm moves upward), space-occupying states such as ascites and pregnancy, atelectasis, pleural effusion in a lower lobe (dull percussion between diaphragm and lung)

Auscultation

The goal of respiratory auscultation is to identify the presence of normal breath sounds, abnormal lung sounds, adventitious (or added) lung sounds, and adventitious pleural sounds. Anterior, posterior, and lateral aspects of the chest are auscultated. If an acoustic stethoscope is used, the diaphragm of the stethoscope, which transmits high-pitched sounds, is the headpiece of choice.

General Auscultation

E To perform anterior thoracic auscultation:

1. Place the patient in an upright sitting position and with the shoulders back.

2. Instruct the patient to breathe only through the mouth and to inhale and exhale deeply and slowly.

3. Place the stethoscope on the apex of the right lung and listen for one complete respiratory cycle (one inhalation and one exhalation).

4. Repeat on the left apex.
5. Note the breath sound auscultated in each area and compare one side with the other.
6. Continue to move the stethoscope down approximately 5 cm, or every other ICS; compare contralateral sides.

E To perform posterior thoracic auscultation:
1. Place the patient in an upright sitting position with a slight forward tilt. Have the patient bend the head down and fold the arms in front at the waist. These actions move the scapula laterally and maximize the lung area that can be auscultated.
2. Firmly place the stethoscope on the patient's right lung apex. Ask the patient to inhale and exhale deeply and slowly every time the stethoscope is felt on the back.
3. Repeat this procedure on the left lung apex.
4. Move the stethoscope down approximately 5 cm, or every other ICS, and auscultate in that area.
5. Auscultate in the same position on the contralateral side.
6. Continue to move inferiorly until the entire posterior lung has been auscultated. Refer to Figure 15-9 from the percussion section for the recommended stethoscope location for each auscultation.

E To perform lateral thorax auscultation:
1. Place the patient in an upright sitting position and with the arms directly overhead.
2. Auscultate either the entire right thorax and then the entire left thorax or alternate right and left; compare side to side. The stethoscope should initially be placed at the ICS directly below the axilla.
3. Instruct the patient to breathe only through the mouth. Have the patient inhale and exhale deeply and slowly every time the stethoscope is felt on the lateral thorax.
4. Note the sound that is auscultated. Continue to move the stethoscope inferiorly approximately every 5 cm, or every other ICS, until the entire thorax has been auscultated.

Breath Sounds

N **Air rushing through the respiratory tract during inspiration and expiration generates different breath sounds in the normal patient. There are three distinct types of normal breath sounds (Table 15-2):**
1. Bronchial (or tubular)
2. Bronchovesicular
3. Vesicular

Breath sounds that are not normal can be classified as either abnormal or adventitious breath sounds. Abnormal breath sounds are characterized as either decreased or absent. Adventitious breath sounds are superimposed sounds on the normal bronchial, bronchovesicular, and vesicular breath sounds. There are six adventitious breath sounds:

1. Fine crackle
2. Coarse crackle
3. Sonorous wheeze
4. Sibilant wheeze
5. Pleural friction rub
6. Stridor

Table 15-3 lists general characteristics of adventitious breath sounds.

A Decreased breath sounds

P Inability to inhale and exhale deeply secondary to emphysema; a large chest; bronchial obstruction; atelectasis

A Absent breath sounds

P Pleural effusion, tumor, pulmonary fibrosis, empyema, hemothorax, hydrothorax, large pneumothorax, pneumonectomy, pulmonary edema, massive atelectasis, complete airway obstruction

Figure 15-10 lists assessment findings frequently associated with common lung conditions.

TABLE 15-2 Characteristics of Normal Breath Sounds

BREATH SOUND	PITCH	INTENSITY	QUALITY	RELATIVE DURATION OF INSPIRATORY AND EXPIRATORY PHASES	LOCATION
Bronchial	High	Loud	Blowing or hollow	I < E 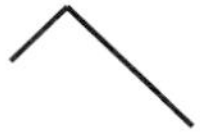	Trachea
Bronchovesicular	Moderate	Moderate	Combination of bronchial and vesicular	I = E 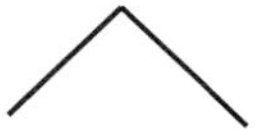	Between scapulae, first and second ICS lateral to the sternum
Vesicular	Low	Soft	Gentle rustling or breezy	I > E 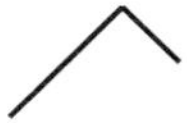	Peripheral lung

TABLE 15-3 Characteristics of Adventitious Breath Sounds

BREATH SOUND	RESPIRATORY PHASE	TIMING	DESCRIPTION	CLEAR WITH COUGH	ETIOLOGY	CONDITIONS
Fine crackle (rale) 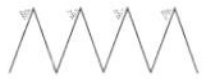	Predominantly inspiration	Discontinuous	Dry, high-pitched crackling, popping, short duration; roll hair near ears between your fingers to simulate this sound	No	Air passing through moisture in small airways that suddenly reinflate	COPD, congestive heart failure (CHF), pneumonia, pulmonary fibrosis, atelectasis
Coarse crackle (coarse rale) 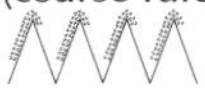	Predominantly inspiration	Discontinuous	Moist, low-pitched crackling, gurgling; long duration	Possibly	Air passing through moisture in large airways that suddenly reinflate	Pneumonia, pulmonary edema, bronchitis, atelectasis
Sonorous wheeze (rhonchi) 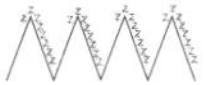	Predominantly expiration	Continuous	Low pitched; snoring	Possibly	Narrowing of large airways or obstruction of bronchus	Asthma, bronchitis, airway edema, tumor, bronchiolar spasm, foreign body obstruction
Sibilant wheeze (wheeze) 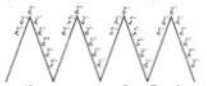	Predominantly expiration	Continuous	High pitched; musical	Possibly	Narrowing of large airways or obstruction of bronchus	Asthma, chronic bronchitis, emphysema, tumor, foreign body obstruction
Pleural friction rub 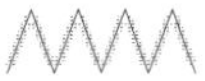	Inspiration and expiration	Continuous	Creaking, grating	No	Inflamed parietal and visceral pleura; can occasionally be felt on thoracic wall as two pieces of dry leather rubbing against each other	Pleurisy, tuberculosis, pulmonary infarction, pneumonia, lung abscess
Stridor 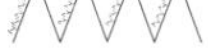	Predominantly inspiration	Continuous	Crowing	No	Partial obstruction of the larynx, trachea	Croup, foreign body obstruction, large airway tumor

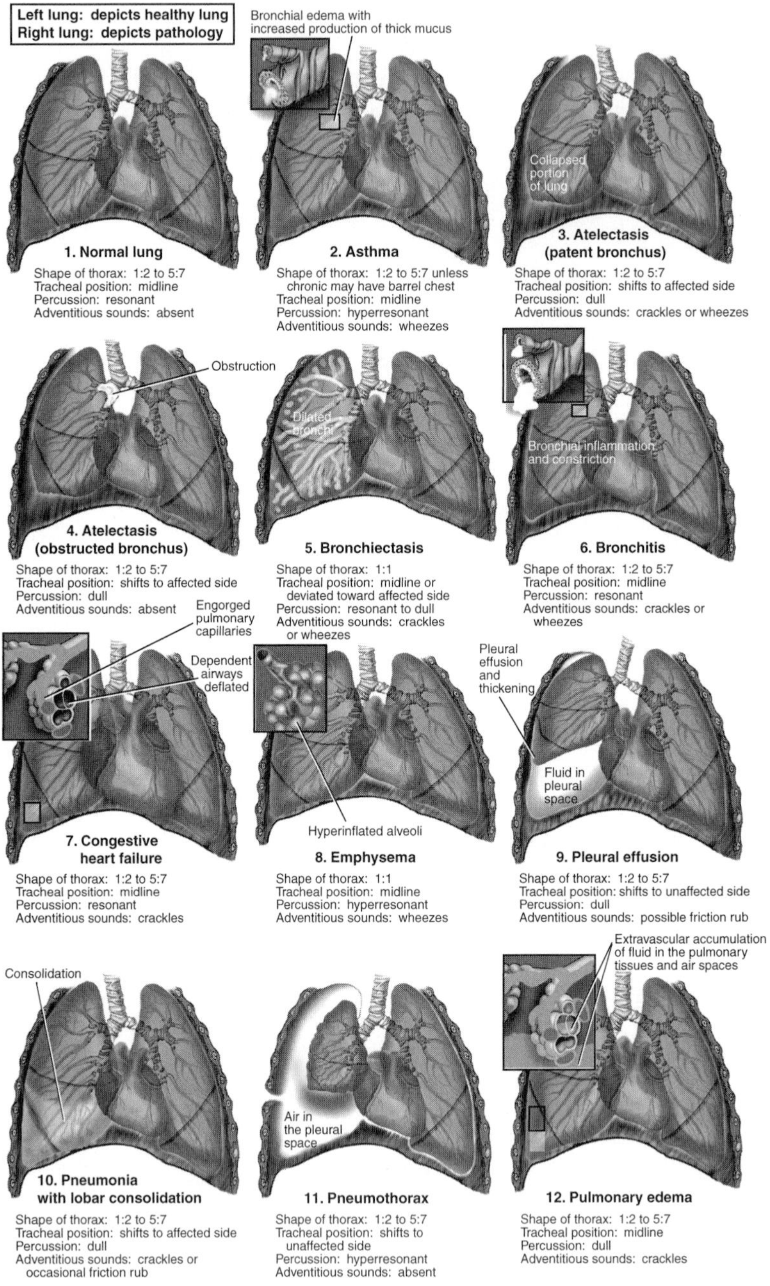

Figure 15-10 Assessment Findings Frequently Associated with Common Lung Conditions

Voice Sounds

The assessment of voice sounds will reveal whether the lungs are filled with air, with fluid, or are solid. This auscultation need be performed only if an abnormality is detected during the general auscultation, percussion, or palpation. There are three techniques by which voice sounds can be assessed:

1. Bronchophony
2. Egophony
3. Whispered pectoriloquy

Only one of these assessments needs to be performed because they all are variations of the same physical principle and assessment technique, and they all provide the same information. The voice sound findings will parallel those obtained during tactile fremitus. Thus, voice sounds will be heard loudest over the trachea and softest in the lung's periphery.

To perform bronchophony:

E **1.** Position the patient for posterior, lateral, or anterior chest auscultation. The area to be auscultated will be that in which an abnormality was found during percussion or palpation or in which adventitious breath sounds were heard.

2. Place the stethoscope in the appropriate location on the patient's chest.

3. Instruct the patient to say the words "99" or "1, 2, 3" every time the stethoscope is placed on the chest or when told to do so.

4. Auscultate the transmission of the patient's spoken word.

To perform egophony:

E **1.** Repeat steps 1 and 2 from the bronchophony procedure.

2. Instruct the patient to say the sound "ee" every time the stethoscope is placed on the chest or when told to do so.

3. Auscultate the transmission of the patient's spoken word.

To perform whispered pectoriloquy:

E **1.** Repeat steps 1 and 2 from the bronchophony procedure.

2. Instruct the patient to whisper the words "99" or "1, 2, 3" every time the stethoscope is placed on the chest or when told to do so.

3. Auscultate the transmission of the patient's spoken word.

N **The normal finding when performing tests for bronchophony, egophony, and whispered pectoriloquy is an unclear transmission or muffled sounds.**

A Positive (or present) voice sounds are:
Bronchophony: clear transmission of "99" or "1, 2, 3" with increased intensity.
Egophony: transformation of "ee" to "ay" with increased intensity; the voice has a bleating or nasal quality.
Whispered pectoriloquy: clear transmission of "99" or "1, 2, 3" with increased intensity.

P Any type of consolidation process, such as pneumonia

A Voice sounds are absent or even more decreased than in the normal lung.

P Air-filled lungs (emphysema, asthma, pneumothorax)

16

Heart and Peripheral Vasculature

Anatomy and Physiology

The heart is located in the thoracic cavity between the lungs and above the diaphragm in an area known as the mediastinum (Figure 16-1). The base of the heart is the uppermost portion, which includes the left and right atria as well as the aorta, the pulmonary arteries, and the superior and inferior venae cavae. The apex, or lower portion of the heart, extends into the left thoracic cavity, causing the heart to appear as if it is lying on its right ventricle.

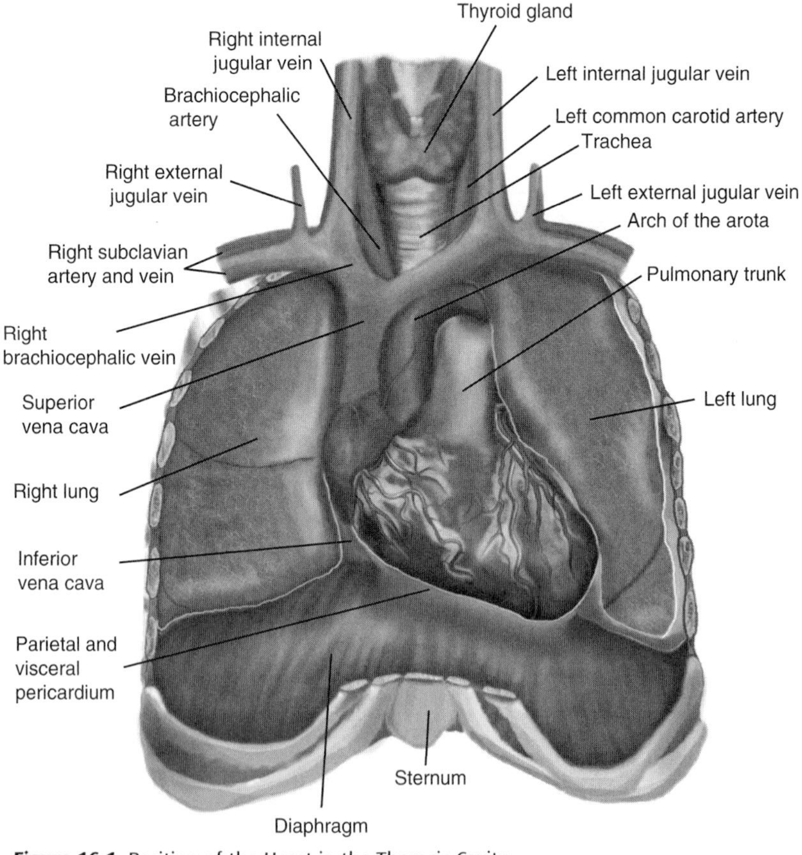

Figure 16-1 Position of the Heart in the Thoracic Cavity

The heart is divided into four chambers: the right and left atria and the right and left ventricles (Figure 16-2).

The A-V (atrioventricular) valve between the right atrium and the right ventricle is known as the tricuspid valve; the A-V valve between the left atrium and the left ventricle is the bicuspid valve, commonly known as the mitral valve. Blood flows from the right ventricle to the pulmonary vasculature for oxygenation by way of the pulmonic valve. Blood is pumped from the left ventricle into the systemic and coronary circulation through the aortic valve. The pulmonic and aortic valves are also known as outflow or semilunar valves.

The myocardium is extremely dependent on a constant supply of oxygen that is delivered through the coronary arterial system. If the coronary blood supply is not sufficient to meet the needs of the heart, the result may be ischemia (local and temporary lack of blood supply to the heart), injury (beyond ischemia but still reversible), or an infarction (necrosis) of the heart muscle itself. Myocardial ischemia is often manifested as chest, jaw, neck, or arm pain known as angina.

The left main coronary artery branches into the left circumflex (LCX) coronary artery and the left anterior descending (LAD) coronary artery. The left main coronary artery may be referred to as the "widowmaker" because of the lethal effect of any obstruction to blood flow before its branch point (Figure 16-3).

Nursing Alert

Warning Signs of Potential Cardiovascular Problems

- Change in color of the lips, face, or nails
- Chest pain
- Extreme diaphoresis
- Dizziness
- Dyspnea
- Edema
- Extremity pain
- Fatigue
- Feelings of doom
- Numbness in the extremities
- Pain that limits self-care
- Palpitations
- Syncope
- Tingling in the extremities

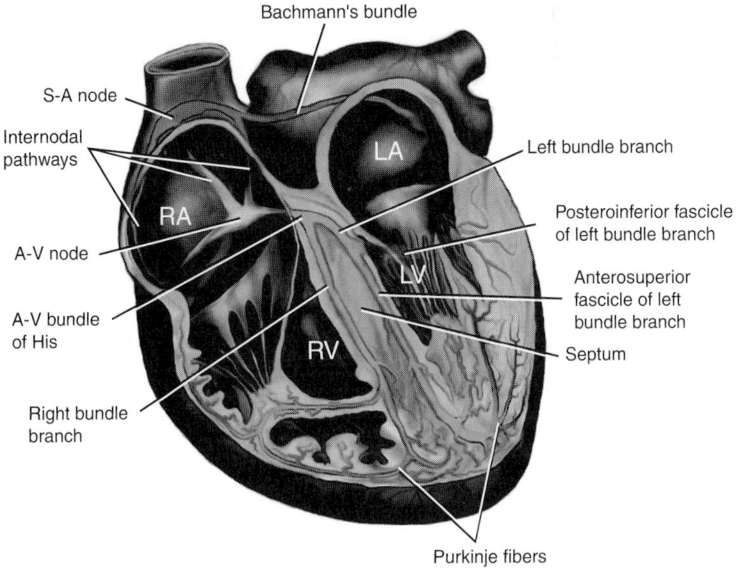

Figure 16-2 The Four Chambers of the Heart

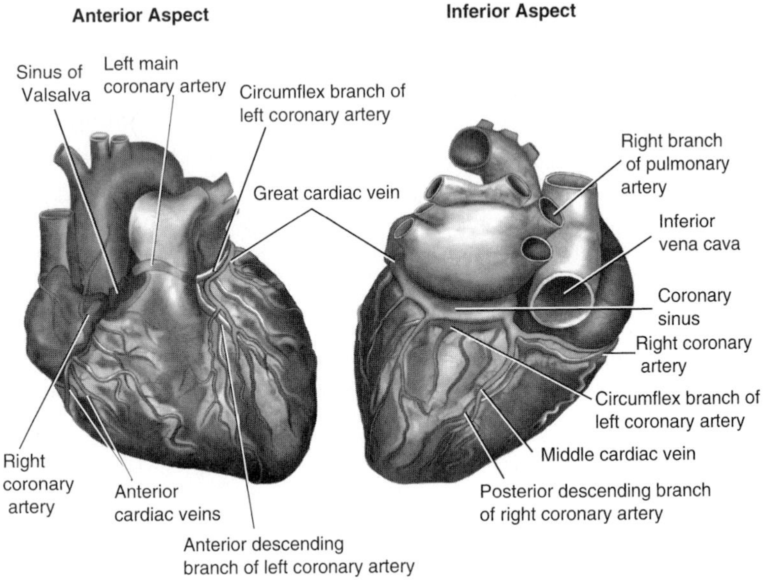

Figure 16-3 The Coronary Arteries and Major Veins of the Heart (Anterior and Inferior Views)

The LAD supplies blood to the anterior wall and apex of the left ventricle as well as to the anterior portion of the interventricular septum. The smaller arterial branches that supply the septum also nourish the ventricular conduction system, including the bundle of His and the right and left bundle branches. The left circumflex branch supplies arterial blood to the left atrium and to the lateral and posterior portions of the left ventricle. In some individuals, the sinoatrial (S-A) node and the A-V node are also supplied by this branch.

The right coronary artery (RCA) supplies nutrients and oxygen to the right atrium, the right ventricle, and the inferior wall of the left ventricle. In most individuals, the RCA supplies the S-A and the A-V nodes as well as the posterior portion of the interventricular septum. In inferior wall infarction, the RCA is most likely the vessel that has been occluded. In anterior wall infarction, the LAD branch would be the most likely source of occlusion with resulting complications in the ventricular conduction system, such as bundle branch blocks or ventricular dysrhythmias.

Venous drainage from the myocardium is carried by the coronary sinus, anterior cardiac veins, and thebesian veins. About 75% of the venous blood empties into the right atrium via the coronary sinus. The thebesian veins carry only a small portion of the unoxygenated blood that is emptied directly into all four chambers of the heart.

The cardiac cycle consists of two phases: systole and diastole. In systole, the myocardial fibers contract and tighten to eject blood from the ventricles. Diastole is a period of relaxation and reflects the pressure remaining in the blood vessels after the heart has pumped.

The electrocardiogram (EKG) shows the P, Q, R, S, and T waves. These waves are electrical voltages produced by the heart and recorded from EKG leads placed on the body. When the atria depolarize, the P wave is produced on the EKG. Approximately 0.16 second after the appearance of the P wave, the QRS complex on the EKG occurs as the ventricles are electrically depolarized. As the ventricles begin to repolarize, the T wave appears on the EKG. The EKG contains an isoelectric line, or flat line, after the T wave, indicating a period of electrical rest.

The sinoatrial node is the normal pacemaker of the heart with a rhythm impulse of 70 beats per minute. The infranodal atrial pathways conduct the impulse from the S-A node to the atrioventricular (A-V) node via the myocardium of the right atrium. The A-V node has an intrinsic rate of 40 to 60 impulses per minute. The impulse travels very rapidly from the A-V node to the bundle branch system via the bundle of His. This system is composed of the left bundle branch (LBB) and right bundle branch (RBB).

The circulatory system consists of arterial pathways, which are the distribution routes, and venous pathways, or the collection system that returns the blood to a central pumping station, the heart. Figure 16-4 demonstrates the journey of the blood through the systemic and pulmonary circuits.

HEALTH HISTORY

Medical History

Abdominal or aortic aneurysm, angina, cardiogenic shock, cardiomyopathy, chest trauma, congenital anomalies, congestive heart failure (CHF), coronary artery disease (CAD), endocarditis, hyperlipoproteinemia, hypertension (HTN), myocardial infarction (MI), myocarditis, pericarditis, peripheral vascular disease (PVD), rheumatic fever, valvular disease, syncope, palpitations

Surgical History

Ablation of accessory pathways, aneurysm repair, cardiac catheterization, chest surgery for trauma, congenital heart repair, coronary artery bypass graft (CABG), coronary stents, directional coronary atherectomy (DCA), electrophysiology studies (EPS), heart transplant, implantable/internal cardioverter/defibrillator (ICD) placement, myotomy/myectomy, percutaneous laser myoplasty, pacemaker insertion, percutaneous transluminal coronary angioplasty (PTCA), pericardial window, pericardiectomy, pericardiotomy, peripheral vascular grafting and bypass, valve replacement

Medications

Antianginals, antidysrhythmics, anticoagulants, antihypertensives, antilipemics, diuretics, inotropics, thrombolytic enzymes, vasodilators

Communicable Diseases

Rheumatic fever (valvular dysfunction), untreated syphilis (aortic regurgitation, aortitis, and aortic aneurysm), viral myocarditis (cardiomyopathy)

Patient Classification

The New York Heart Association has outlined four classifications for patients with cardiac pathologies. Class I indicates that the patient has no symptoms with ordinary physical activity. Class II means that the patient has some symptoms with normal activity and may have a slight limitation of activity. Class III indicates that the patient has symptoms with less than ordinary activity and has a marked limit of activity. Class IV indicates that the patient has symptoms with any physical activity or even at rest.

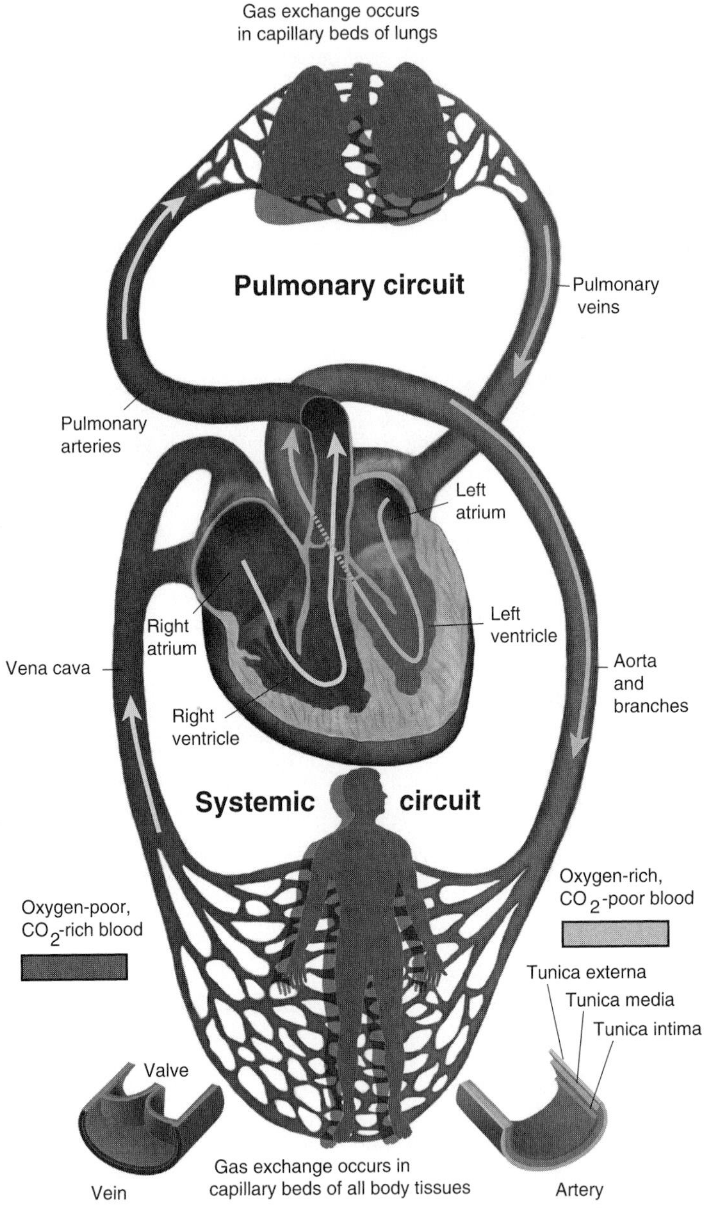

Figure 16-4 The Systemic and Pulmonary Circuits. The systemic pump consists of the left side of the heart, and the pulmonary circuit pump represents the right side of the heart.

Equipment

- Stethoscope
- Sphygmomanometer
- Watch with second hand
- Tape measure

Nursing Alert

Risk Factors for Cardiovascular Disease

Fixed (patient cannot alter)
Age, gender, race, family history

Major Modifiable (patient can significantly reduce risk of cardiovascular disease by controlling these factors)
Hypertension (HTN), hyperlipidemia, tobacco use, glucose intolerance, physical inactivity, diet, lack of estrogen in postmenopausal women

Minor Modifiable (patient can decrease risk of cardiovascular disease to a lesser degree)
Psychophysiological stress, sedentary living, obesity

Assessment of the Precordium

The cardiac landmarks (Figure 16-5) are defined as follows:

1. The aortic area is the second intercostal space (ICS) to the right of the sternum.
2. The pulmonic area is the second ICS to the left of the sternum.
3. The midprecordial area, Erb's point, is located in the third ICS to the left of the sternum.

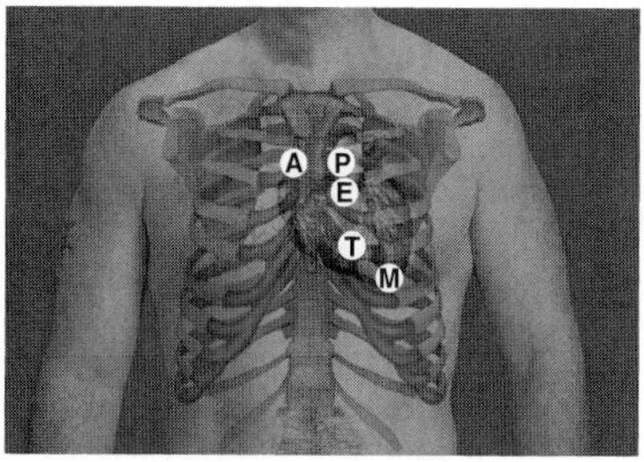

Figure 16-5 The Cardiac Landmarks. A = Aortic Area; P = Pulmonic Area; E = Erb's Point; T = Tricuspid Area; and M = Mitral Area.

4. The tricuspid area is the fifth ICS to the left of the sternum. Other names for this area are the right ventricular area and the septal area.
5. The mitral area is the fifth ICS at the left midclavicular line. Other names for this area are the left ventricular area and the apical area.

These cardiac landmarks are the locations where the heart sounds are heard best, not where the valves are actually located. The mitral area is correlated anatomically with the apex of the heart; the aortic and pulmonic areas are correlated anatomically with the base of the heart. Assessment of the heart should proceed in an orderly fashion from the base of the heart to the apex or from the apex of the heart to the base.

Inspection

Aortic Area

E 1. Lightly place your index finger on the angle of Louis.
2. Move your finger laterally to the right of the sternum and to the rib. This is the second rib.
3. Move your finger down beneath the second rib to the ICS. The aortic

Nursing Checklist

General Approach to Heart Assessment

1. Ensure that the room is warm, quiet, and well lit.
2. Expose the patient's chest only as much as is needed for the assessment.
3. Position the patient in a supine or sitting position.
4. Stand to the patient's right side. The light should come from the opposite side of where you are standing in order to accentuate shadows,

area is located in the second ICS to the right of the sternum.

N **No pulsations should be visible.**

A Pulsation

P Aortic root aneurysm

Pulmonic Area

E 1. Lightly place your index finger on the left second ICS.
2. The pulmonic area is located at the second ICS to the left of the sternum.

N **No pulsations should be visible.**

A Pulsation or bulge

P Pulmonary stenosis

Midprecordial Area

E 1. Lightly place your index finger on the left second ICS.
2. Continue to move your finger down the left rib cage, counting the third rib and the third ICS.
3. The midprecordial area, or Erb's point, is located at the third ICS, left of the sternal border. Both aortic and pulmonic murmurs may be heard here.

N **No pulsations should be visible.**

A Pulsation or systolic bulge

P Left ventricular aneurysm

A Retraction

P Pericardial disease

Tricuspid Area

E 1. Lightly place your index finger on the left third ICS.
2. Continue to move your finger down the left rib cage counting the fourth rib, the fourth ICS, the fifth rib, and the fifth ICS.
3. The tricuspid area is located at the fifth ICS, left of the sternal border.

N **No pulsations should be visible.**

A Systolic pulsation

P Right ventricular enlargement (increased stroke volume related to anxiety, hyperthyroidism, fever, and pregnancy)

Mitral Area

E 1. Lightly place your index finger on the left fifth ICS.
2. Move your finger laterally to the midclavicular line. This is the mitral landmark. In a large-breasted patient, have the patient displace the left breast upward and to the left so you can locate the mitral landmark.

N **There is normally no movement in the precordium except at the mitral area, where the left ventricle lies close enough to the skin's surface that it visibly pulsates during systole. The apical impulse at the mitral landmark is generally visible in about one-half of the adult population. This pulsation is also known as the point of maximal impulse (PMI) and occurs simultaneously with the carotid pulse.**

A Hypokinetic (decreased movement) pulsations

P Conditions that place more fluid between the left ventricle and the chest wall (pericardial effusion, cardiac tamponade), excess subcutaneous tissue, low-output states such as shock, may be absent in half of the adult population

A Hyperkinetic (increased movement) pulsations

P High-output states (mitral regurgitation, thyrotoxicosis, severe anemia, left-to-right heart shunts)

Palpation

During palpation, assess for the apical impulse, pulsations, thrills (vibrations that feel similar to what one feels when a hand is placed on a purring cat), and heaves (lifting of the cardiac area secondary to increased workload and force of left ventricular contraction; also referred to as *lift*). The patient must be in a supine position for palpation of the heart.

E Palpate the cardiac landmarks for:
1. Pulsations: using the finger pads, locate the cardiac landmark and palpate the area for pulsations.

2. Thrills: using the palmar surface of the hand at the base of the fingers (also known as the ball of the hand), locate the cardiac landmark and palpate the area for thrills.
3. Heaves: follow step 2 and palpate the area for heaves.

Aortic Area

E Palpate the aortic area for pulsations, thrills, and heaves.

N **No pulsations, thrills, or heaves are palpated.**

A Thrill

P Turbulent blood flow in the left ventricle (aortic stenosis and aortic regurgitation)

Pulmonic Area

E Palpate the pulmonic area for pulsations, thrills, and heaves.

N **No pulsations, thrills, or heaves are palpated.**

A Thrill

P Turbulent blood flow in the right ventricle (pulmonic stenosis and pulmonic regurgitation)

Midprecordial Area

E Palpate the midprecordial area for pulsations, thrills, and heaves.

N **No pulsations, thrills, or heaves are palpated.**

A Pulsations

P Left ventricular aneurysm, enlarged right ventricle

Tricuspid Area

E Palpate the tricuspid area for pulsations, thrills, and heaves.

N **No pulsations, thrills, or heaves are palpated.**

A Thrill

P Tricuspid stenosis and tricuspid regurgitation

A Heave

P Right ventricular enlargement (secondary to increased workload)

Mitral Area

E Palpate the mitral area for pulsations, thrills, and heaves. If a pulsation (apical impulse) is not palpable, turn the patient to the left side and palpate in this position. This position facilitates palpation because the heart shifts closer to the chest wall.

N **The apical impulse is palpable in approximately one-half of the adult population. It is felt as a light, localized tap that is 1 to 2 cm in diameter. The amplitude is small. The apical impulse can be felt immediately after the first heart sound and lasts for approximately one-half of systole. Neither a heave nor a thrill is present in the normal adult population.**

A Thrill

P Mitral stenosis and mitral regurgitation

A A heave, or sustained apex beat, visible though displaced laterally to the left sixth ICS at the anterior axillary line

P Left ventricular hypertrophy related to increased size of the left ventricle in the thorax and subsequent shifting of the heart (aortic stenosis, systemic hypertension, idiopathic hypertrophic subaortic stenosis)

A Hypokinetic pulsations

P Pericardial effusion, cardiac tamponade, obesity, hypovolemia, decreased myocardial contractility

A Hyperkinetic pulsations greater than 1 to 2 cm in diameter

P High-output states (mitral regurgitation, thyrotoxicosis, severe anemia, left-to-right heart shunts)

Auscultation

Aortic Area

E Place the diaphragm of the stethoscope on the aortic landmark and listen for S_2.

NURSING CHECKLIST

General Approach to Heart Auscultation

1. Explain to the patient what you are going to do.
2. Expose the patient's chest only as much as is needed for the assessment. Do not auscultate through clothing.
3. Position the patient in a supine or sitting position. The left lateral position can be used for auscultation of the mitral and tricuspid areas.
4. Use the correct headpiece of the stethoscope. The diaphragm transmits high-frequency sounds, whereas the bell transmits low-frequency sounds. Keep in mind when using the bell that it should rest lightly on the skin. If too much pressure is applied, the bell will act like a diaphragm.
5. Warm the headpiece in your hands before placing it on the patient.
6. Listen to all four of the valvular cardiac landmarks at least twice. During the first auscultation, identify S_1 and S_2, and then listen for a possible S_3 and S_4. During the second auscultation, listen for murmurs and friction rubs. As you gain expertise, you may be able to listen for S_1, S_2, S_3, S_4, murmurs, and friction rubs all at the same time.
7. Listen for at least several cardiac cycles (10 to 15 seconds) in each area.

N **S_2 is caused by the closure of the semilunar valves. S_2 corresponds to the "dub" sound in the phonetic "lub-dub" representation of heart sounds. S_2 heralds the onset of diastole. S_2 is louder than S_1 at this landmark.**

A Greatly intensified or diminished A_2 (aortic component of S_2)

P Intensified A_2: arterial hypertension; diminished A_2: aortic stenosis

A Ejection click (high-pitched sound that is created by the opening of the valve after S_1, does not vary with the respiratory cycle, and can radiate)

P Aortic stenosis (calcified valve)

Pulmonic Area

E Place the diaphragm of the stethoscope on the chest wall at the pulmonic landmark and listen for S_2.

N **S_2 is heard in the pulmonic area. S_2 is louder than S_1 at this landmark. It is softer than the S_2 auscultated in the aortic area because the pressure on the left side of the heart is greater than that on the right. A normal physiological splitting of S_2 is heard best at the pulmonic area. The components of a split S_2 are A_2 (aortic) and P_2 (pulmonic). The aortic component occurs slightly before the pulmonic component during inspiration. The physiology of a split S_2 is that during inspiration, because of the more negative intrathoracic pressure, the venous return to the right side of the heart increases. Thus, pulmonic closure is delayed because of the extra time needed for the increased blood volume to pass through the valve. The A_2 component of the split S_2 is normally louder than the P_2 component because of the greater pressures in the left side of the heart.**

A Abnormally wide S_2 split (aortic valve closes early and pulmonic valve closes late; present on both inspiration and expiration, but wider on inspiration)

P Delay in electrical stimulation of the right ventricle (right bundle branch block)

A Fixed splitting: wide splitting that does not change with inspiration or expiration; pulmonic valve consistently closes later than aortic valve

P Right ventricular failure, large atrial septal defect

A Paradoxical splitting: aortic valve closes after pulmonic valve because of the delay in left ventricular systole; occurs during expiration, disappears with inspiration

P Left bundle branch block, aortic stenosis, patent ductus arteriosus, severe hypertension, left ventricular failure

A Pulmonic ejection click that does not radiate and is loudest on expiration and quieter on inspiration

P Opening of a diseased pulmonic valve

A P_2 louder than or equal in volume to A_2

P Pulmonary hypertension

Midprecordial Area

Erb's point is where both aortic and pulmonic murmurs may be auscultated. Refer to the discussion on murmurs later in this chapter for additional information.

Tricuspid Area

E Place the diaphragm of the stethoscope on the chest wall at the tricuspid landmark to listen for S_1.

N **S_1 in the tricuspid area is softer than the S_1 auscultated in the mitral area because the pressure in the left side of the heart is greater than that in the right. S_1 is louder than S_2 at this landmark. A normal physiological splitting of S_1 is best heard in the tricuspid area. This split occurs because the mitral valve closes slightly before the tricuspid valve because of greater pressures in the left side of the heart. The components of a split S_1 are M_1 (mitral) and T_1 (tricuspid). Physiological splitting disappears when the patient holds his or her breath.**

A Abnormally wide split S_1 (wider than usual during inspiration and still heard on expiration)

P Electrical malfunctions (right bundle branch block), mechanical problems (mitral stenosis)

Mitral Area

E 1. Place the diaphragm of the stethoscope over the mitral area to identify S_1.
2. If you are unable to distinguish S_1 from S_2, use the hand closest to the head to palpate the carotid artery while auscultating the mitral landmark. You will hear S_1 with each carotid pulse beat.

N **S_1 is heard loudest in the mitral area. S_1 is caused by the closure of the mitral and tricuspid valves. S_1 corresponds to the "lub" sound in the phonetic "lub-dub" representation of heart sounds. S_1 is louder than S_2 at this landmark. S_1 also heralds the onset of systole. At normal or slow heart rates, systole (the time occurring between S_1 and S_2) is usually shorter than diastole. Diastole constitutes two-thirds of the cardiac cycle; systole constitutes the other third. The intensity of S_1 depends on:**
1. The adequacy of the A-V cusps in halting the ventricular blood flow
2. The mobility of the cusps
3. The position of the cusps and the rate of ventricular contraction.

A An abnormally loud S_1

P Mitral stenosis, short PR interval syndrome (0.11–0.13 second), high-output states such as tachycardia, hyperthyroidism, and exercise

A A soft S_1

P Mitral valve limited in motion (rheumatic fever)

A A variable (loud and soft) S_1

P Complete heart block, atrial fibrillation

A A high-pitched opening snap in early diastole

P Mitral stenosis

A Tachycardia (increased heart rate, shortened diastole, systole and diastole difficult to distinguish)

P Exercise, fever, anxiety, pregnancy, heart failure

Nursing Tip

S_3 Heart Sound

Phonetically, an S_3 heart sound is thought to resemble the pronunciation of the word *Kentucky*:

S_1 S_2 S_3
Ken túc ky

Mitral and Tricuspid Areas (S_3)

Auscultation of the mitral and tricuspid areas is repeated for low-pitched sounds, specifically S_3 (otherwise known as a ventricular diastolic gallop, or extra heart sound). An S_3 is an early diastolic filling sound that originates in the ventricles and is therefore heard best at the apex of the heart. A right-sided S_3 sound (tricuspid area) is heard more loudly during inspiration because the venous return to the right side of the heart increases with a more negative intrathoracic pressure. An S_3 sound occurs just after an S_2 sound.

E 1. Place the bell of the stethoscope over the mitral landmark. When an S_3 originates in the left ventricle, it is heard best with the patient in a left lateral decubitus position and exhaling.
2. When originating in the right ventricle, an S_3 can best be heard by lightly placing the bell of the stethoscope over the third or fourth ICS, left of the sternal border.
3. Auscultate for 10 to 15 seconds for a left- or right-sided S_3.

N **An S_3 can be a normal physiological sound in children and young adults. After the age of 30, however, a physiological S_3 occurs very infrequently. An S_3 can also be normal in high-output states such as the third trimester of pregnancy.**

A S_3 in a nongravid adult

P Ventricular dysfunction, excessively rapid early diastolic ventricular filling, restrictive myocardial or pericardial disease; possible congestive heart failure and fluid overload

Mitral and Tricuspid Areas (S_4)

An S_4, or atrial diastolic gallop, is a late diastolic filling sound associated with atrial contraction. An S_4 can be either left or right sided and is therefore heard best in the mitral and tricuspid areas. An S_4 sound occurs just before an S_1 sound.

Sometimes, the S_3 and S_4 sounds can occur simultaneously in mid-diastole, thus creating one loud diastolic filling sound. This is known as a summation gallop.

E 1. Lightly place the bell of the stethoscope over the mitral area.
2. Lightly place the bell of the stethoscope over the tricuspid area.
3. Auscultate for 10 to 15 seconds for a left- or right-sided S_4.

N **An S_4 sound may occur with or without any evidence of cardiac decompensation. A left-sided S_4 is usually louder on expiration. A right-sided S_4 is usually louder on inspiration.**

A Presence of an S_4 sound

P Conditions that increase the resistance to filling because of a poorly compliant ventricle (MI, CAD, heart failure, cardiomyopathy), conditions that result in systolic overload (hypertension, aortic stenosis, hyperthyroidism)

Nursing Tip

S_4 Heart Sound

Phonetically, an S_4 heart sound is thought to resemble the pronunciation of the word *Tennessee*:

S_4 S_1 S_2
Ten nes sée

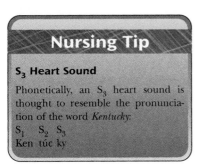

Murmurs

Murmurs are distinguished from heart sounds by their longer duration. Murmurs may be classified as innocent (always systolic and not associated with any other abnormalities), functional (associated with high-output states), or pathological (related to structural abnormalities). Murmurs are produced by turbulent blood flow in the following situations:

1. Flow across a partial obstruction
2. Increased flow through normal structures
3. Flow into a dilated chamber
4. Backward or regurgitant flow across incompetent valves
5. Shunting of blood out of a high-pressure chamber or artery through an abnormal passageway

When assessing for a murmur, analyze the murmur according to the following seven characteristics:

1. Location: area where the murmur is heard the loudest (e.g., mitral or pulmonic)
2. Radiation: transmission of sounds from the specific valves to other adjacent anatomic areas (e.g., mitral murmurs often radiate to the axilla)
3. Timing: phase of the cardiac cycle during which the murmur is heard. Murmurs can be either systolic or diastolic. If the murmur occurs simultaneously with the pulse, it is a systolic murmur. If it does not, it is a diastolic murmur. Murmurs can further be characterized as pansystolic or holosystolic, meaning that the murmur is heard throughout all of systole. Murmurs can also be characterized as early, mid, or late systolic or diastolic.
4. Intensity: see Table 16-1 for the six grades of loudness, or intensity. The murmur is recorded with the grade over the roman numeral VI to show the scale being used (e.g., III/VI).
5. Quality: harsh, rumbling, blowing, or musical
6. Pitch: high, medium, or low. Low-pitched murmurs should be auscultated using the bell of the stethoscope, whereas high-pitched murmurs should be auscultated using the diaphragm of the stethoscope.
7. Configuration: pattern that the murmur makes over time (Figure 16-6). The configuration of a murmur can be described as crescendo (soft to loud), decrescendo (loud to soft), crescendo-decrescendo (soft to loud to soft), or plateau (sustained sound).

TABLE 16-1

Grading Heart Murmurs

GRADE	CHARACTERISTICS
I	Very faint; heard only after a period of concentration
II	Faint; heard immediately
III	Moderate intensity
IV	Loud; may be associated with a thrill
V	Loud; stethoscope must remain in contact with the chest wall in order to hear; thrill palpable
VI	Very loud; heard with stethoscope off of chest wall; thrill palpable

E 1. Have the patient remain in the same position as was used for the first auscultation (i.e., supine or sitting).

2. Auscultate each of the following cardiac landmarks for 10 to 15 seconds:

   a. Aortic and pulmonic areas, using the diaphragm of the stethoscope

   b. Mitral and tricuspid areas, using the diaphragm of the stethoscope

   c. Mitral and tricuspid areas, using the bell of the stethoscope

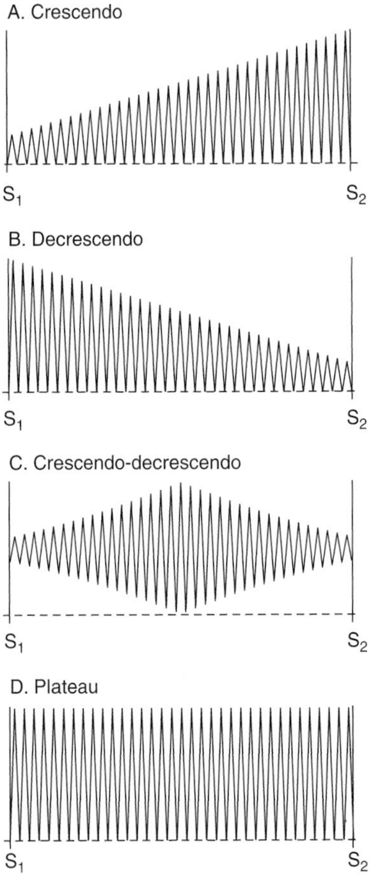

Figure 16-6 Characteristic Patterns of Murmurs

3. Using the characteristics of location, radiation, timing, configuration, intensity, pitch, and quality, label the murmur.

N **No murmur should be heard; however, a physiological, or functional murmur in children and adolescents may be innocent. These murmurs are usually systolic, short, grade I or II, vibratory, and heard at the left sternal border, and they do not radiate. No cardiac symptoms accompany the murmur.**

A Murmurs of stenosis (Table 16-2)

P Valve that should be open remains partially closed, producing an increased afterload (rheumatic fever, congenital defects of the valves, calcification of the valve)

A Murmurs of regurgitation or insufficiency (see Table 16-2)

P Valve that should be closed remains partially open, leading to increased preload (rheumatic fever, congenital defects of the valves)

Pericardial Friction Rub

E **1.** Position the patient reclining in the sitting position, in the knee-chest position, or leaning forward.

2. Using the diaphragm of the stethoscope, auscultate from the sternum (third to fifth ICS) to the apex (mitral area) for 10 to 15 seconds.

3. Characterize any sound according to its location, radiation, timing, quality, and pitch.

Nursing Tip

Pericardial Friction Rub Versus Pleural Friction Rub

- A pericardial friction rub produces a *high*-pitched, multiphasic, scratchy (may be leathery or grating) sound that *does not* change with respiration. It is a sign of pericardial inflammation.
- A pleural friction rub produces a *low*-pitched, coarse, grating sound that *does* change with respiration. When the patient holds his or her breath, the sound disappears. The patient may also complain of pain upon breathing. It is a sign of visceral and parietal pleural inflammation.

TABLE 16-2 Murmurs and Pericardial Friction Rub

HEART SOUND	LOCATION/RADIATION	QUALITY/ PITCH	CONFIGURATION
Systolic Murmurs			
Aortic stenosis	Second right ICS; may radiate to neck or left sternal border	Harsh/medium	Crescendo/decrescendo
Pulmonic stenosis	Second or third left ICS; radiates toward shoulder and neck	Harsh/medium	Crescendo/decrescendo
Mitral regurgitation	Apex; fifth ICS, left midclavicular line; may radiate to left axilla and back	Blowing/high	Holosystolic/plateau
Tricuspid regurgitation	Lower left sternal border; may radiate to right sternum	Blowing/high	Holosystolic/plateau
Diastolic Murmurs			
Aortic regurgitation	Second right ICS and Erb's point; may radiate to left or right sternal border	Blowing/high	Decrescendo
Pulmonic regurgitation	Second left ICS; may radiate to left lower sternal border	Blowing/high	Decrescendo
Mitral stenosis	Apex; fifth ICS, left midclavicular line; may get louder with patient on left side; does not radiate	Rumbling/low	Crescendo/decrescendo
Tricuspid stenosis	Fourth ICS, at sternal border	Rumbling/low	Crescendo/decrescendo
Pericardial Friction Rub	Third to fifth ICS, left of sternum; does not radiate	Leathery, scratchy, grating/high	Three components: **1.** Ventricular systole **2.** Ventricular diastole **3.** Atrial systole

Note: Timing is described as systolic or diastolic; intensity is described in Table 16-1.

N **No pericardial friction rub is auscultated.**

A Pericardial friction rub (see Table 16-2)

P Inflamed visceral and parietal layers of the pericardium rub together to produce the friction rub (pericarditis, renal failure)

Prosthetic Heart Valves

E/N **Prosthetic heart valves can be located in any of the four heart valves, though mitral and aortic valve replacements are the most common. Refer to the sections on aortic and mitral valve auscultations.**

A Prosthetic heart valves produce abnormal heart sounds; mechanical prosthetic valve sounds can be heard without the use of a stethoscope.

P Mechanical prosthetic valves (caged-ball, tilting disk, and bileaflet valves) produce "clicky" sounds; homograft (human tissue) and heterograft (animal tissue) valves sound similar to human valves but usually also produce a murmur.

Assessment of the Peripheral Vasculature

Inspection of the Jugular Venous Pressure

Identify the internal and external jugular veins (Figure 16-7) with the patient in a supine position and the patient's head elevated to 30° or 45° so that the jugular veins are visible. The external jugular veins are more superficial than the internal jugular (IJ) veins and traverse the neck diagonally from the center of the clavicle to the angle of the jaw. The IJ veins are larger and are located deep below the sternocleidomastoid muscle and adjacent to the carotid arteries. The pulsations of the IJ veins can be difficult to visualize because the veins are deep and the pulsations can be confused with those of the adjacent carotid arteries.

Information about central venous pressure (CVP) can be obtained directly via a catheter inserted into one of the jugular veins (the IJ veins are the veins of choice for cannulation because they do not have

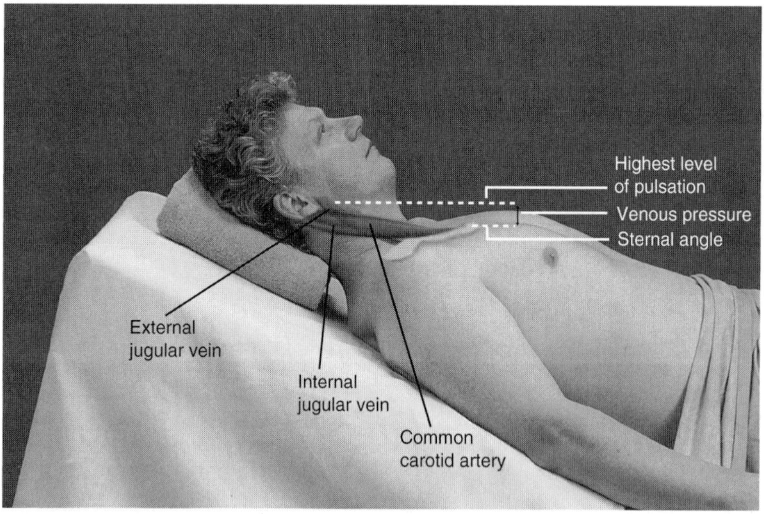

Figure 16-7 Inspection of Jugular Venous Pressure

valves and they provide a more direct route to the right atrium) or indirectly.

E To indirectly estimate a patient's JVP:

1. Place the patient at a 30° to 45° angle (the highest position where the neck veins remain visible).
2. Measure the vertical distance in centimeters from the patient's sternal angle to the top of the distended neck vein. This measurement will give you the JVP.
3. Knowing that the sternal angle is roughly 5 cm above the right atrium, take the JVP measurement obtained in the previous step and add 5 cm to get an estimate of the CVP. For example, a JVP of 2 cm at a 45° angle estimated on a patient's right side is equivalent to a CVP of 5 + 2, or 7, cm.

N **A JVP reading less than 4 cm is considered normal. Normally, the jugular veins are:**

1. **Most distended when the patient is flat, because gravity is eliminated and the jugular veins fill.**

2. **One to 2 cm above the sternal angle when the head of the bed is elevated to a 45° angle.**

3. **Absent when the head of the bed is elevated to a 90° angle.**

A JVP greater than 4 cm

P Increased right ventricular pressure, increased blood volume, obstruction to right ventricular flow

A Bilateral jugular venous distension (JVD)

P Increased JVP

A Unilateral JVD

P Local vein blockage

A JVD when the head of the bed is elevated to a 90° angle

P Severe right ventricular failure, constrictive pericarditis, cardiac tamponade

Inspection of the Hepatojugular Reflux

Hepatojugular reflux is a sensitive indicator of right ventricular failure. Hepatojugular reflux is evaluated if CVP is normal but right ventricular failure is suspected.

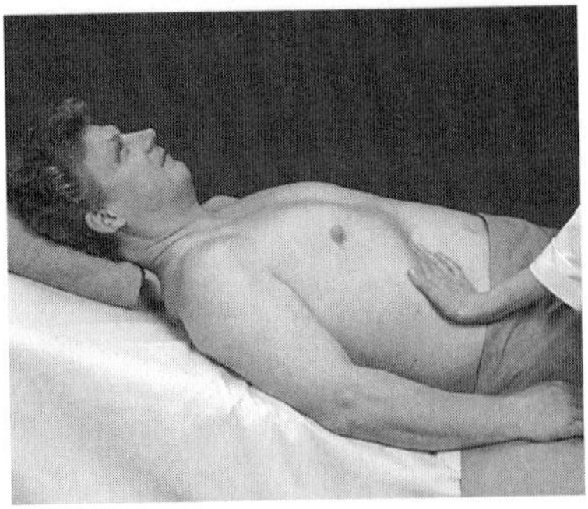

Figure 16-8 Hepatojugular Reflux

E 1. Place the patient flat in bed or elevated to a 30° angle if the jugular veins are visible. Remind the patient to breathe normally.

2. Using single or bimanual deep palpation, press firmly on the right upper quadrant for 30 to 60 seconds. If this area is tender, press on another part of the abdomen.

3. Observe the neck for an elevation in JVP (Figure 16-8).

N **The applied pressure does not normally elicit any change in the jugular veins.**

A A rise of more than 1 cm in JVP

P Right-sided congestive heart failure, fluid overload

Palpation and Auscultation of Arterial Pulses

E 1. The arterial pulse assessment is best facilitated by having the patient in a supine position with the head of the bed elevated 30° to 45°. If the patient cannot tolerate such a position, then the supine position alone is acceptable.

2. Using the finger pads of the index and middle fingers of your dominant hand, palpate the pulses. The number of fingers used depends on the amount of space where the pulse is located.

> **Nursing Alert**
>
> **Palpation of Carotid Pulses**
>
> The carotid pulses should not be palpated together because excessive stimulation can elicit a vagal response and slow the heart. Palpating both carotid pulses at the same time can also cut off circulation to the patient's head.

3. Evaluate the pulse in terms of:
   a. Rate.
   b. Rhythm: if there is an irregularity in the pulse rate, auscultate the heart.
   c. Amplitude: see Figure 16-9.

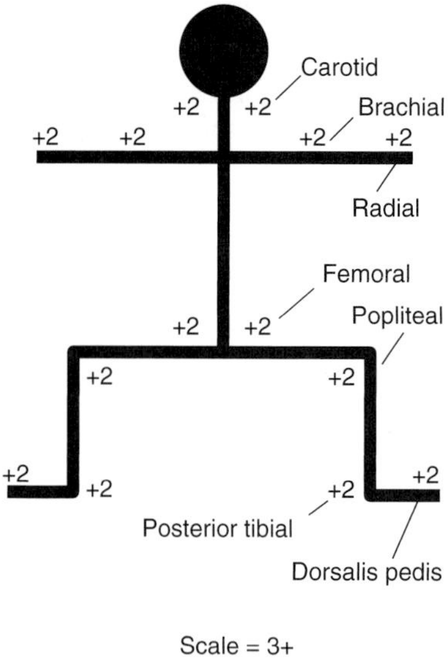

Figure 16-9 Stick Figure Depicting Arterial Pulse Assessment. (Temporal pulse is not routinely shown on the stick figure. 0 = absent; +1 = weak; +2 = within normal limits; +3 = bounding.)

   d. Symmetry: palpate the pulses on both sides of the patient's body simultaneously (with the exception of the carotid pulses).

4. Using the bell of the stethoscope, auscultate the carotid and femoral pulses for bruits, which are blowing sounds heard when blood flow becomes turbulent as it rushes past an obstruction. Ask the patient to hold his or her breath during auscultation of the carotid pulse because respiratory sounds can interfere with auscultation.

N **Refer to Chapter 9 for normal pulse rate, rhythm, and amplitude. When symmetry is being assessed, the pulses should be equal bilaterally. No bruits should be auscultated in the carotid or femoral pulses.**

A/P Figure 16-10 illustrates abnormal pulses and lists characteristics and possible etiologies.

A Bruits at the temporal, carotid, and femoral areas

P Obstruction (atherosclerotic plaque formation), jugular-vein-carotid-artery fistula, high-output states such as anemia or thyrotoxicosis

Inspection and Palpation of Peripheral Perfusion

E Inspect the fingers, toes, or points of trauma on the feet and legs for ulceration. Inspect the sides of the ankles for ulceration.

> **Nursing Tip**
>
> **Peripheral Perfusion**
>
> Refer to Chapter 10 for **E**, **N**, **A**, and **P** on color, clubbing, capillary refill, skin temperature, edema, skin texture, and hair distribution.

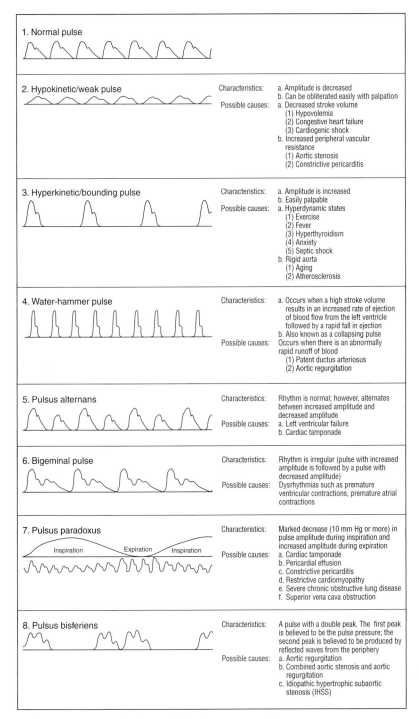

1. Normal pulse

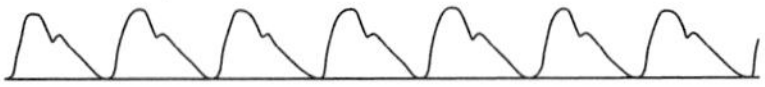

2. Hypokinetic/weak pulse

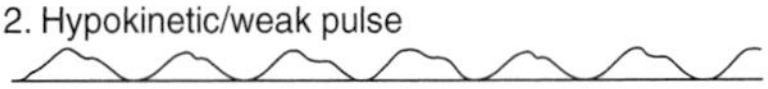

Characteristics:
a. Amplitude is decreased
b. Can be obliterated easily with palpation

Possible causes:
a. Decreased stroke volume
(1) Hypovolemia
(2) Congestive heart failure
(3) Cardiogenic shock
b. Increased peripheral vascular resistance
(1) Aortic stenosis
(2) Constrictive pericarditis

3. Hyperkinetic/bounding pulse

Characteristics:
a. Amplitude is increased
b. Easily palpable

Possible causes:
a. Hyperdynamic states
(1) Exercise
(2) Fever
(3) Hyperthyroidism
(4) Anxiety
(5) Septic shock
b. Rigid aorta
(1) Aging
(2) Atherosclerosis

4. Water-hammer pulse

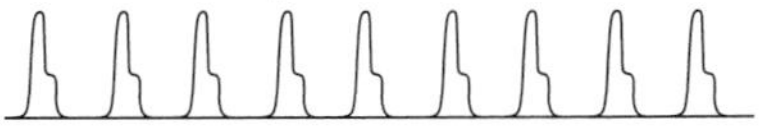

Characteristics:
a. Occurs when a high stroke volume results in an increased rate of ejection of blood flow from the left ventricle followed by a rapid fall in ejection
b. Also known as a collapsing pulse

Possible causes:
Occurs when there is an abnormally rapid runoff of blood
(1) Patent ductus arteriosus
(2) Aortic regurgitation

5. Pulsus alternans

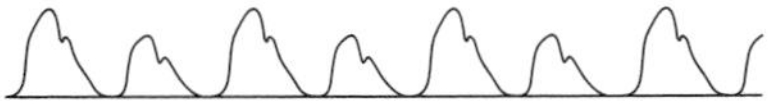

Characteristics:
Rhythm is normal; however, alternates between increased amplitude and decreased amplitude

Possible causes:
a. Left ventricular failure
b. Cardiac tamponade

6. Bigeminal pulse

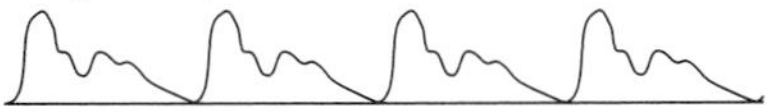

Characteristics:
Rhythm is irregular (pulse with increased amplitude is followed by a pulse with decreased amplitude)

Possible causes:
Dysrhythmias such as premature ventricular contractions, premature atrial contractions

7. Pulsus paradoxus

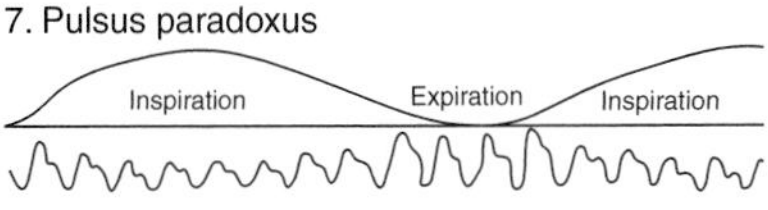

Characteristics:
Marked decrease (10 mm Hg or more) in pulse amplitude during inspiration and increased amplitude during expiration

Possible causes:
a. Cardiac tamponade
b. Pericardial effusion
c. Constrictive pericarditis
d. Restrictive cardiomyopathy
e. Severe chronic obstructive lung disease
f. Superior vena cava obstruction

8. Pulsus bisferiens

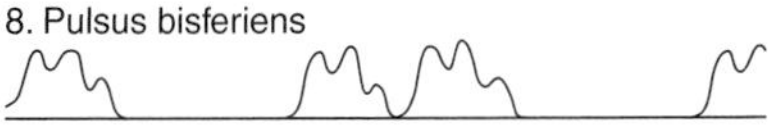

Characteristics:
A pulse with a double peak. The first peak is believed to be the pulse pressure; the second peak is believed to be produced by reflected waves from the periphery

Possible causes:
a. Aortic regurgitation
b. Combined aortic stenosis and aortic regurgitation
c. Idiopathic hypertrophic subaortic stenosis (IHSS)

Figure 16-10 Alterations in Arterial Pulses

N **No ulcerations are present.**

A Arterial ulcerations

1. Location: occur at toes or points of trauma on the feet or legs

2. Characteristics: well-defined edges; black or necrotic tissue; deep, pale bases; lack of bleeding; hairlessness or disruption of the hair in conjunction with shiny, thick, waxy skin

3. Pain: exceedingly painful; claudication related to arterial disease relieved via rest; pain at rest relieved via dependency (lowering the affected extremity)

P Inadequate arterial flow (peripheral vascular disease, diabetes mellitus); pain caused by ischemia; Raynaud's disease

A Venous ulcerations:

1. Location: sides of the ankles

2. Characteristics: uneven edges; ruddy, granulated tissue; thin, shiny skin that lacks the support of subcutaneous tissue; hairlessness or disruption of hair pattern

3. Pain: deep muscular pain with acute deep vein thrombosis (DVT); aching and cramping relieved via elevation

P Inadequate venous flow

Palpation of the Epitrochlear Node

The epitrochlear node drains lymph from the ulnar surface of the forearm and hand and from the middle, ring, and little fingers.

E 1. Place the patient in a sitting position.

2. Support the patient's hand with your hand.

3. With your other hand, reach behind the patient's elbow and place your finger pads in the groove between the biceps and triceps muscles, superior to the medial condyle of the humerus.

4. Palpate the epitrochlear node for size, shape, consistency, tenderness, and mobility.

N **The epitrochlear node is normally not palpable.**

A Enlarged lymph node

P Infection, malignancy

REFERENCE

New York Heart Association Criteria Committee. (1964). *Diseases of the heart and blood vessels: Nomenclature and criteria for diagnosis* (6th ed.). Boston: Little, Brown.

17

Abdomen

Anatomy and Physiology

The abdomen is the largest cavity of the body and is located between the diaphragm and the symphysis pubis (Figure 17-1).

Anatomic maps serve as a frame of reference during assessment of the abdomen (Figure 17-2 and Tables 17-1 and 17-2). The epigastrium, the region around the stomach, and the periumbilical region, the region around the umbilicus, span more than one quadrant. The organs of the abdomen include the stomach, small intestine, large intestine, liver, gallbladder, bile duct, pancreas, spleen, vermiform appendix, kidneys, ureters, and bladder.

Nursing Tip

7 Fs of Abdominal Distension

Seven possible causes for abdominal distension are:

- Fat
- Fluid (ascites)
- Flatus
- Feces
- Fetus
- Fatal growth (malignancy)
- Fibroid tumor

Nursing Tip

Referred Abdominal Pain

Abdominal pain can be difficult to assess because the location of abdominal pain may not be directly attributive to the area of the causative factors. In referred pain, the sensory cortex perceives pain via nerve fibers where the internal abdominal organs were located in fetal development. Pain originating from the liver, spleen, pancreas, stomach, and duodenum may be referred.

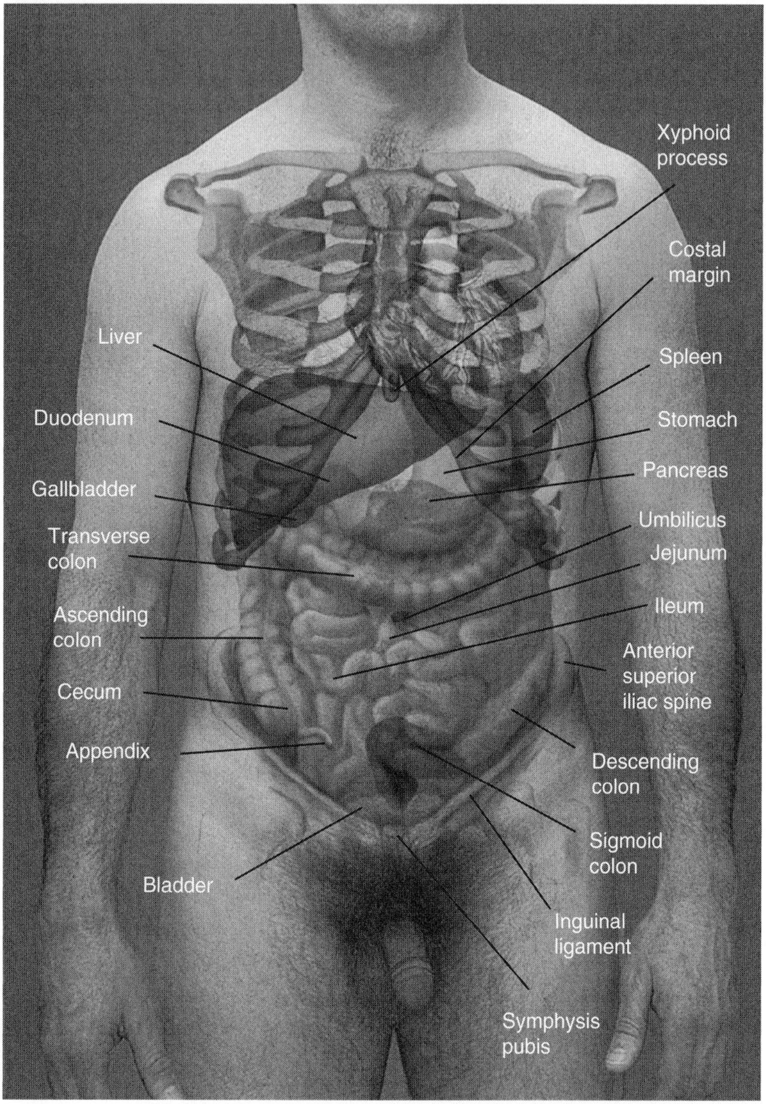

Figure 17-1 Structures of the Abdomen: Anterior View

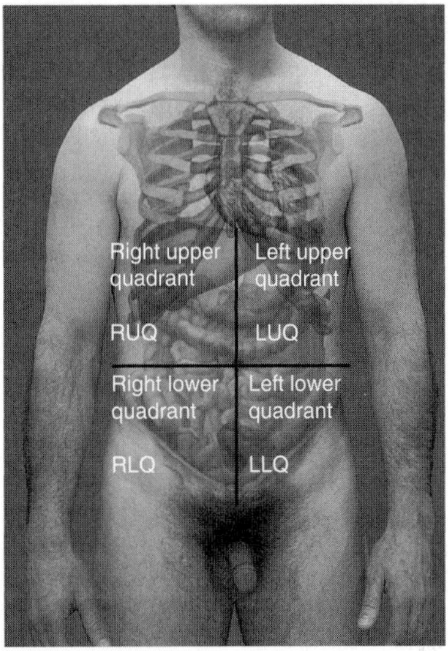

Figure 17-2 Abdominal Quadrants

TABLE 17-1 Four-Quadrant Anatomic Map

RIGHT UPPER QUADRANT (RUQ)

- Liver
- Gallbladder
- Pylorus
- Duodenum
- Pancreas (head)
- Portion of right kidney and adrenal gland
- Hepatic flexure of colon
- Section of ascending and transverse colons

LEFT UPPER QUADRANT (LUQ)

- Left lobe of liver
- Stomach
- Spleen
- Pancreas (body)
- Portion of left kidney and adrenal gland
- Splenic flexure of colon
- Sections of transverse and descending colons

RIGHT LOWER QUADRANT (RLQ)

- Appendix
- Cecum
- Lower pole of right kidney
- Right ureter
- Right ovary (female)
- Right spermatic cord (male)

LEFT LOWER QUADRANT (LLQ)

- Sigmoid colon
- Section of descending colon
- Lower pole of left kidney
- Left ureter
- Left ovary (female)
- Left spermatic cord (male)

TABLE 17-2 Etiologies of Abdominal Pain: Anatomical Regions Where They Are Perceived

RIGHT UPPER QUADRANT	LEFT UPPER QUADRANT	RIGHT LOWER QUADRANT	LEFT LOWER QUADRANT
Biliary stone	Gastric ulcer	Appendicitis	Diverticulitis
Cholecystitis	Gastritis	Crohn's disease	Ectopic pregnancy (ruptured)
Cholelithiasis	Myocardial infarction	Diverticulitis	Endometriosis
Duodenal ulcer	Pneumonia	Ectopic pregnancy (ruptured)	Hernia (strangulated)
Gastric ulcer	Splenic enlargement	Endometriosis	Irritable bowel syndrome
Hepatic abscess	Splenic rupture	Hernia (strangulated)	Mittelschmerz
Hepatitis		Irritable bowel syndrome	Ovarian cyst
Hepatomegaly		Mittelschmerz	Pelvic inflammatory disease
Pancreatitis		Ovarian cyst	Renal calculi
Pneumonia		Pelvic inflammatory disease	Salpingitis
		Renal calculi	Ulcerative colitis
		Salpingitis	

EPIGASTRIUM	PERIUMBILICAL	DIFFUSE
Abdominal aortic aneurysm	Abdominal aortic aneurysm	Gastroenteritis
Appendicitis (early)	Appendicitis (early)	Peritonitis
Biliary stone	Diverticulitis	
Cholecystitis	Intestinal obstruction	
Diverticulitis	Irritable bowel syndrome	
Gastroesophageal reflux disease	Pancreatitis	
Hiatal hernia	Peptic ulcer	
	Recurrent abdominal pain (in children)	
	Volvulus	

HEALTH HISTORY

Medical History

Malignancies, peritonitis, cholecystitis, appendicitis, pancreatitis, small bowel obstruction, colitis, hepatitis, diverticulosis, diverticulitis, hiatal hernia, peptic ulcer disease, Crohn's disease, acute renal failure, chronic renal failure, gallstones, kidney stone, parasitic infections, food poisoning, cirrhosis, infectious mononucleosis, hyper- or hypoadrenalism, irritable bowel disease, gastroesophageal reflux disease, urinary tract infection, malabsorption syndromes

Surgical History

Cholecystectomy, gastrectomy, Bilroth I or II, ileostomy, colostomy, appendectomy, colectomy, nephrectomy, pancreatectomy, ileal conduit, portal caval shunt, splenectomy, hiatal hernia repair, umbilical hernia repair, femoral or inguinal repair, removal of renal calculi, liver transplant, renal transplant

Social History

Alcohol use: altered nutrition, impaired gastric absorption, at risk for upper and lower gastrointestinal bleeding, cirrhosis of liver

Equipment

- Drapes
- Small pillow for under knees
- Tape measure or small ruler with centimeter markings
- Marking pencil
- Gooseneck lamp for tangential lighting
- Stethoscope
- Sterile safety pin or sterile needle

NURSING CHECKLIST

General Approach to Abdominal Assessment

1. Ensure that the room is at a warm, comfortable temperature to prevent patient chilling and shivering, and make sure the room is quiet and free of interruptions.
2. Use an adequate light source. This includes both a bright, overhead light and a freestanding lamp for tangential lighting.
3. Ask the patient to urinate before the examination.
4. Drape the patient from the xiphoid process to the symphysis pubis, then expose the patient's abdomen.
5. To ensure abdominal relaxation, position the patient comfortably in a supine position with knees flexed over a pillow, or position the patient so that the arms are either folded across the chest or at the sides.
6. Have patient point to tender areas; assess these last. Mark these and other significant findings (e.g., scars, dullness) on the body diagram in the patient's chart.
7. Watch the patient's face closely for signs of discomfort or pain.

Assessment of the Abdomen

The order of abdominal assessment is inspection, auscultation, percussion, and palpation. Auscultation is performed second because palpation and percussion can alter bowel sounds.

Inspection

Contour

E View the contour of the patient's abdomen, from the costal margin to the symphysis pubis both from overhead and on a plane horizontal to the patient's abdomen.

N **In the normal adult, the abdominal contour is flat (straight horizontal line from costal margin to symphysis pubis) or slightly rounded (convex from costal margin to symphysis pubis).**

A A highly convex (rounded) or protuberant, symmetric profile from costal margin to symphysis pubis

P Secondary to one of the 7 *F*s (refer to Nursing Tip)

A A concave (scaphoid), symmetric profile from costal margin to symphysis pubis

P Decreased fat deposits, malnourished state, flaccid muscle tone

Symmetry

E **1.** View the symmetry of the patient's abdomen, from the costal margin to the symphysis pubis.
2. Move to the foot of the examination table, and recheck the symmetry of the patient's abdomen.

N **The abdomen should be bilaterally symmetric.**
A Asymmetric abdomen
P Tumor, cyst, bowel obstruction, enlargement of abdominal organs, scoliosis; bulging at umbilicus secondary to umbilical hernia

Rectus Abdominis Muscles

E 1. Instruct the patient to raise the head and shoulders off the examination table.
2. Observe the rectus abdominis muscles for separation.
N **The symmetry of the abdomen remains uniform, and no ridge is observed parallel to the umbilicus or between the rectus abdominis muscles.**
A Diastasis recti abdominis: ridge between the rectus abdominis muscles
P Marked obesity, past pregnancy; not considered harmful

Pigmentation and Color

E Inspect the color of the patient's abdomen, from the costal margin to the symphysis pubis.
N **The abdomen should be uniform in color and pigmentation.**
A Uneven skin color or pigmentation
P Jaundice: liver dysfunction; Cullen's sign (blue tint at the umbilicus), suggesting free blood in the peritoneal cavity; rupture of the fallopian tube secondary to an ectopic pregnancy or with acute hemorrhagic pancreatitis; café au lait spot (irregular patches of tan skin): Von Recklinghousen's disease
A Caput medusae: engorged abdominal veins
P Circulatory obstruction of the superior or inferior vena cava, portal vein emaciation

Scars

E Inspect the abdomen for scars, from the costal margin to the symphysis pubis.

> **Nursing Tip**
>
> **Abdominal Scars**
>
> The most common sources of abdominal scarring are appendectomy, hysterectomy, and cesarean section. On the body diagram in the patient's chart, document the location, size, and condition of all scars.

N **There should be no abdominal scars.**
A Scar(s)
P Traumatic injuries, burns, surgery

Striae

E Observe the abdominal skin for striae, or atrophic lines or streaks.
N **No striae are present.**
A Striae
P Rapid or prolonged stretching of the skin (pregnancy, tumors, ascites, obesity)

Respiratory Movement

E Observe the abdomen for smooth, even, respiratory movement.
N **There are no respiratory retractions. Normally, the abdomen rises on inspiration and falls on expiration.**
A Abnormal respiratory movements and retractions
P Appendicitis with local peritonitis, pancreatitis, biliary colic, or perforated ulcer

Masses and Nodules

E Observe the abdominal skin for masses and nodules.
N **No masses or nodules are present.**
A Abdominal masses or nodules
P Pregnancy, metastases of an internal malignancy

Visible Peristalsis

E Observe the abdominal wall for surface motion.

N **Ripples of peristalsis may be observed in thin patients. Peristalsis movement slowly traverses the abdomen in a slanting downward direction.**

A Strong, observable peristaltic contractions

P Intestinal obstruction

Pulsation

E Inspect the epigastric area for pulsations.

N **In the patient with a normal build, a nonexaggerated pulsation of the abdominal aorta may be visible in the epigastric area. In heavier patients, pulsation may not be visible.**

A Marked, strong abdominal pulsation

P Aortic aneurysm, aortic regurgitation, right ventricular hypertrophy

Umbilicus

E 1. Observe the umbilicus in relation to the abdominal surface.
2. Ask the patient to flex the neck and perform the valsalva maneuver.
3. Observe for protrusion of intestine through the umbilicus.

N **The umbilicus is depressed and beneath the abdominal surface.**

A Protrusion of the umbilicus above the abdominal surface

P Umbilical hernia, ascites, masses, pregnancy, metastasis of abdominal carcinoma to the umbilicus (Sister Mary Joseph's nodule)

Auscultation

Bowel Sounds

E 1. Lightly place the diaphragm of the stethoscope on the abdominal wall, beginning at the RLQ.
2. Listen to the frequency and character of the bowel sounds. It is necessary to listen for at least 5 minutes in each abdominal quadrant before concluding that bowel sounds are absent.
3. Move the diaphragm to the RUQ, the LUQ, and the LLQ.

N **Bowel sounds are heard as intermittent gurgling sounds throughout the abdominal quadrants. They are usually high pitched, and they typically occur 5 to 30 times per minute. Bowel sounds result from the movement of air and fluid through the gastrointestinal tract. Normally, bowel sounds are always present at the ileocecal valve area (RLQ).**

Normal hyperactive bowel sounds are called borborygmi. They are loud, audible, gurgling sounds. Borborygmi may be due to hyperperistalsis ("stomach growling") or the sound of flatus in the intestines.

A Absent bowel sounds

P Late intestinal obstruction

A Hypoactive bowel sounds

P Decreased motility of the bowel (peritonitis, nonmechanical obstruction, inflammation, gangrene, electrolyte imbalances, intraoperative manipulation of the bowel)

A Hyperactive bowel sounds

P Increased motility of the bowel (gastroenteritis, diarrhea, laxative use, subsiding ileus); partial obstruction

A High-pitched tinkling

P Partial obstruction

Vascular Sounds

E 1. Place the bell of the stethoscope over the abdominal aorta, renal arteries, iliac arteries, and femoral arteries (Figure 17-3).
2. Listen for bruits over each area.

> **Nursing Alert**
>
> **Palpation Contraindication**
>
> Never palpate over areas where bruits are auscultated. Palpation may cause rupture. Immediately refer the patient to a physician.

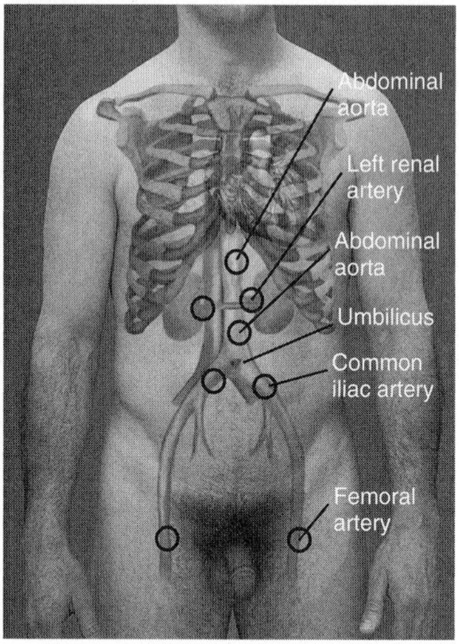

Figure 17-3 Stethoscope Placement for Auscultating Abdominal Vasculature

N **No bruits are auscultated.**

A Bruits: turbulent blood flow suggesting a partial obstruction

P Abdominal aortic aneurysm, renal stenosis, femoral stenosis

Venous Hum

E Using the bell of the stethoscope, listen for a venous hum (a continuous, medium-pitched sound) in all four quadrants.

N **Venous hums are normally not present in adults.**

A A continuous pulsing or fibrillary sound in the periumbilical area

P Portal hypertension secondary to cirrhosis of the liver causing obstructed portal circulation

Friction Rubs

E 1. Using the diaphragm of the stethoscope, listen for friction rubs over the right and left costal margins, the liver, and the spleen.
2. Listen for friction rubs in all four quadrants.

N **No friction rubs are present.**

A Friction rubs: high-pitched sounds that resemble the sound produced by two pieces of sandpaper being rubbed together and that increase on inspiration

P Rubbing together of the visceral layers of the peritoneum over the liver and spleen secondary to tumors, inflammation, or infarct

Percussion

General Percussion

E 1. Percuss all four quadrants in a systematic manner. Begin percussion in the RLQ, move upward to the RUQ, cross over to the LUQ, and move downward to the LLQ.
2. Visualize each organ in the corresponding quadrant; note when tympany changes to dullness.

N **Tympany is the predominant sound heard because air is present in the stomach and intestines. It is a high-pitched sound of long duration. In obese patients, adipose tissue may decrease tympany. Dullness is normally heard over organs such as the liver or a distended bladder. Dull sounds are high-pitched and of moderate duration.**

A Dullness over areas where tympany normally occurs, such as over the stomach and intestines

P Mass, tumor, pregnancy, ascites, full intestine

Nursing Alert

Risk Factors for Hepatitis A

- Overcrowded living quarters
- Poor personal hygiene (poor handwashing especially after defecation)
- Poor sanitation (sewage disposal)
- Food and water contamination
- Ingestion of shellfish caught in contaminated water

> **Nursing Alert**
>
> **Risk Factors for Hepatitis B/C**
>
> - IV drug use with shared needles
> - Receipt of possibly contaminated blood transfusion
> - Homosexual or bisexual males
> - Receipt of multiple transfusions of blood and blood products (oncology and hemodialysis patients, hemophiliacs)
> - Frequent contact with blood (health care workers such as nurses, doctors, phlebotomists, and laboratory personnel)

Liver Span

E **1.** Stand to the right side of the patient.
2. Beginning at the right midclavicular line below the umbilicus, percuss upward to find the lower border of the liver.
3. With a marking pen, mark where the sound changes from tympany to dullness.
4. Percuss down the right midclavicular line to find the area where lung resonance changes to dullness. Mark that area.
5. With a tape measure or ruler, measure the distance between the two marks in centimeters.

N **The distance between the two marks is normally 6 to 12 cm in the midclavicular line. There is a direct correlation between body size and the size of the liver. The mean span is 10.5 cm for a man and 7.0 cm for a woman.**

A Hepatomegaly: liver span greater than 12 cm

P Hepatitis, cirrhosis, cardiac or renal congestion, cyst, metastatic tumor

P A false increased liver border can be caused by lung consolidation or pleural effusion.

A A liver span of less than 6 cm

P Late stages of cirrhosis (liver atrophy)

P A false decreased liver border can be caused by gas, tumors, or pregnancy displacing the liver.

Liver Descent

E **1.** Percuss the liver descent by asking the patient to take a deep breath and to hold it (the diaphragm moves downward on inspiration).
2. Again, find the lower border of the liver by percussing from tympany to dullness along the right midclavicular line. Have the patient exhale.
3. Repercuss the liver-lung border.
4. Mark where the percussed sound changes.
5. Measure the difference in centimeters between the two lower borders of the liver.

N **Lower border dullness normally descends 2 to 3 cm.**

A Liver descent greater or less than 2 to 3 cm

P Liver descent greater than 2 to 3 cm: hepatomegaly; liver descent less than 2 cm: abdominal tumor, pregnancy, ascites

Spleen

E **1.** Percuss the lower level of the left lung slightly posterior to the midaxillary line and continue percussing downward (Figure 17-4).
2. Percuss downward until dullness is ascertained. In some individuals, the spleen is positioned too deeply to be discernible via percussion.

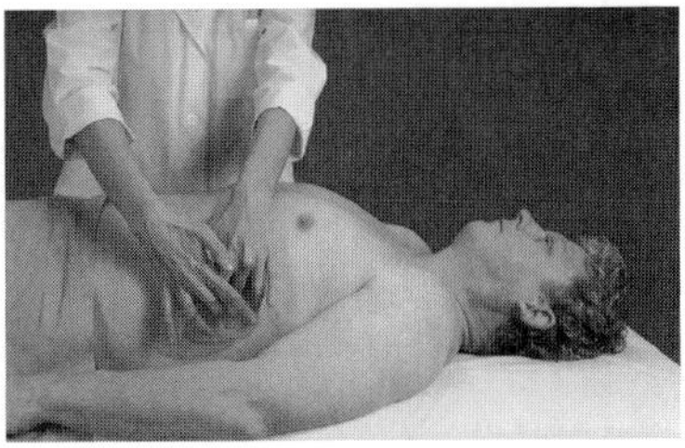

Figure 17-4 Percussion of the Spleen

N **The upper border of dullness normally is found 6 to 8 cm above the left costal margin. Splenic dullness may be heard from the 6th to the 10th rib.**

A Splenomegaly: dullness occurring more than 8 cm above the left costal margin

P Portal hypertension resulting from liver disease; thrombosis; stenosis; atresia; angiomatous deformities of the portal or splenic vein; cyst; aneurysm of the splenic artery

Stomach

E Percuss for a gastric air bubble in the LUQ at the left lower anterior rib cage and left epigastric region.

N **The tympany of the gastric air bubble is lower in pitch than the tympany of the intestine.**

A An increase in size of the gastric air bubble

P Gastric dilation

Fist Percussion

Fist percussion is done over the kidneys and liver to check for tenderness.

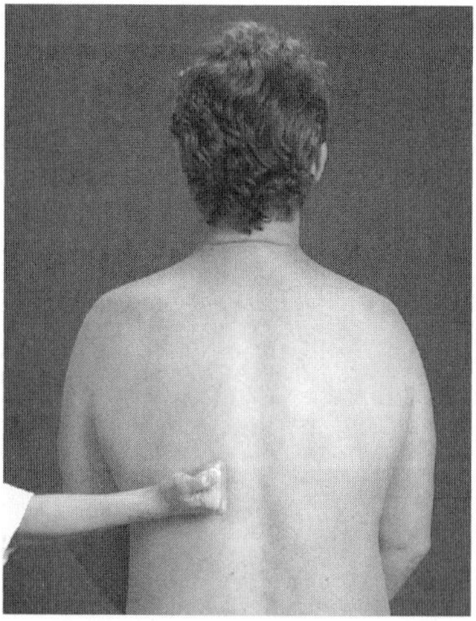

Figure 17-5A Direct Fist Percussion of the Left Kidney

> **Nursing Alert**
>
> **Risk Factors for Stomach Cancer**
>
> - Diet high in smoked foods and lacking significant quantities of fruits and vegetables
> - Pernicious anemia
> - Possibly heredity
> - Chronic stomach inflammation

Kidney

E **1.** Place the patient in a sitting position.

2. Using a closed fist, strike the right costovertebral angle (direct fist percussion, see Figure 17-5A) *or*

2A. Place the palmar surface of one hand over the right costovertebral angle. Strike that hand using the ulnar surface of the fist of the other hand (indirect fist percussion, see Figure 17-5B).

3. Ask the patient what was felt. Observe the patient's reaction.

4. Repeat on the left side.

N **No tenderness should be elicited.**

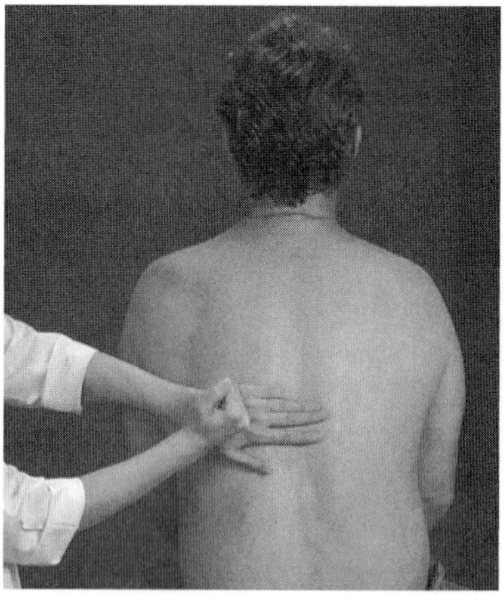

Figure 17-5B Indirect Fist Percussion of the Left Kidney

A Tenderness over the costovertebral angle

P Pyelonephritis

Liver

E **1.** Place the patient in a supine position.
2. Place the palmar surface of one hand over the lower right rib cage (i.e., where the liver was percussed).
3. Strike that hand using the ulnar surface of the fist of the other hand (Figure 17-6).
4. Ask the patient what was felt. Observe the patient's reaction.

N **Tenderness is not normally elicited via either maneuver.**

A Tenderness or pain elicited over the costovertebral angle or the liver

P Costovertebral angle tenderness: pyelonephritis; liver tenderness: cholecystitis, hepatitis

Bladder

E **1.** Percuss upward from the symphysis pubis to the umbilicus.
2. Note where the percussion sound changes from dullness to tympany.

N **A urine-filled bladder is dull to percussion. A recently emptied bladder is not normally percussable above the symphysis pubis.**

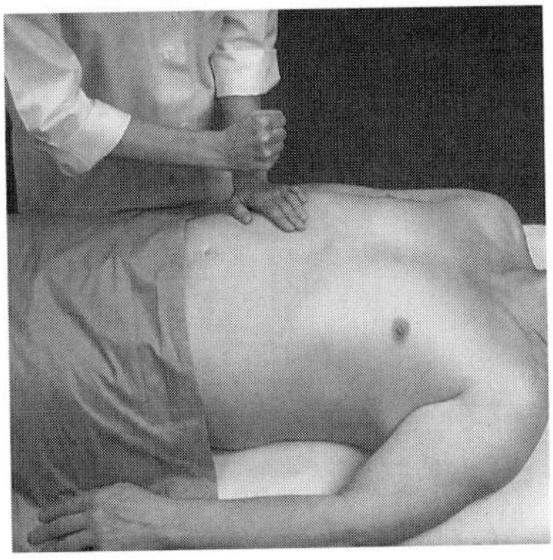

Figure 17-6 Indirect Fist Percussion of the Liver

A Percussable bladder that was recently emptied

P Inability to empty the bladder completely, elderly, postoperative patients, neurogenic bladder dysfunction, benign prostatic hypertrophy, medications, bedridden patients, acutely ill patients

Palpation

Light Palpation

E **1.** With your hands and forearms on a horizontal plane, use the pads of the approximated fingers to depress the abdominal wall 1 cm (Figure 17-7).
2. Avoid using short, quick jabs.
3. Lightly palpate all four quadrants in a systematic manner.

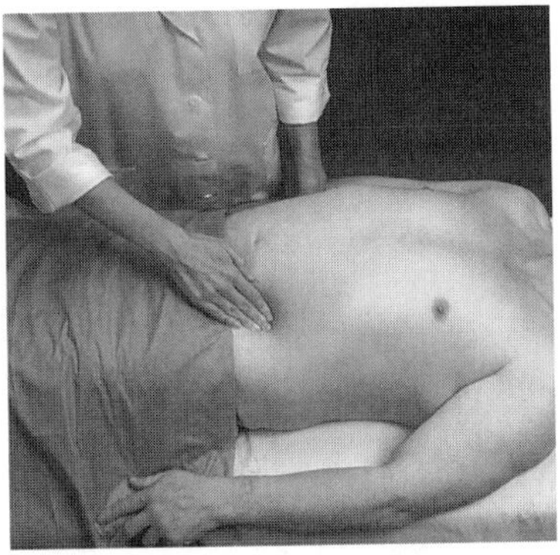

Figure 17-7 Light Palpation of the Abdomen

> **Nursing Tip**
>
> **Abdominal Pain Assessment**
>
> Before beginning the palpation assessment, ask the patient to cough. Coughing can elicit a sharp twinge of pain in the involved area if peritoneal irritation is present. Palpate the involved area last.

N **The abdomen normally feels smooth and consistently soft.**

A Skin temperature changes, tenderness, large masses

P Tenderness and increased skin temperature: inflammation; large masses: tumor, feces, enlarged organs

Abdominal Muscle Guarding

To determine whether muscle guarding is involuntary:

E **1.** Perform light palpation of the rectus muscles during expiration.
2. Note muscle tensing.

N **Guarding or tensing of the abdominal musculature is absent during expiration. The abdomen is soft. During expiration the patient normally cannot exercise voluntary muscle tensing.**

A Muscle guarding of the rectus muscles on expiration

P Irritation of the peritoneum (peritonitis)

Deep Palpation

To perform deep palpation of all four quadrants, you can use either a one-handed or a two-handed method.

E **1.** With the one-handed method, use the palmar surfaces of the extended fingers to depress the skin approximately 5–8 cm (2 to 3 inches) in the RLQ (Figure 17-8A).
2. The two-handed method is best used when palpation is difficult because of obesity or muscular resistance. With the two-handed method, the nondominant hand is placed on top of the dominant hand. The bottom hand is used for sensation, and the top hand is used to apply pressure (Figure 17-8B).
3. Identify any masses and note location, size, shape, consistency, tenderness, pulsation, and degree of mobility.
4. Continue palpation of the RUQ, LUQ, and LLQ.

N **No organ enlargement should be palpable, nor should there be any abnormal masses, bulges, or swellings. Normally, only the aorta and the edge of the liver are palpable. When the large colon or bladder is full, palpation is possible.**

A Palpable gallbladder, liver, spleen, fecal-filled colon, flatus-filled cecum, masses, bulges, or swellings

P Organomegaly (e.g., cholecystitis, hepatitis, or cirrhosis); masses, bulges, or swelling: tumors, fluids, feces, flatus, fat

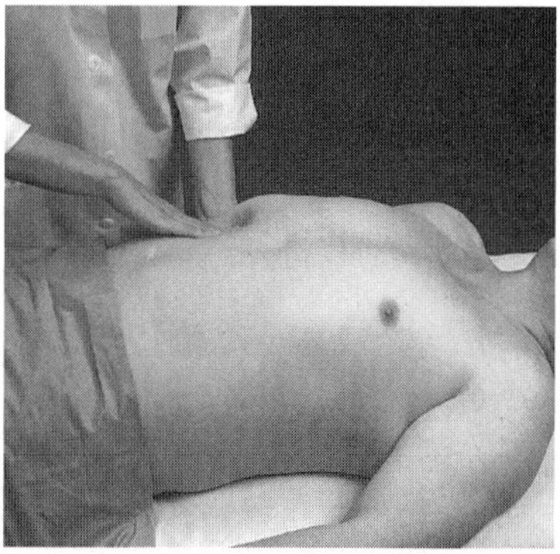

A. One-Handed Method

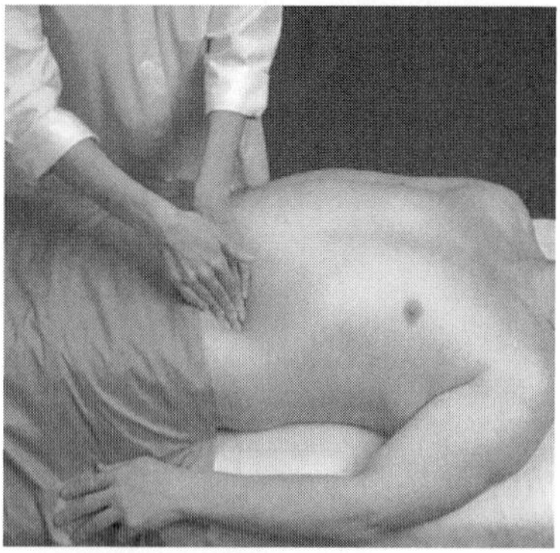

B. Bimanual Method

Figure 17-8 Deep Palpation

Liver

Liver palpation can be performed via one of two methods: the bimanual method or the hook method.

Bimanual Method

E **1.** Stand to the patient's right side and facing the patient's head.
2. Place your left hand under the patient's right flank and near the 11th or 12th rib.
3. Press upward with the left hand to elevate the liver toward the abdominal wall.
4. Place your right hand parallel to the midline in the right midclavicular line and below the right costal margin or the level of liver dullness.
5. Instruct the patient to take a deep breath.
6. On expiration, use your fingers to push down and under the costal margin. On inspiration, the liver will descend and contact the hand (Figure 17-9A).
7. Note the level of the liver.
8. Note masses, size, shape, consistency, and tenderness.

Hook Method

E **1.** Stand to the patient's right side and facing the patient's feet.
2. Place your hands side by side on the right costal margin and below the level of liver dullness.
3. Hook the fingers in and up toward the costal margin and ask the patient to take a deep breath and to hold it.
4. Palpate the liver's edge as the liver descends (see Figure 17-9B).
5. Note the level of the liver.
6. Note size, shape, consistency, masses, and tenderness.

N **A normal liver edge presents as a firm, sharp, regular ridge with a smooth surface. Normally, the liver is not palpable, although it may be felt in extremely thin adults.**

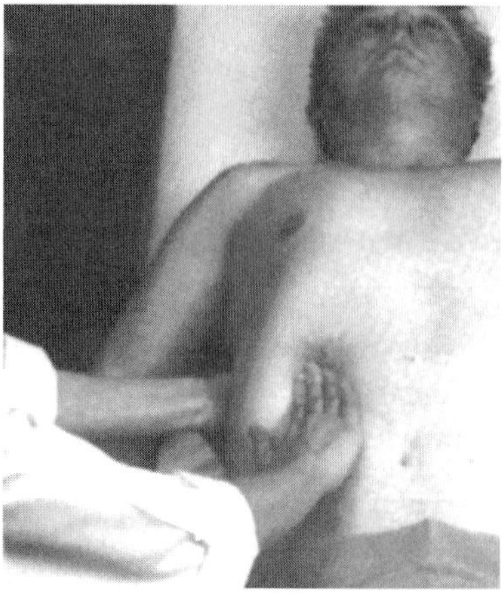

A. Bimanual Method

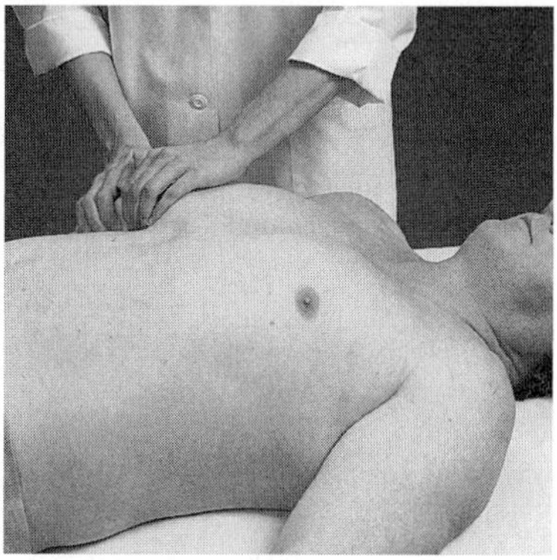

B. Hook Method

Figure 17-9 Palpation of the Liver

Nursing Alert

Risk Factors for Liver Cancer

- Cirrhosis
- Hepatitis B
- Cigarette smoking
- Alcohol use
- Exposure to toxic substances such as arsenic or vinyl chloride
- Primary malignancy

A Liver palpable below the costal margin both medially and laterally

P Congestive heart failure, hepatitis, encephalopathy, cirrhosis, cyst, cancer

A Enlarged, hard liver with nodules and an irregular border

P Liver malignancy

A Pain on palpation; cessation of inhalation with palpation due to pain is Murphy's sign.

P Cholecysitis

Spleen

Use the bimanual technique to palpate the spleen.

E **1.** Stand to the patient's right side.
2. Reach across and place your left hand beneath the patient and over the left costovertebral angle. Press upward to lift the spleen anteriorly toward the abdominal wall. Because an enlarged spleen is very tender and may rupture, palpate gently.
3. With your right hand, press inward along the left costal margin while asking the patient to take a deep breath (Figure 17-10).
3A. The procedure can be repeated with the patient lying on the right side and flexing the hips and knees. Because the spleen is located retroperitoneally, this position facilitates the spleen's coming forward and to the right.
4. Note size, shape, consistency, and masses.

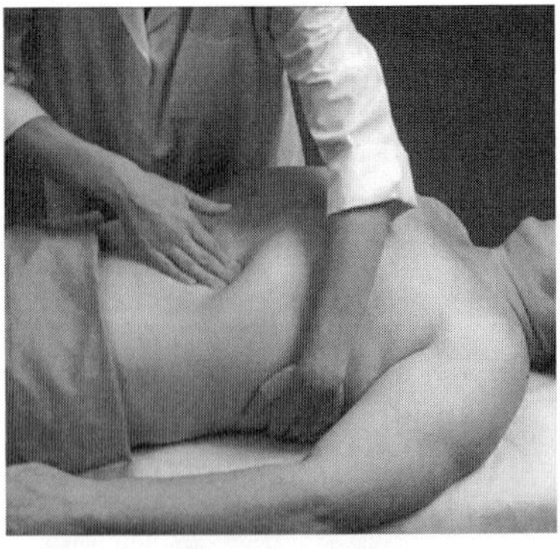

Figure 17-10 Palpation of the Spleen

N **The spleen is normally not palpable.**

A Splenomegaly: enlarged, usually very tender spleen

P Inflammation, congestive heart failure, cancer, cirrhosis, mononucleosis

Kidneys

E **1.** Stand to the patient's right side.
2. Place one hand on the right costovertebral angle.
3. Place the other hand below and parallel to the costal margin.
4. As the patient takes a deep breath, firmly press your hands together and try to feel the lower pole of the kidney (Figure 17-11).
5. At the peak of inspiration, press your fingers together with greater pressure from above than from below.

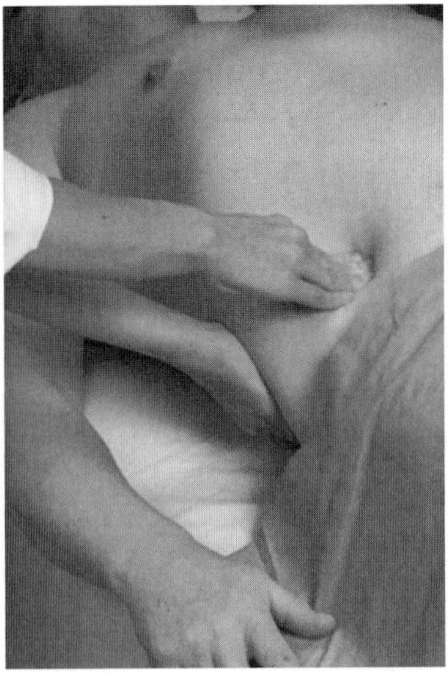

Figure 17-11 Palpation of the Right Kidney

> **Nursing Tip**
>
> **Differentiating Kidney Palpation**
>
> Features that distinguish an enlarged liver from an enlarged kidney are:
> 1. The edge of the liver is typically sharper and extends medially and laterally; the pole of the kidney is more rounded.
> 2. The edge of the liver cannot be "captured"; an enlarged kidney can be captured.
>
> Features that distinguish an enlarged left kidney from an enlarged spleen are:
> 1. A palpable notch on the medial edge of the spleen.
> 2. Percussion of the spleen produces dullness because the bowel is displaced downward; percussion of the left kidney yields resonance because of the intervening bowel.

6. Ask the patient to exhale and to briefly hold the breath.
7. Release the pressure of your fingers.
8. If the kidney has been "captured," it can be felt as it slips back into place.
9. Note size, shape, consistency, and masses.
10. For the left kidney, reach across the patient and place your left hand under the patient's left flank.
11. With your right hand, apply downward pressure below the left costal margin and repeat steps 4 through 9.

N **The kidneys are not palpable in the normal adult. However, the lower pole of the right kidney may be felt in very thin individuals. Kidneys are more readily palpable in the elderly because of decreased muscle tone and bulk.**

A Enlarged kidneys

P Hydronephrosis, neoplasm, polycystic kidney disease

Aorta

E 1. With one hand on each side of the abdominal aorta and slightly to the left of midline, press the upper abdomen.
2. Assess the width of the aorta (Figure 17-12).

N **The aorta normally is 2.5 to 4.0 cm in width and pulsates in an anterior direction.**

A Aorta greater than 4.0 cm in width and pulsating laterally

P Abdominal aortic aneurysm

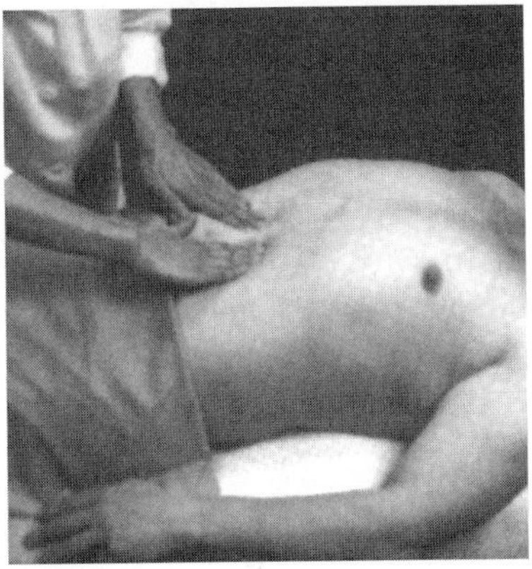

Figure 17-12 Palpation of the Aorta

> **Nursing Alert**
>
> **Risk for Aortic Rupture**
>
> Do not palpate an aorta that you suspect has an aneurysm. Notify the patient's physician immediately if you suspect an abdominal aortic aneurysm because the aneurysm may dissect and cause renal failure, loss of limbs, and, eventually, death if left untreated.

Bladder

E 1. Using deep palpation, palpate the abdomen in the midline starting at the symphysis pubis and progressing upward to the umbilicus (Figure 17-13).

2. If bladder is located, palpate the shape, size, and consistency.

N **An empty bladder is not usually palpable. A moderately full bladder is smooth and round and is palpable above the symphysis pubis. A full bladder is palpated above the symphysis pubis and may be close to the umbilicus.**

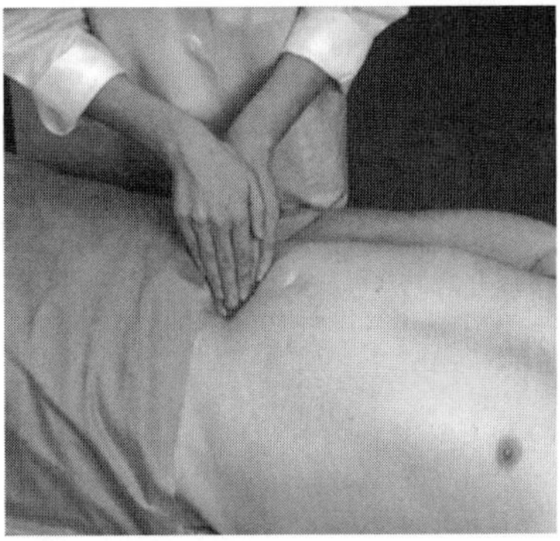

Figure 17-13 Palpation of the Bladder

A Nodular or asymmetric bladder

P Malignancy (either a tumor in the bladder or an abdominal tumor that is compressing the bladder), benign prostatic hypertrophy

Inguinal Lymph Nodes

E 1. Place the patient in a supine position and with the knees slightly flexed.

2. Drape the genital area.

3. Using the finger pads of the second, third, and fourth fingers, apply firm pressure and use a rotary motion to palpate in the right inguinal area.

4. Palpate for lymph nodes in the left inguinal area.

N **It is normal to palpate small, movable nodes less than 1 cm in diameter. Palpable nodes are nontender.**

A Lymph nodes greater than 1 cm in diameter or nonmovable, tender lymph nodes

P Localized or systemic infections, malignancy, lymphoma

18

Musculoskeletal System

Anatomy and Physiology

The musculoskeletal system supports body position, promotes mobility, protects underlying soft organs, allows for mineral storage, and produces select blood components (platelets, red blood cells, and white blood cells). The system consists of an intricate framework of bones, joints, skeletal muscles, and supportive connective tissue (cartilage, tendons, and ligaments).

The adult human skeleton is composed of 206 bones (Figure 18-1). Bone is ossified connective tissue. The skeleton is divided into the central axial skeleton (facial bones, skull, auditory ossicles, hyoid bone, ribs, sternum, and vertebrae) and the peripheral appendicular skeleton (limbs, pelvis, scapula, and clavicle).

There are over 600 muscles in the human body, and they can be characterized as one of three types. Cardiac and smooth muscles are involuntary, meaning that the individual has no conscious control over the initiation and termination of muscle contraction. The largest type of muscle, and the only type of voluntary muscle, is called skeletal muscle. Skeletal muscle provides for mobility by exerting a pull on the bones near a joint. Figure 18-2 illustrates the major muscles.

Bursae are sacs filled with fluid that act as cushions between two adjacent surfaces (i.e., between tendon and bone or between tendon and ligament) to reduce friction. Joints secure the bones firmly together but allow for some degree of movement between bones. Table 18-1 lists terms used to describe joint range of motion (ROM).

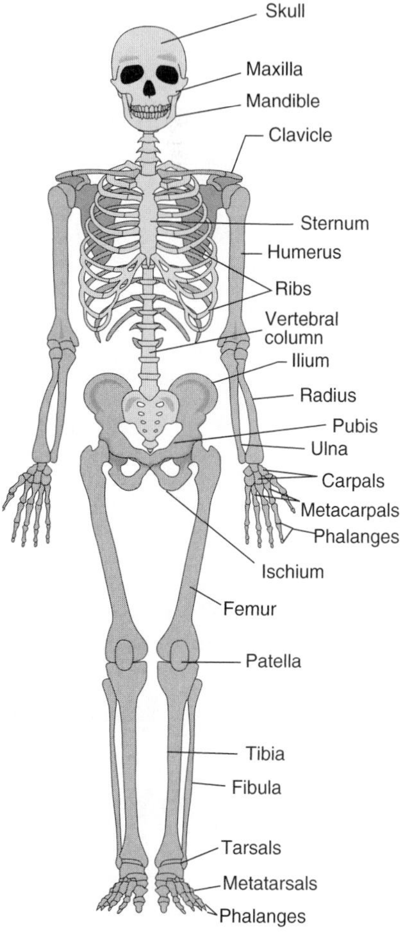

Figure 18-1 Adult Skeleton: Anterior View

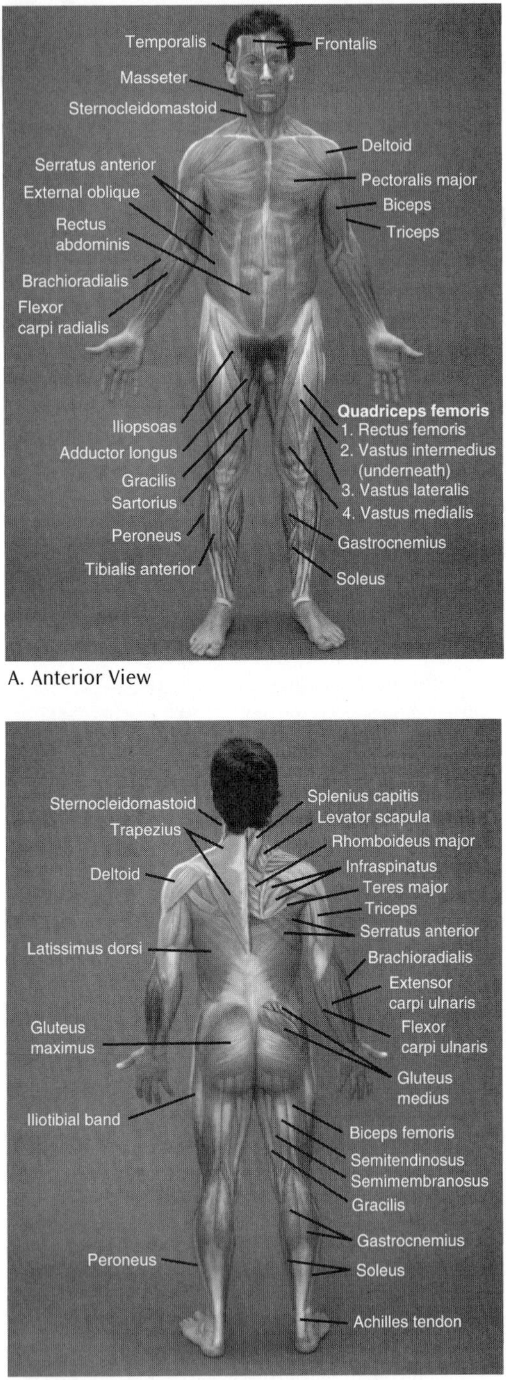

A. Anterior View

B. Posterior View

Figure 18-2 Muscles of the Body

TABLE 18-1 Descriptive Terms for Joint Range of Motion

TERM	DESCRIPTION	CHANGE IN JOINT ANGLE
Flexion	Bending of a joint so that the articulating bones on either side of the joints are moved closer together	Decreased
Extension	Bending the joint so that the articulating bones on either side of the joint are moved farther apart	Increased
Hyperextension	Extension beyond the neutral position	Increased beyond the angle of extension
Adduction	Moving the extremity medially and toward the midline of the body	Decreased
Abduction	Moving the extremity laterally and away from the midline of the body	Increased
Internal rotation	Rotating the extremity medially along its own axis	No change
External rotation	Rotating the extremity laterally along its own axis	No change
Circumduction	Moving the extremity in a conical fashion so that the distal aspect of the extremity moves in a circle	No change
Supination	Rotating the forearm laterally at the elbow so that the palm of the hand turns laterally to face upward	No change
Pronation	Rotating the forearm medially at the elbow so that the palm of the hand turns medially to face downward	No change
Opposition	Moving the thumb outward to touch the little finger of the same hand	No change
Inversion	Tilting the foot outward, with the lateral side of the foot lowered	No change
Eversion	Tilting the foot inward, with the medial side of the foot lowered	No change
Dorsiflexion	Flexing the foot at the ankle so that the toes move toward the chest	Decreased
Plantar flexion	Moving the foot at the ankle so that the toes move away from the chest	Increased
Elevation	Raising a body part in an upward direction	No change
Depression	Lowering a body part	No change
Protraction	Moving a body part anteriorly along its own axis (parallel to the ground)	No change
Retraction	Moving a body part posteriorly along its own axis (parallel to the ground)	No change
Gliding	One joint surface moves over another joint surface in a circular or angular nature	No change

Ligaments connect bones to each other at the joint level and encase the joint capsule. Ligaments act to support purposeful joint movement and to prevent detrimental joint movement.

HEALTH HISTORY

Medical History

Rheumatoid arthritis, osteoarthritis, osteoporosis, Paget's disease, gout, ankylosing spondylitis, osteogenesis imperfecta, joint prosthesis loosening or malfunction, aseptic necrosis, chronic low back pain, herniated nucleus pulposus, chronic muscle spasms or cramps, scoliosis, poliomyelitis, polymyalgia rheumatica, osteomalacia, rickets, Marfan's syndrome, scleroderma, spina bifida, congenital deformity, muscular dystrophy (MD), multiple sclerosis (MS), myasthenia gravis, amyotrophic lateral sclerosis (ALS), Guillain-Barré syndrome, Reiter's syndrome, carpal tunnel syndrome, paralysis

Surgical History

Joint aspiration, therapeutic joint arthroscopy, joint arthroplasty, joint replacement, synovectomy, meniscectomy, arthrodesis, open reduction and internal fixation (ORIF), discectomy, laminectomy, spinal fusion, Harrington rod placement or other spinal instrumentation, torn rotator cuff repair, debridement, limb or digit amputation, limb or digit reattachment

Injuries and Accidents

Fracture, dislocation, subluxation, tendon tear, tendonitis, muscle contusion, joint strain or sprain, spinal cord injury, torn rotator cuff, traumatic amputation of a digit or limb, crush injury, back injury (including herniated vertebral disc), sports-related injury (e.g., golf elbow, pitcher's shoulder), cartilage damage

Special Needs

Amputation, hemiplegia, paraplegia, quadriplegia, need for brace or splint, limb in a cast, need for supportive devices, muscle atrophy

Work Environment

Manual movement of heavy objects (lifting, pushing, pulling), duties requiring repetitive motions (e.g., keyboard use), duties requiring prolonged standing or ambulation, use of hazardous equipment, availability and use of safety equipment (e.g., lifting equipment, back support vest or brace)

Health Check-ups

Immunizations up to date (especially polio and tetanus), DEXA scan

Equipment

- Measuring tape (cloth type that will not stretch)
- Goniometer (protractor-type instrument with two movable arms to measure the angle of a skeletal joint when assessing range of motion)
- Sphygmomanometer and blood pressure cuff
- Felt-tip marker

NURSING CHECKLIST

General Approach to Musculoskeletal Assessment

1. Assist the patient into a position of comfort.
2. Be clear in your instructions to the patient if you are asking the patient to perform a certain body movement to or to assume a certain position. Demonstrate the desired movement if necessary.
3. Notify the patient before touching or manipulating a painful body part.
4. Inspection, palpation, ROM, and muscle testing are performed on the major skeletal muscles and joints of the body in a cephalocaudal, proximal-to-distal manner. Always compare paired muscles and joints.
5. Examine nonaffected body parts before affected body parts.
6. Avoid unnecessary or excessive manipulation of a painful body part. If the patient complains of pain, stop the aggravating motion.
7. Some musculoskeletal disorders affect the patient more during certain times of the day. Arrange for the follow-up appointment to be during the patient's time of optimal function.

Assessment of the Musculoskeletal System

General Assessment

Overall Appearance

E 1. Obtain height and weight (see Chapter 7).
2. Observe the patient's ability to tolerate weight bearing; assess the amount of weight bearing placed on each of the lower limbs.
3. Identify obvious structural abnormalities (e.g., atrophy, scoliosis, kyphosis, amputated limbs, contractures).
4. Note indications of discomfort (e.g., restricted weight bearing or movement, frequent shifting of position, facial grimacing, excessive fatigue).

N **Body height and weight should be appropriate for age and gender (see Chapter 7). Structural defects should be absent. There should be no outward indications of discomfort during rest, weight bearing, or joint movement. There should be a distinct and symmetrical relationship between the limbs, torso, and pelvis.**

A Excessively tall, short, overweight, or underweight

P Marfan's syndrome, dwarfism, obesity, malnutrition

A Height loss

P Severe osteoporosis, ankylosing spondylitis

A Structural defects

P Acromegaly, congenital defect, surgery, trauma, scoliosis, kyphosis

Posture

E 1. Stand in front of the patient.
2. Instruct the patient to stand with the feet together.
3. Observe the structural and spatial relationship of the head, torso, pelvis, and limbs. Assess for symmetry of the shoulders, scapulae, and iliac crests.
4. Ask the patient to sit; observe the patient's posture.

N **In the standing position, the torso and head are upright. The head is midline and perpendicular to the horizontal line of the shoulders and pelvis. The shoulders and hips are level, the scapulae and iliac crests symmetric. The arms hang freely from the shoulders. The feet are aligned, and the toes point forward.**

The extremities are proportional to overall body size and shape, and like limbs are symmetric. The knees face forward and are symmetric and level. There is usually less than a 2-inch space between the knees when the patient stands with the feet together and facing forward. When full growth is reached, arm span is equal to height. In the sitting position, both feet should be placed firmly on the floor surface, and the toes should point forward.

A Forward slouching of the shoulders

P Poor postural habits resulting in false thoracic kyphosis

Gait and Mobility

E 1. Instruct the patient to walk normally across the room, then to walk on the toes, and then to walk on the heels.
2. Instruct the patient to walk in a heel-to-toe fashion (tandem walking).
3. Instruct the patient to walk first forward and then backward.
4. Instruct the patient to side step first to the left and then to the right.
5. Instruct the patient to close the eyes and to ambulate forward several steps.
6. Observe the patient during transfer between the standing and sitting positions.

N **Walking is initiated in one smooth, rhythmic action, with the heel and then the ball of the same foot striking the floor. The patient remains erect and balanced during all stages of gait. Step height and length are symmetric for each foot. The arms swing freely at the side of the torso but in opposite direction to the movement of the legs. The lower limbs are able to bear full body weight during standing and ambulation. The patient should be able to transfer easily to various positions.**

A/P See Table 18-2.

Inspection

Muscle Size and Shape

E 1. Survey the overall appearance of the muscle mass.
2. Instruct the patient to contract the muscle without inducing movement (isometric muscle contraction), relax the muscle, and contract the muscle again.
3. Observe for any obvious muscle contraction.

N **Muscle contour is affected by the exercise and activity patterns of the individual. Muscle shape may be accentuated in certain body areas (e.g., the limbs and upper torso) but should be symmetric. There may be hypertrophy in the dominant hand. During muscle contraction, you should be able to see sudden tautness of the muscle area. Termination of muscle tautness should be associated with muscle relaxation. There is no involuntary movement.**

A Atrophy: a reduction in muscle size and shape

P Immobility (disuse atrophy), sedentary lifestyle (generalized atrophy), hemiparesis, paraplegia, quadriplegia (local atrophy), following removal of a limb cast or splint

A Involuntary muscle movement

P See Table 18-3.

Joint Contour and Periarticular Tissue

E 1. Observe the shape of the joint when the joint is in its neutral anatomic position.
2. Visually inspect the 5 to 7.5 cm (2 to 3 inches) of skin and subcutaneous tissue surrounding the joint. Assess the periarticular area for erythema, swelling, bruising, nodules, deformities, masses, skin atrophy, and skin breakdown.

N **Joint contour should be somewhat flat in extension and smooth and**

TABLE 18-2 Examples of Abnormal Gait Patterns

TYPE OF ABNORMAL GAIT	ETIOLOGY	DESCRIPTION
Antalgic	Degenerative joint disease of the hip or knee	Limited weight bearing is placed on an affected leg in an attempt to limit discomfort.
Short leg	Discrepancy in leg length, flexion contracture of the hip or knee, congenital hip dislocation	A limp is present during ambulation unless shoes have been adapted to compensate for length discrepancy.
Spastic hemiplegia	Cerebral palsy, unilateral upper motor neuron lesion (e.g., stroke)	Extension of one lower extremity with plantar flexion and foot inversion; arm is flexed at the elbow, wrist, and fingers. The patient walks by swinging the affected leg in a semicircle. The foot is not lifted off the floor. The affected arm does not swing with the gait.
Scissors	Multiple sclerosis, bilateral upper motor neuron disease	Adduction at the knee level produces short, slow steps. Gait is uncoordinated, stiff, and jerky. The foot is dragged across the floor in a semicircle.
Cerebellar ataxia	Cerebellar disease	Gait is broad based and uncoordinated, and the patient appears to stagger and sway during ambulation.
Sensory ataxia	Disorders of peripheral nerves, dorsal roots, and posterior column that interfere with proprioceptive input	Stance is broad based. Patient lifts feet up too high and abruptly slaps them on the floor, heel first. The patient watches the floor carefully to help ensure correct foot placement because the patient is unaware of position in space.

continues

TABLE 18-2 Examples of Abnormal Gait Patterns *continued*

TYPE OF ABNORMAL GAIT	ETIOLOGY	DESCRIPTION
Festinating	Parkinson's disease	Decreased step height and length, but increased step speed, resulting in "shuffling" (feet barely clearing the floor). Patient's posture is stooped, and patient appears to hesitate both in initiation and in termination of ambulation. Rigid body position, with flexion of the knees during standing and ambulation.
Steppage or footdrop	Peroneal nerve injury, paralysis of the dorsiflexor muscles, damage to spinal nerve roots L5 and S1 from poliomyelitis	Hip and knee flexion are needed for step height in order to lift the foot off the floor. Instead of placing the heel of the foot on the floor first, the whole sole of the foot is slapped on the floor at once. May be unilateral or bilateral.
Apraxic	Alzheimer's disease, frontal lobe tumors	Patient has difficulty with walking despite intact motor and sensory systems. The patient is unable to initiate walking, as if stuck to the floor. After walking is initiated, the gait is slow and shuffling.
Trendelenburg	Developmental dysplasia of hip, muscular dystrophy	During ambulation, pelvis of the unaffected side drops when weight bearing is performed on the affected side. When both hips are affected, a "waddling" gait may be evident.

TABLE 18-3 Involuntary Muscle Movements

TYPE	DESCRIPTION
Fasciculation	Visible twitching of a group of muscle fibers that may be stimulated by the tapping of a muscle.
Fibrillation	Ineffective, uncoordinated muscle contraction that resembles quivering.
Spasm	Sudden muscle contraction. A cramp is a muscle spasm that is strong and painful. Clonic muscle spasms are contractions that alternate with a period of muscle relaxation. A tonic muscle spasm is a sustained contraction with a period of relaxation.
Tetany	Paroxysmal tonic muscle spasms, usually of the extremities. The face and jaw may also be affected by spasm. Tetany may be associated with discomfort.
Chorea	Rapid, irregular, and jerky muscle contractions of random muscle groups. It is unpredictable and without purpose. It can involve the face, upper trunk, and limbs. Sometimes, the patient tries to incorporate the movement into voluntary movement, which may appear grotesque and exaggerated. The patient may have difficulty with chewing, speaking, and swallowing.
Tremors	A period of continuous shaking due to muscle contractions. Although the quality of the tremors will be influenced by the cause, the amplitude and the frequency should remain the same. Tremors may be fine or coarse, rapid or slow, continuous or intermittent. They may be exacerbated during rest and attempts at purposeful movements, or by certain body positions.
Tic	Sudden, rapid muscle spasms of the upper trunk, face, or shoulders. The action is often repetitive and may decrease during purposeful movement. It can be persistent or limited in nature.
Ballism	Jerky, twisting movements due to strong muscle contraction.
Athetosis	Slow, writhing, twisting type of movement. The patient is unable to sustain any part of the body in one position. The movements are most often in the fingers, hands, face, throat, and tongue, although any part of the body can be affected. The movements are generally slower than in chorea.
Dystonia	Similar to athetosis but differing in the duration of the postural abnormality, and involving large muscles such as the trunk. The patient may present with an overflexed or overextended posture of the hand, pulling of the head to one side, torsion of the spine, inversion of the foot, or closure of the eyes along with a fixed grimace.
Myoclonus	A rapid, irregular contraction of a muscle or group of muscles, such as the type of jerking movement that occurs when drifting off to sleep.
Tremors at rest	Asymmetrical and coarse movements that disappear or diminish with action. They tend to diminish or cease with purposeful movement.
Action tremors	Symmetrical or asymmetrical movements that increase in states of fatigue, weakness, drug withdrawal, hypocalcemia, uremia, or hepatic disease. This type of tremor may be induced in a normal individual when he or she is required to maintain a posture that demands extremes of power or precision. Action tremors are also called postural tremors.
Intention tremors	These tremors may appear only on voluntary movement of a limb and may intensify on termination of movement.
Asterixis	This is a variant of a tremor. The rate of limb flexion and extension is irregular, slow, and of wide amplitude. The outstretched limb temporarily loses muscle tone.

rounded in flexion. Bilateral joints should be symmetric in position and appearance. There should be no observable erythema, swelling, bruising, nodules, deformities, masses, skin atrophy, or skin breakdown.

A Joint enlargement (inflammation)

P Rheumatoid arthritis, gout, sepsis, trauma

A Joint deformity

P Immobility (contractures), joint dislocation (complete dislodgment of bone from its joint cavity) or subluxation (partial dislodgment of a bone from its joint cavity)

A Alteration in periarticular skin and subcutaneous tissue

P Strain, sprain, contusion, dislocation, fracture within or near the joint capsule, trauma

Palpation

Muscle Tone

E **1.** Palpate the muscle by applying light pressure with the finger pads of the dominant hand.
2. Note the change in muscle shape as the muscle belly (the wide, central aspect of the muscle) tapers off to become a tendon.
3. Instruct the patient to alternately perform muscle relaxation and isometric muscle contraction. Note the change in palpable muscle tone between relaxation and isometric contraction.
4. Palpate the muscle belly during contraction induced by voluntary movement of a nearby joint.
5. Perform passive ROM to all extremities and note whether these movements are smooth and sustained.

N **On palpation, the muscle should feel smooth and firm, even during muscle relaxation. Normal muscle tone provides light resistance to passive stretch. Muscle tone increases in response to anxiety and excitable states and decreases during rest and sleep. The wide central aspect of the muscle (the muscle belly) should be palpable, and you should detect a change in its shape as it tapers down to become a tendon. The hypertrophied muscle has a distinctive contour and displays muscle tautness even during relaxation.**

A Hypotonicity (flaccidity): decrease in muscle tone

P Diseases involving the muscles, anterior horn cells, or peripheral nerves

A Spasticity: increase in muscle tension on passive stretching

P Upper motor neuron dysfunction

A Muscle spasm: persistent muscle contraction without relaxation

P Postfracture, paralysis, electrolyte imbalance, peripheral vascular disease, cerebral palsy

A Crepitus: grating or crackling sensation caused by two rough musculoskeletal surfaces rubbing together

P Shaft fracture due to trauma or loss of bone density

A Muscle masses

P Muscle rupture, tendon rupture, displaced fracture, complete dislocation

Joints

E **1.** With the joint in its neutral anatomic position, use the finger pads of the dominant hand to palpate the joint by applying light pressure beginning 5 to 7 cm (2 to 3 inches) away from the center of the joint.
2. Palpate from the periphery inward to the center of the joint.
3. Note any swelling, pain, tenderness, warmth, and nodules.

N **When the major skeletal joints are palpated in their neutral anatomic positions, external joint contour feels smooth, strong, and firm. The area surrounding the joint (periarticular tissue) is free of swelling, pain, tenderness, warmth, and nodules. As the joint is moved through its normal range of motion, it**

articulates in proper alignment and without any visible or palpable deformity. Palpation of joint movement yields a smooth sensation without grating or popping.

A Bony enlargement or bony deformities

P Urate deposits associated with gout, synovitis

A Subcutaneous nodules

P Rheumatoid arthritis, tophi nodules secondary to gout

A Periarticular warmth

P Joint inflammation, gout, trauma, infection

A Crepitus

P Degenerative joint disease (DJD), rheumatoid arthritis

Range of Motion (ROM)

E **1.** Instruct the patient to move the joint through each of its various ROM movements.

2. Note the angle of each joint movement.

3. Note any pain, tenderness, and crepitus.

4. If the patient is unable to perform active ROM, then passively move each joint through its ROM.

5. Always stop if the patient complains of pain, and never push a joint beyond its anatomic angle.

N **Refer to the specific sections on joints for the ROM for each joint movement (see Table 18-1).**

A Inability to voluntarily and comfortably move a joint in the directions and to the degrees that are considered normal

P Degenerative joint disease, rheumatoid arthritis, joint trauma; also refer to specific muscle joint sections

Muscle Strength

Each muscle group is assessed for strength via the same movements used to assess ROM.

E **1.** Note whether muscle groups are strong and equal.

2. Always compare right and left sides of paired muscle groups.

3. Note involuntary movements.

N **Normal muscle strength allows for complete, voluntary joint ROM against both gravity and moderate to full resistance. Muscle strength is equal bilaterally. There is no observed involuntary muscle movement. See Table 18-4 for muscle strength grading.**

TABLE 18-4 Muscle Strength Grading Scale

FUNCTIONAL ABILITY DESCRIPTION	SCALE (%)	0–5/5 SCALE
Complete range of joint motion against both gravity and full manual resistance from the nurse.	100%	5/5 Normal (N)
Complete range of joint motion against both gravity and moderate manual resistance from the nurse.	75%	4/5 Good (G)
Complete range of joint motion possible only without manual resistance from the nurse.	50%	3/5 Fair (F)
Complete range of joint motion possible only with the joint supported by the nurse to eliminate the force of gravity and without any manual resistance from the nurse.	25%	2/5 Poor (P)
Muscle contraction detectable but insufficient to move the joint even when the forces of both gravity and manual resistance have been eliminated.	10%	1/5 Trace (Tr)
Complete absence of visible and palpable muscle contraction.	0%	0/5 None (0)

A Significant decrease in skeletal muscle strength (complete joint ROM impossible or possible only without resistance or gravity)

P General atrophy, severe fatigue, malnutrition, muscle relaxant medications (e.g., Valium), long-term steroid use, deteriorating neuromuscular disorders (ALS, MD, MS, myasthenia gravis, Guillain-Barré syndrome)

A One-sided muscle weakness or paralysis (hemiplegia)

P Cerebrovascular accident, brain tumor, head trauma

Examination of Joints

Temporomandibular Joint

E **1.** Stand in front of the patient.
2. Inspect the right and left temporomandibular joints.
3. Palpate the temporomandibular joints.
- **a.** Place your index and middle fingers over the joints.
- **b.** Ask the patient to open and close the mouth.
- **c.** Feel the depressions into which your fingers move when the patient's mouth is open.
- **d.** Note the smoothness with which the mandibles move.
- **e.** Note any audible or palpable clicking as the mouth opens.

4. Assess ROM. Ask the patient to:
- **a.** Open the mouth as wide as possible.
- **b.** Push out the lower jaw.
- **c.** Move the jaw from side to side.

5. Palpate the strength of the masseter and temporalis muscles as the patient clenches the teeth to assess cranial nerve (CN) V.

N **It is normal to hear or palpate a click when the mouth opens. The mouth can normally open 3 to 6 cm with ease. The lower jaw protrudes without deviating to the side and can move 1 to 2 cm laterally.**

A Pain, limited ROM, crepitus

P Malocclusion, arthritis, dislocation, poorly fitting dentures, myofacial dysfunction, trauma

Cervical Spine

E **1.** Stand behind the patient.
2. Inspect the position of the cervical spine.
3. Palpate the spinous processes of the cervical spine and the muscles of the neck.
4. Stand in front of the patient.
5. Assess ROM of the cervical spine. Ask the patient to:
- **a.** Touch the chin to the chest (flexion).
- **b.** Look up at the ceiling (hyperextension).
- **c.** Move each ear to the shoulder on its respective side without elevating the shoulder (lateral bending).
- **d.** Turn the head to each side to look at the shoulder (rotation).

6. Assess the strength of the cervical spine by having the patient repeat the movements outlined in step 5 while you apply opposing force. This process also assesses the function of CN XI.

N **The cervical spine's alignment is straight, and the head is held erect. Normal ROM of the cervical spine is—flexion: 45°; hyperextension: 55°; lateral bending: 40° to each side; and rotation: 70° to each side.**

A Neck that is not erect and straight

P Degenerative joint disease of the cervical vertebrae, torticollis

A A change in neck size

P Klippel-Feil syndrome: congenital absence of one or more cervical vertebrae and fusion of the upper cervical vertebrae resulting in bilateral elevation of the scapulae and a shortened neck appearance and possibly accompanied by a low hairline, neck webbing, and decreased neck mobility

A Inability to perform ROM and pain and tenderness on palpation

P Osteoarthritis, neck injury, disc degeneration (in aging patients and occupational stress), degenerative joint disease, spondylosis

Shoulders

E **1.** Stand in front of the patient.
2. Inspect the size, shape, and symmetry of the shoulders.
3. Move behind the patient and inspect the scapula for size, shape, and symmetry.
4. Palpate the shoulders and surrounding muscles.
a. Move from the sternoclavicular joint along the clavicle to the acromioclavicular joint.
b. Palpate the acromion process, the subacromial area, the greater tubercle of the humerus, the anterior aspect of the glenohumeral joint, and the biceps groove.
5. Assess ROM of the shoulders. Instruct the patient to:
a. Place the arms at the sides, elbows extended, and move the arms forward in an arc (forward flexion).
b. Move the arms backward in an arc as far as possible (hyperextension).
c. Place the arms at sides, elbows extended, and move both arms out to the side in an arc until the palms touch together overhead (abduction).
d. Move one arm at a time in an arc toward the midline and cross it as far as possible (adduction).
e. Place the hands behind the back and reach up trying to touch the scapula (internal rotation).
f. Place both hands behind the head and flex the elbows (external rotation).
g. Shrug the shoulders. Shrugging assesses CN XI function.
6. Assess the strength of the shoulders by applying opposing force while the patient performs the ROM movements outlined in step 5.

N **The shoulders are equal in height. There is no fluid palpable in the shoulder area. Crepitus is absent. Normal ROM of the shoulder is—forward flexion: 180°; hyperextension: 50°; abduction: 180°; adduction: 50°; internal rotation: 90°; and external rotation: 90°.**

A Increased outward prominence of the scapula (winging)

P Serratus anterior muscle injury or weakness

A Decreased movement, pain with movement, swelling from fluid, and asymmetry

P Degenerative joint disease, bursitis, osteoarthritis, injury, acromioclavicular joint separation (separated shoulder), shoulder subluxation, dislocation, immobility

Elbows

E **1.** Stand to the side of the elbow being examined.
2. Support the patient's forearm on the side that is being examined (at an angle of approximately 70°).
3. Inspect the elbow in flexed and extended positions. Note the olecranon process and the grooves on each side of the olecranon process.
4. Using your thumb and middle fingers, palpate the elbow. Note the olecranon process, the olecranon bursa, the groove on each side of the olecranon process, and the medial and lateral epicondyles of the humerus.
5. Assess ROM of the elbows. Instruct the patient to:
a. Bend the elbow (flexion).
b. Straighten the elbow (extension).
c. Hold the arm straight out, bend at the elbow, and turn the palm upward toward the ceiling (supination).
d. Turn the palm downward toward the floor (pronation).

6. Assess the strength of the elbow:
   a. Use your nondominant hand to stabilize the patient's arm at the elbow. With your dominant hand, grasp the patient's wrist.
   b. Instruct the patient to flex the elbow (i.e., pull it toward the chest) while you apply opposing resistance.
   c. Instruct the patient to extend the elbow (i.e., push it away from the chest) while you apply opposing resistance.
   d. Repeat with other arm.

N **The elbows are at the same height and are symmetric in appearance. Normal ROM of the elbow is—flexion: 160°; extension: 0°; supination: 90°; and pronation: 90°.**

A Dislocation or subluxation of the elbow: asymmetric elbows, forearm not in usual alignment, associated pain

P Sports-related injuries, falls, motor vehicle accidents

A Localized tenderness and pain on elbow flexion, extension, or both

P Epicondylitis from repetitive motions of the forearm (e.g., swinging a tennis racquet, hammering, using a screwdriver); radial head fractures; flexion contracture of the elbow

A Red, warm, swollen, tender areas in the grooves beside the olecranon process; palpable synovial fluid

P Inflammatory processes (gouty arthritis, bursitis, rheumatoid arthritis, SLE)

A Flexion contracture of the elbow

P Seen with hemiparesis following a CVA

Wrists and Hands

E 1. Stand in front of the patient.

2. Inspect the wrists and the palmar and dorsal aspects of the hands. Note shape, position, contour, and number of fingers.

3. Inspect the thenar eminence (the rounded prominence at the base of the thumb).

4. Support the patient's hand in your two hands, with your fingers underneath the patient's hands and your thumbs on the dorsa of the patient's hands.

5. Palpate the joints of the wrists by moving your thumbs from side to side. Feel the natural indentations.

6. Palpate the joints of the hand:
   a. Use your thumbs to palpate the metacarpophalangeal joints, which are immediately distal to and on each side of the knuckles.
   b. Between your thumb and index finger, gently pinch the sides of the proximal and distal interphalangeal joints.

7. Assess ROM of the wrists and hands. Ask the patient to:
   a. Straighten the hand (extension) and bend it up at the wrist toward the ceiling (hyperextension).
   b. Bend the wrist toward the palmar surface (flexion).
   c. Bend the fingers up toward the ceiling at the metacarpophalangeal joints (hyperextension).
   d. Bend the fingers toward the floor at the metacarpophalangeal joints (flexion).
   e. Place the hands on a flat surface and move them side to side (radial deviation is movement toward the thumb, and ulnar deviation is movement toward the little finger) without moving the elbow.
   f. Make a fist with the thumb on the outside of the clenched fingers.
   g. Spread the fingers apart.
   h. Touch the thumb to each fingertip. Touch the thumb to the base of the little finger.

8. Assess the strength of the wrists. Ask the patient to:
   a. Place the arm on a table and supinate the forearm. (Stabilize the forearm by placing your nondominant hand on it.)

b. Flex the wrist while you apply resistance with your dominant hand.

c. Extend the wrist while you apply resistance.

9. Assess the strength of the fingers. Ask the patient to:

a. Spread the fingers apart while you apply resistance.

b. Push the fingers together while you apply resistance.

10. Assess the strength of the hand grasp. Ask the patient to:

a. Grasp your dominant index and middle fingers in his or her dominant hand and grasp your nondominant index and middle fingers in his or her nondominant hand.

b. Squeeze your fingers as hard as possible.

c. Release the grasps.

N **There are five fingers on each hand. Normal ROM of the wrists is—extension: 0°; hyperextension: 70°; flexion: 90° radial deviation: 20°; and ulnar deviation: 55°; Normal ROM for the metacarpophalangeal joints is—hyperextension: 30° and flexion: 90°.**

A Polydactyly (extra fingers), syndactyly (webbing between the fingers), loss of fingers

P Congenital (polydactyly and syndactyly), traumatic amputation

A Bony enlargement or bony deformities of the joints of the hand

P Osteoarthritis: bony enlargement of the proximal interphalangeal joint (Bouchard's node) and the distal interphalangeal joint (Heberden's node) of the finger; rheumatoid arthritis; ulnar deviation; swan neck deformities

A Ganglion cyst: round growth near the tendons or joint capsule of the wrist

P Benign growth of unknown etiology

A Muscular atrophy of the thenar eminence

P Medial nerve compression seen in carpal tunnel syndrome

A Flexion of fingers

P Dupuytren's contracture

A Severe flexion ankylosis of the wrist

P Rheumatoid arthritis or extended disuse

A Wrist drop, inability to flex wrist

P Radial nerve damage

A Inability to prevent spreading of fingers

P Ulnar nerve damage

A Weakness of opposition of thumb

P Median nerve damage

Hips

E 1. While the patient is standing, inspect the iliac crests, the size and symmetry of the buttocks, and the number of gluteal folds.

2. Observe the patient's gait.

3. Assist the patient to a supine position on the examination table, with the patient's legs straight and the feet pointing toward the ceiling.

4. Palpate the hip joints.

5. Assess ROM of the hips. Ask the patient to:

a. Raise a straight leg (i.e., with the knee extended) off the examination table (hip flexion with knee straight). The other leg should remain on the table.

b. With the knee flexed, raise the leg off the examination table and toward the chest as far as possible (hip flexion with knee flexed). The other leg should remain on the table. This is called the Thomas test.

c. Flex the hip and knee. Move the flexed leg medially while moving the foot outward (internal rotation).

d. Flex the hip and knee. Move the flexed leg laterally while moving the foot medially (external rotation).

e. With the knee straight, swing the leg away from the midline (abduction).

f. With the knee straight, swing the leg toward the midline (adduction).

g. Roll over onto the abdomen and assume a prone position.

h. From the hip, move the leg back as far as possible while keeping the pelvis on the table (hyperextension). This can also be performed while the patient is standing.

6. Assist the patient to a supine position.

7. Assess the strength of the hips.

a. Place the palm of your hand on the anterior thigh and above the knee. Instruct the patient to raise the leg against your resistance. Repeat on the other leg.

b. Place the palm of your hand behind and above the knee. Instruct the patient to lower the leg against your resistance. Repeat on the other leg.

c. Place your hands on the lateral aspects of the patient's legs at the level of the knees. Instruct the patient to move the legs apart against your resistance.

d. Place your hands on the medial aspects of the patient's legs just above the knees. Instruct the patient to move the legs together against your resistance.

N **Normal ROM of the hips is—flexion with knee straight: 90°; flexion with knee flexed: 120°; internal rotation: 40°; external rotation: 45°; abduction: 45°; adduction: 30°; and hyperextension: 15°.**

A Leg that is externally rotated and painful on movement

P Hip fracture, which usually results from a fall (affected leg may also be shorter)

A Positive Thomas test: inability to flex one knee and hip while simultaneously maintaining the other leg in full extension

P Flexion contractures of the hip joint (degenerative joint diseases)

Knees

E **1.** With the patient standing, note the position of the knees in relation to each other as well as to the hips, thighs, ankles, and feet.

2. Ask the patient to sit on the examination table and to flex and rest the knees at the edge of the table.

3. Inspect the contour of the knees. Note the normal depressions around each patella.

4. Inspect the suprapatellar pouches and prepatellar bursae.

5. Note the quadriceps muscles (located on the anterior thighs).

6. Palpate the knees. The patient may assume a supine position if it is more comfortable.

a. With your thumb on one side of the knee, and the other four fingers on the other side of the knee, grasp the anterior thigh approximately 10 cm above the patella.

b. As you palpate, gradually move your hand down the suprapatellar pouch.

7. Palpate the tibiofemoral joints. It is best to flex the patient's knee 90° when performing this palpation.

a. Place both thumbs on the knee and wrap the fingers around the knee posteriorly.

b. Press in with the thumbs as you palpate the tibial margins.

c. Palpate the lateral collateral ligament.

8. Assess ROM of the knees. Ask the patient to stand and:

a. Bend the knee (flexion)

b. Straighten the knee (extension). (The patient may also be able to hyperextend the knee.)

9. With the patient seated and the patient's legs hanging off table, assess the strength of the knees.

a. Ask the patient to bend the knee. Place your nondominant hand under the knee and place your dominant hand over the ankle.

b. Instruct the patient to straighten the leg against your resistance.

> **Nursing Tip**
>
> **Remembering Genu Varum versus Genu Valgum**
>
> Genu varum: Let the *r* remind you that there is **r**oom between the patient's knees or that the knees are apart.
>
> Genu valgum: Let the *g* remind you that the patient's knees are together or that they are stuck together like glue.

c. Ask the patient to flex the knee to approximately 45° and to place the foot on the examination table. Place one hand under the knee and place the other hand over the ankle.

d. Instruct the patient to keep the foot on the examination table despite your attempts to straighten the leg.

N **The knees are in alignment with each other and do not protrude medially or laterally. Normal ROM of the knees is—flexion: 130° and extension: 0°. In some cases, hyperextension up to 15° is possible.**

A Alteration in lower limb alignment

P Genu valgum (knock knees), genu varum (bow legs)

A Knee effusion

P Baker's cyst

Ankles and Feet

E **1.** Inspect the ankles and feet as the patient stands, walks, and sits (bearing no weight).

2. Inspect the alignment of the feet and toes in relation to the lower legs.

3. Inspect shape and position of the toes.

4. Assist the patient to a supine position on the examination table.

5. Stand at the foot of the patient.

6. Palpate the ankles and feet.

a. Grasp the heel with the fingers of both hands. Palpate the posterior aspect of the heel at the calcaneus.

b. Use your thumbs to palpate the medial malleolus (bony prominence on the distal medial aspect of the tibia) and the lateral malleolus (bony prominence on the distal lateral aspect of the fibula).

c. Move your hands forward and palpate the anterior aspects of the ankle and foot, particularly at the joints.

d. Palpate the inferior aspect of the foot over the plantar fascia.

e. Use your finger pads to palpate the Achilles tendon.

f. With your thumb and index finger, palpate each metatarsophalangeal joint.

g. Between your thumb and index finger, palpate the medial and lateral surfaces of each interphalangeal joint.

7. Assess ROM of the ankles and feet. Ask the patient to:

a. Point the toes toward the chest by moving the ankle (dorsiflexion).

b. Point the toes toward the floor by moving the ankle (plantar flexion).

c. Turn the soles of the feet outward (eversion).

d. Turn the soles of the foot inward (inversion).

e. Curl the toes toward the floor (flexion).

f. Spread the toes apart (abduction).

g. Move the toes together (adduction).

8. Assess the strength of the ankles and feet.

a. Assist the patient to a supine position on the examination table, with the patient's legs extended and feet slightly apart.

b. Stand at the foot of the examination table.

c. Place your left hand on top of the patient's right foot and place your right hand on top of the patient's left foot.
d. Ask the patient to point the toes toward the chest (dorsiflexion) despite your resistance.
e. Place your left hand on the sole of the patient's right foot and place your right hand on the sole of the patient's left foot.
f. Ask the patient to point the toes downward (plantar flexion) despite your resistance.

N **The foot is in alignment with the lower leg. Normal ROM of the ankles and feet is—dorsiflexion: 20°; plantar flexion: 45°; eversion: 20°; inversion: 30°; abduction: 30°; and adduction: 10°.**

A Alteration in the shape and position of the foot

P Pes varus: foot turned inward (toward the midline); pes valgus: foot turned laterally (away from the midline); pes planus (flat foot): foot with a low longitudinal arch; pes cavus: foot with an exaggerated arch; hallux valgus (bunion): laterally deviated big toe, medially deviated first metatarsal, enlarged metatarsophalangeal joint inflamed from the pressure; hammer toe: flexion of the proximal interphalangeal joint and hyperextension of the distal metatarsophalangeal joint

A Pain over the plantar fascia

P Plantar fasciitis (heel-spur syndrome) is an inflammation of the plantar fascia where it attaches to the calcaneus. The pain tends to be worse first thing in the morning and with prolonged standing, sitting, or walking.

A Swollen, red, painful metatarsophalangeal joint

P Gouty arthritis

A Decreased ROM of ankle

P Ankle sprain, fracture, or trauma

Spine

E 1. Ask the patient to stand and to leave the back of the gown open.
2. Stand behind the patient so that you can visualize the posterior anatomy.
3. Inspect the position and alignment of the spine from a posterior position and a lateral position.
4. Draw an imaginary line:
   a. From the head down through the spinous processes.
   b. Across the top of the scapulae.
   c. Across the top of the iliac crests.
   d. Across the bottom of the gluteal folds.
5. Use your thumb to palpate the spinous processes.
6. Palpate the paravertebral muscles.
7. Assess ROM of the spine. If necessary, use your hands to stabilize the patient's pelvis during the ROM assessment. Ask the patient to:
   a. Bend forward from the waist and touch the toes (flexion).
   b. Bend to each side (lateral bending).
   c. Bend backward (hyperextension).
   d. Twist the shoulders to each side (rotation).

N **The normal spine has cervical concavity, thoracic convexity, and lumbar concavity (Figure 18-3). An imaginary line can be drawn from the head straight down the spinous processes to the gluteal cleft. The imaginary lines drawn from the scapulae, iliac crests, and gluteal folds are symmetric with each other. Normal ROM of the spine is—flexion: 90°; lateral bending: 35°; hyperextension: 30°; and rotation: 30°. As the patient flexes forward, the concavity of the lumbar spine disappears, and the entire back assumes a convex C shape.**

A Abnormal curvature or flattening of the spinal processes

P Scoliosis: lateral curvature of the thoracic or lumbar vertebrae (congenital defect); kyphosis: excessive convexity of the thoracic spine (osteoporosis, ankylosing spondylitis, Paget's dis-

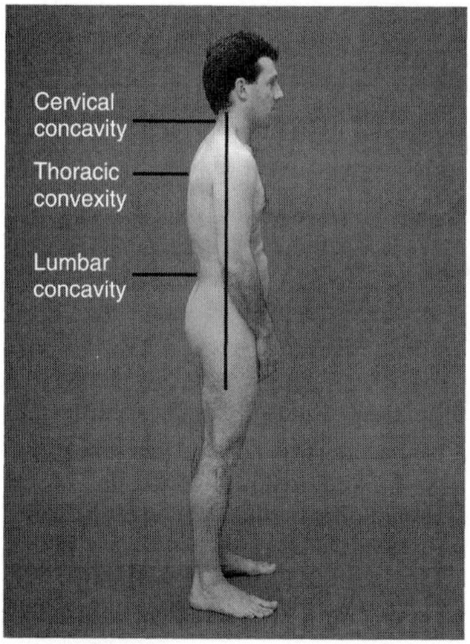

A. Lateral View

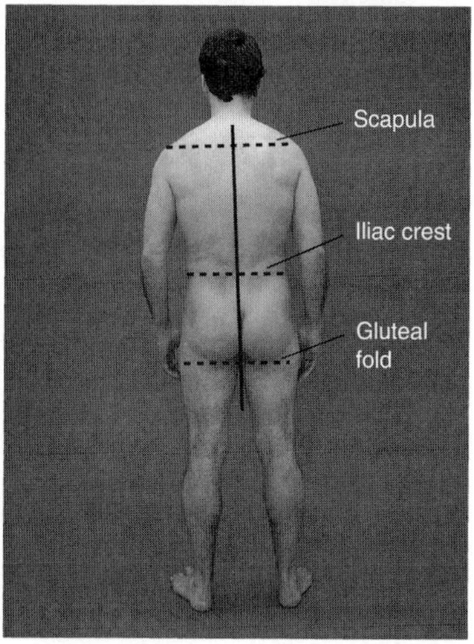

B. Posterior View

Figure 18-3 Alignment of Spinal Landmarks

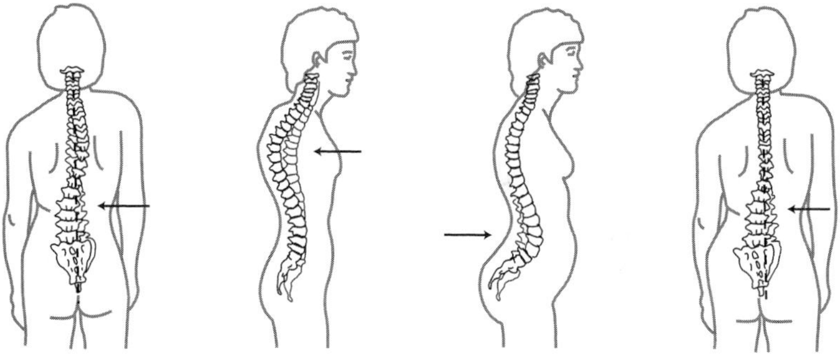

A. Scoliosis B. Kyphosis C. Lordosis D. List

Figure 18-4 Abnormalities of the Spine

ease); lordosis: excessive concavity of the lumbar spine (obesity, pregnancy); list: leaning of the spine (herniated vertebral disc; painful, paravertebral muscle spasms) (Figure 18-4).

A Unequal iliac crests

P Scoliosis, congenital or acquired limb-length discrepancies

A Decreased ROM

P Back injury, osteoarthritis, ankylosing spondylitis

A A list, leaning of the spine

P Herniated vertebral disc, paravertebral muscle spasm

19

Mental Status and Neurological Techniques

Anatomy and Physiology

The nervous system controls all body functions and thought processes. The complex interrelationships among the various divisions of the nervous system permit the body to maintain homeostasis; to receive, interpret, and react to stimuli; and to control voluntary and involuntary processes, including cognition.

Meninges

There are three layers of meninges (protective membranes) between the brain and the skull. The outer layer is the dura mater; underneath this membrane is the subdural space. The second layer is the arachnoid mater. Below the arachnoid mater is the subarachnoid space, where cerebrospinal fluid (CSF) is circulated. The third layer is the pia mater.

Central Nervous System

The brain and the spinal cord compose the central nervous system. The brain is divided into four main components: the cerebrum, the diencephalon, the cerebellum, and the brain stem (Figure 19-1).

The cerebrum is incompletely divided into right and left hemispheres connected by the corpus callosum, which serves as a communication link. The cerebral cortex, or the outermost layer of the cerebrum, is involved in memory storage and recall; conscious understanding of sensation; vision, hearing, and motor function.

The diencephalon, a relay center for the brain, is composed of the thalamus, epithalamus, and hypothalamus. The hypothalamus controls body temperature regulation, pituitary hormone control, autonomic nervous system responses, and affects behavior via its connections with the limbic system.

The cerebellum is divided into two lateral lobes and a medial part called the vermis. The vermis is the part of the cerebellum concerned primarily with maintenance of posture and equilibrium. Each cerebellar hemisphere is responsible for coordination of movement of the ipsilateral side of the body.

The brain stem is divided into the midbrain, the pons, and the medulla oblongata. The midbrain contains the nuclei of cranial nerves III (oculomotor) and IV (trochlear), which are associated with control of eye movements. Sensory and motor nuclei of cranial nerves V (trigeminal), VI (abducens), VII (facial), and VIII (acoustic) are located in the pons. The medulla oblongata contains the nuclei of cranial nerves IX (glossopharyngeal), X (vagus), XI (spinal accessory), and XII (hypoglossal).

The spinal cord is a continuation of the medulla oblongata (Figure 19-2). A cross section of the spinal cord will show gray matter in the shape of an H, and white matter surrounding the gray matter.

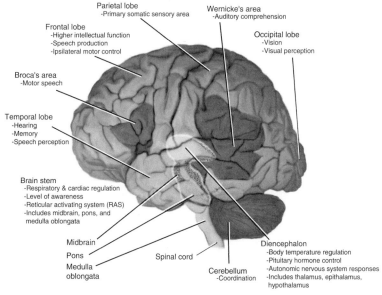

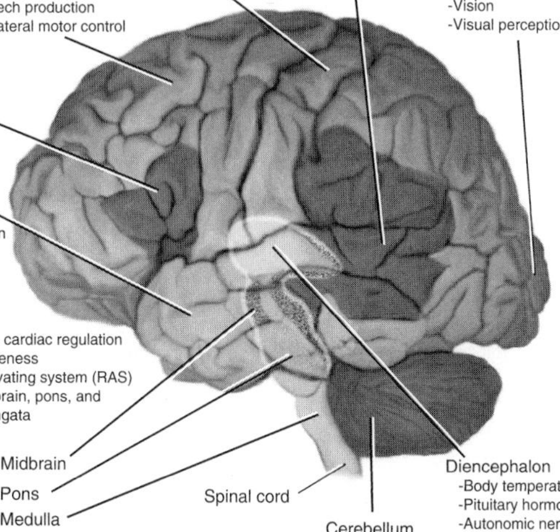

Figure 19-1 The Locations and Functions of the Cerebral Lobes, Brain Stem, Cerebellum, and Diencephalon

Peripheral Nervous System

The peripheral nervous system consists of nervous tissue found outside the central nervous system, including the spinal nerves, cranial nerves, and the autonomic nervous system (ANS).

The 31 pairs of spinal nerves include 8 cervical, 12 thoracic, 5 lumbar, 5 sacral, and 1 coccygeal.

There are 12 pairs of cranial nerves. Table 19-1 summarizes the functions of the cranial nerves.

The ANS is divided into two functionally different subdivisions: the sympathetic and parasympathetic nervous systems. The ANS functions without voluntary control to maintain the body in a state of homeostasis. See Table 19-2 for sympathetic versus parasympathetic responses.

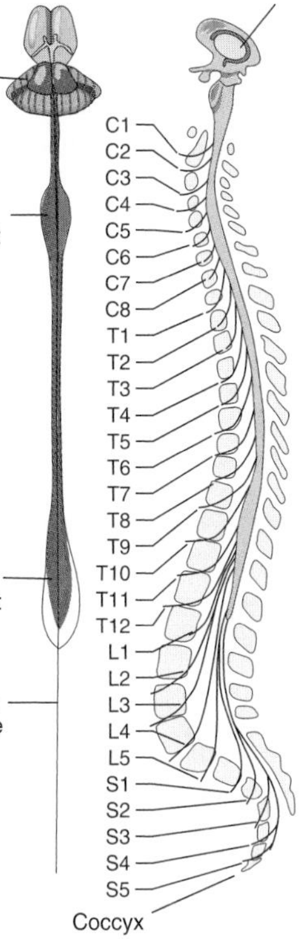

Figure 19-2 The Spinal Cord and Spinal Nerves

TABLE 19-1 The 12 Cranial Nerves and Their Functions

NAME AND NUMBER	FUNCTION
Olfactory (I)	Smell
Optic (II)	Visual acuity, visual fields, funduscopic examination
Oculomotor (III)	Cardinal fields of gaze (EOM movement), eyelid elevation, pupil reaction, doll's eyes phenomenon
Trochlear (IV)	EOM movement
Trigeminal (V)	Motor: strength of temporalis and masseter muscles Sensory: light touch, superficial pain, temperature to face, corneal reflex
Abducens (VI)	EOM movement
Facial (VII)	Motor: facial movements Sensory: taste anterior two-thirds of tongue *Parasympathetic: tears and saliva secretion
Acoustic (VIII)	Cochlear: gross hearing, Weber and Rinne tests Vestibular: vertigo, equilibrium, nystagmus
Glossopharyngeal (IX)	Motor: soft palate and uvula movement, gag reflex, swallowing, guttural and palatal sounds Sensory: taste posterior one-third of tongue *Parasympathetic: carotid reflex, chemoreceptors
Vagus (X)	Motor and Sensory: same as CN IX *Parasympathetic: carotid reflex, stomach and intestinal secretions, peristalsis, involuntary control of bronchi, heart innervation
Spinal Accessory (XI)	Sternocleidomastoid and trapezius muscle movements
Hypoglossal (XII)	Tongue movement, lingual sounds

**Cannot be directly assessed.*
EOM = extraocular muscle; CN = cranial nerve.

The sympathetic nervous system, sometimes called the thoracolumbar system, controls "fight or flight" actions. The parasympathetic nervous system (craniosacral) is responsible for "general housekeeping" of the body.

Reflexes

Reflexes are classified into three main categories: muscle stretch, or deep tendon reflexes (DTRs); superficial reflexes; and pathological reflexes.

TABLE 19-2 Sympathetic versus Parasympathetic Response

SYSTEM	SYMPATHETIC RESPONSE	PARASYMPATHETIC RESPONSE
Neurological	Pupils dilated Heightened awareness	Pupils normal size
Cardiovascular	Increased heart rate Increased myocardial contractility Increased blood pressure	Decreased heart rate Decreased myocardial contractility
Respiratory	Increased respiratory rate Increased respiratory depth Bronchial dilation	Bronchial constriction
Gastrointestinal	Decreased gastric motility Decreased gastric secretions Increased glycogenolysis Decreased insulin production Sphincter contraction	Increased gastric motility Increased gastric secretions Sphincter dilatation
Genitourinary	Decreased urine output Decreased renal blood flow	Normal urine output

Nursing Tip

Cranial Nerve Mnemonics

Mnemonics can help you remember the name of each cranial nerve and whether each nerve has a sensory function, a motor function, or both.

First Letter of Cranial Nerve	Number of Cranial Nerve	Function of Cranial Nerve*
On (olfactory)	I	**S**ome
Old (optic)	II	**S**ay
Olympus's (oculomotor)	III	**M**arry
Towering (trochlear)	IV	**M**oney
Tops (trigeminal)	V	**B**ut
A (abducens)	VI	**M**y
Finn (facial)	VII	**B**rother
And (acoustic)	VIII	**S**ays
German (glossopharyngeal)	IX	**B**ad
Viewed (vagus)	X	**B**usiness
Some (spinal accessory)	XI	**M**arry
Hops (hypoglossal)	XII	**M**oney

*__S__ = sensory nerve; **M** = motor nerve; **B** = both sensory and motor nerve.

HEALTH HISTORY

Medical History

Amyotrophic lateral sclerosis (ALS), multiple sclerosis (MS), tumors, Guillain-Barré syndrome, cerebral aneurysm, arteriovenous malformations (AVM), stroke (CVA), migraines, Alzheimer's disease, myasthenia gravis, congenital defects, metabolic disorders, childhood seizures, head trauma, neuropathies, peripheral vascular disease

Surgical History

Craniotomy, laminectomy, carotid endarterectomy, transsphenoidal hypophysectomy, cordotomy, aneurysmectomy or repair

Medications

Antidepressants, antiseizure medications, narcotics, antianxiety medications

Injuries and Accidents

Closed head injury, chronic subdural hematoma, spinal cord injury, peripheral nerve damage

Family Health History

Congenital defects such as neural tube defects, hydrocephalus, arteriovenous malformations, headaches, epilepsy, Alzheimer's disease

Social History

Alcohol use: patients suffering from chronic alcoholism may exhibit the following abnormal findings:

- Korsakoff's psychosis
- Wernicke's encephalopathy
- Polyneuropathy
- Tremor

Tobacco use: increased risk of stroke

Drug use: seizures

Nursing Alert

Risk Factors for Stroke

Significant risk factors for stroke include:

- Hypertension
- Diabetes mellitus
- Cocaine use
- Cigarette smoking
- Hyperlipidemia
- Atrial fibrillation and flutter
- Sickle cell disease
- IV drug abuse
- Alcohol abuse
- Obesity
- Oral contraceptive use, especially in women who are over age 35 who smoke and have hypertension

Equipment

- Cotton wisp
- Cotton-tipped applicators
- Penlight
- Tongue blade
- Tuning fork (128 Hz or 256 Hz)
- Reflex hammer
- Sterile, 22-gauge needle or sterile safety pin
- Familiar small objects (coins, key, paper clip)
- Vials containing odorous materials (coffee, orange extract, vinegar)
- Vials containing hot and cold water
- Vials containing solutions for tasting: quinine (bitter), glucose solution (sweet), lemon or vinegar (sour), saline (salty)
- Snellen chart or Rosenbaum pocket screener
- Pupil gauge in millimeters

NURSING CHECKLIST

General Approach to Neurological Assessment

1. Greet the patient and explain the assessment techniques that you will be using.
2. Provide a warm, quiet, and well-lit environment.
3. After the mental status examination, instruct the patient to remove all street clothing; provide an examination gown for the patient to put on.
4. Begin the assessment with the patient in a comfortable, upright, sitting position, or, for the patient on bedrest, position the patient comfortably, preferably with the head of the bed elevated, or flat.

Assessment of the Neurological System

A complete neurological assessment includes an assessment of mental status, sensation, cranial nerves (CN), motor functioning, cerebellar function, and reflexes. For patients with minor or intermittent symptoms, a rapid screening assessment may be used as outlined in Table 19-3.

Mental Status

Much of the mental status assessment should be done during the interview. Mental status may also be assessed throughout the neurological assessment. Assess physical appearance and behavior, communication, level of consciousness (LOC), cognitive abilities, and mentation while conversing with the patient.

Physical Appearance and Behavior

Posture and Movements

E 1. Observe the patient's ability to wait patiently.
2. Note whether the patient's posture is relaxed, slumped, or stiff.
3. Observe the patient's movements for control and symmetry.
4. Observe the patient's gait (see Chapter 18).

N **The patient should appear relaxed and display the appropriate amount of concern for the assessment. The patient should exhibit erect posture, a smooth gait, and symmetric body movements.**

A Restlessness, tenseness, pacing

P Anxiety, metabolic disturbances

A Poor eye contact, slow responses, slow gait, slumped posture

P Depression

A Stooped, flexed, or rigid posture; drooping neck; deformities of the spine; tics

P Kyphosis, scoliosis, Parkinson's disease, cerebral palsy, schizophrenia, muscular atrophy, myasthenia gravis, stroke, osteoporosis

Dress, Grooming, and Personal Hygiene

E 1. Note the appearance of the patient's clothing, specifically:
   a. Cleanliness
   b. Condition
   c. Age appropriateness
   d. Weather appropriateness
   e. Appropriateness for the patient's socioeconomic group
2. Observe the patient's personal grooming (hair, skin, nails, and teeth) for:
   a. Adequacy
   b. Symmetry
   c. Odor

N **The patient should be clean and well groomed and should wear appropriate clothing for age, weather, and socioeconomic status.**

TABLE 19-3 Neurological Screening Assessment

ASSESSMENT PARAMETER	ASSESSMENT SKILL	COMMENTS
Mental status	Note general appearance, affect, speech content, memory, logic, judgment, and speech patterns during the history.	If any abnormalities or inconsistencies are evident, perform full mental status assessment.
	Perform Glasgow Coma Scale (GCS) with motor assessment component and pupil assessment.	If GCS <15, perform full assessment of mental status and consciousness. If motor assessment is abnormal or asymmetric, perform complete motor and sensory assessment.
Sensation	Assess pain and vibration in the hands and feet, light touch on the limbs.	If deficits are identified, perform a complete sensory assessment.
Cranial nerves	Assess CN II, III, IV, VI: visual acuity, gross visual fields, funduscopic examination, pupillary reactions, and extraocular movements. Assess CN VII, VIII, IX, X, XII: facial expression, gross hearing, voice, and tongue.	If any abnormalities exist, perform complete assessment of all 12 cranial nerves.
Motor system	• Muscle tone and strength • Abnormal movements • Grasps	If deficits are noted, perform a complete motor system assessment.
Cerebellar function	Observe the patient's: 1. Gait on arrival 2. Ability to: • Walk heel-to-toe • Walk on toes • Walk on heels • Hop in place • Perform shallow knee bends 3. Check Romberg's sign. 4. Finger-to-nose test 5. Fine repetitive movement with hands	If any abnormalities exist, perform complete cerebellar assessment.
Reflexes	Assess the deep tendon reflexes and the plantar reflex.	If an abnormal response is elicited, perform a complete reflex assessment.

A Poor personal hygiene, such as uncombed hair or body odor, and unkempt clothing
P Depression, schizophrenia, dementia
A One-sided differences in grooming
P Cerebrovascular accident (CVA)

Facial Expression

E Observe for appropriateness of, variations in, and symmetry of facial expressions.
N **Facial expressions should be appropriate to the content of the conversation and should be symmetric.**
A Extreme, inappropriate, or unchanging facial expressions or asymmetric facial movements
P Anxiety, depression, Parkinson's disease (unchanging facial expression), lesion in the facial nerve (CN VII)

Affect

E 1. Observe the patient's interaction with you, paying particular attention to both verbal and nonverbal behaviors.
2. Note whether the patient's affect appears labile, blunted, or flat.
3. Note variations in the patient's affect when discussing a variety of topics.
4. Note any extreme emotional responses during the interview.
N **The appropriateness and degree of affect should vary with the topics discussed and the patient's cultural norms and should be reasonable, or eurhythmic (normal).**
A Unresponsive, inappropriate, or blunted affect
P Depression, schizophrenia
A Anger, hostility, paranoia
P Paranoid schizophrenia
A Euphoric, dramatic, disruptive, irrational, or elated behaviors
P Mania

Communication

E 1. Note voice quality including voice volume and pitch.
2. Assess articulation, fluency, and rate of speech by engaging the patient in normal conversation. Ask the patient to repeat words and sentences after you or to name objects you point out.
3. Note the patient's ability to carry out requests during the assessment, such as pointing to objects within the room as requested. Ask questions that require "yes" and "no" responses.
4. Write simple commands for the patient to read and perform: for example, "point to your nose" or "tap your right foot." Reading ability may be influenced by the patient's educational level or by visual impairment.
5. Ask the patient to write his or her own name and birthday and a sentence composed by the patient or dictated by you. Note the patient's spelling, grammatical accuracy, and logical thought process.
N **The patient should be able to produce spontaneous, coherent speech. The speech should have an effortless flow and normal inflections, volume, pitch, articulation, rate, and rhythm. Content of the message should make sense. Comprehension of language should be intact. The patient's ability to read and write should match educational level. Non-native speakers may exhibit some hesitancy or inaccuracy in written and spoken language.**
A Aphasia: impairment of language functioning
P See Table 19-4.
A Dysarthria: disturbance in muscular control of speech
P Ischemia affecting motor nuclei of CN X and CN XII; defects in the premotor or motor cortices, which provide motor input for the face, throat, and mouth; cerebellar disease
A Dysphonia: difficulty making laryngeal sounds, possibly progressing to aphonia (total loss of voice)
P CN X lesions, swelling and inflammation of the larynx

TABLE 19-4 Classification of Aphasia

APHASIA	PATHOPHYSIOLOGY	EXPRESSION	CHARACTERISTICS
Broca's aphasia	Motor cortex lesion, Broca's area	Expressive Nonfluent	Speech slow and hesitant, the patient has difficulty in selecting and organizing words. Naming, word and phrase repetition, and writing impaired. Subtle defects in comprehension.
Wernicke's aphasia	Left hemisphere lesion in Wernicke's area	Receptive Fluent	Auditory comprehension impaired, as is content of speech. Patient unaware of deficits. Naming severely impaired.
Anomic aphasia	Left hemisphere lesion in Wernicke's area	Amnesic Fluent	Patient unable to name objects or places. Comprehension and repetition of words and phrases intact.
Conduction aphasia	Lesion in the arcuate fasciculus, which connects and transports messages between Broca's and Wernicke's areas	Central Fluent	Patient has difficulty repeating words, substitutes incorrect sounds for another (e.g., *dork* for *fork*).
Global aphasia	Lesions in the frontal-temporal area	Mixed Fluent	Both oral and written comprehension severely impaired, naming, repetition of words and phrases, ability to write impaired.
Transcortical sensory aphasia	Lesion in the periphery of Broca's and Wernicke's areas (watershed zone)	Fluent	Impairment in comprehension, naming, and writing. Word and phrase repetition intact.
Transcortical motor aphasia	Lesion anterior, superior, or lateral to Broca's area	Nonfluent	Comprehension intact. Naming and ability to write impaired. Word and phrase repetition intact.

Level of Consciousness (LOC)

E **1.** Observe the patient's eyes when entering the room (environmental stimuli). Note whether the patient's eyes are already open or whether they open when you enter the room (before any verbalization). Note the patient's response to any general environmental stimuli such as noises and lights.

2. If the patient's eyes are closed, call out the patient's name (verbal stimuli). Observe whether the patient's eyes open, whether he or she responds verbally and appropriately, and whether he or she follows verbal commands.

3. If the patient does not respond to verbal stimuli, lightly touch the patient's hand or gently shake the patient awake.

4. If the patient does not respond to environmental or verbal stimuli, proceed to the application of a painful stimulus:

a. With a pen, apply pressure to the nailbed of each extremity

b. Firmly pinch the trapezius muscle, or

c. Apply pressure to the supraorbital ridge or the manubrium.

5. Observe the patient's reaction to the painful stimulus. Note whether the patient's eyes open.

6. Observe whether the patient can localize the painful stimulus (e.g., reaches for the area being stimulated). Strength of the patient's extremities can be evaluated by assessing the strength and distance of movement in the patient's attempt to reach the painful stimulus. Note any abnormal motor responses.

7. Compare the motor responses and response strength of the right versus left sides of the patient.

8. Note whether the patient responds verbally to the painful stimulus.

9. Assess orientation by asking questions related to person, place, and time:

a. Person: name of the patient, name of spouse or significant other

b. Place: where the patient is now (e.g., what town and state), where the patient lives

c. Time: the time of day, the month, the year, the season

10. Determine the Glasgow Coma Scale (GCS) rating. The GCS is an international scale used in grading neurological responses of injured or severely ill patients. It is monitored in patients who have the potential for rapid deterioration in level of consciousness. The GCS assesses three parameters of consciousness: eye opening, verbal response, and motor response (Figure 19-3).

N **The patient's best response to each of these categories is what is recorded. The sum of the three categories is the total GCS score. The highest score of responsiveness is 15, and the lowest is 3. A score of 15 indicates a fully alert, oriented individual.**

A/P See Table 19-5.

Cognitive Abilities and Mentation

Assessment of cognitive function includes testing for attention, memory, judgment, insight, spatial perception, calculation, abstraction, thought processes, and thought content.

Attention

E **1.** Slowly pronounce a series of numbers (approximately 1 second apart), starting with a series of two numbers and progressing to a series of five or six numbers: for example, 2, 5; 3, 7, 8; 1, 9, 4, 3; 1, 5, 4, 9, 0.

2. Ask the patient to repeat the numbers in correct order, both forward and backward.

3. If the patient is unable to repeat the first series correctly, give the patient a different series of the same

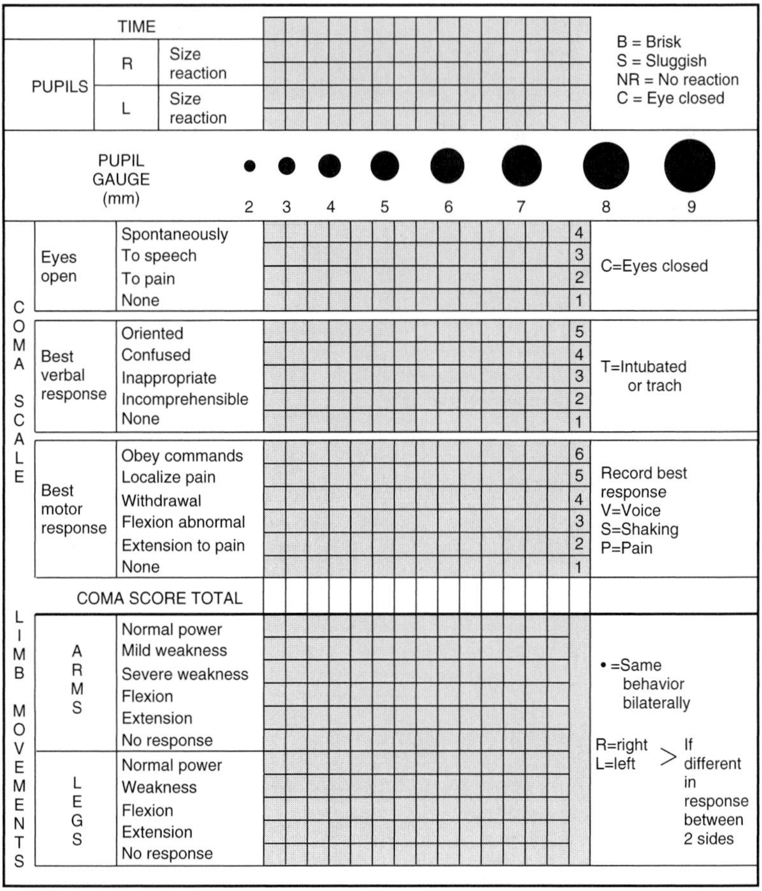

Figure 19-3 Neurological Flow Sheet, including Glasgow Coma Scale

number of digits. Stop after two misses of any length series.

4. "Serial 7s" is another way of assessing attention and concentration. Instruct the patient to begin with the number 100 and to count backward by subtracting 7 each time (i.e., 100, 93, 86, 79, 72, 65, etc).

N **The patient should be able to correctly repeat the series of numbers up to a series of five numbers. The patient should be able to accurately recite serial 7s or serial 3s to at least the 40s or 50s from 100 within 1 minute.**

A Short attention span

P Dementia, neurological injury or disease, mental retardation

Memory

E **1.** Assess immediate recall in conjunction with attention span.

2. Give a list of three items the patient is to remember and to repeat in 5 minutes.

3. If the patient is unable to remember one or more of the items, show the patient a list containing the items along with other items, and check recognition.

TABLE 19-5 Levels of Consciousness: Abnormalities and Pathophysiology

LOC	GCS	RESPONSE TO STIMULI	PUPIL RESPONSE	PATHOPHYSIOLOGY	PROGNOSIS
Confusion	14	Spontaneous but may be inappropriate Memory faulty Reflexes intact	Normal	Metabolic derangements Diffuse brain dysfunction	Good chance of recovery Must treat primary cause
Lethargy	13–14	Requires stimulus to respond (verbal, touch) Reflexes intact	Normal to unequal	Metabolic derangements Medications Increased ICP	Good chance of recovery Must treat primary cause
Stupor	12–13	Requires vigorous, continuous stimuli to respond Reflexes intact	Normal, unequal, or sluggish	Metabolic derangements Medications Increased ICP	Good chance of recovery Must treat primary cause
Permanent vegetative state	8–10	Responds to pain No cognitive response Reflexes abnormal	Normal	Anoxic ischemic insults	Irreversible
Locked-in syndrome	6	Awake and aware Responds with eyes only	Normal	Lesion in ventral pons All four extremities and lower cranial nerves paralyzed Myasthenia gravis Acute polyneuritis	Poor prognosis
Coma	3–6	Abnormal Varied response to pain Reflexes abnormal or absent	Abnormal Dilated or pinpoint	Anoxia Traumatic injury Space-occupying lesion Cerebral edema	Prognosis dependent on length of time in coma
Brain death	3	No response Reflexes abnormal or absent	Abnormal Dilated or pinpoint	Anoxia Structural damage	Irreversible

LOC = level of consciousness; GCS = Glasgow Coma Scale; ICP = intracranial pressure.

4. Record the number of items remembered over the number of items given.
5. Long-term memory is memory that is retained for at least 24 hours. In a test of long-term memory, the patient is typically asked to identify spouse's name, spouse's birthday, mother's maiden name, president's name, and the patient's own birthday.

N **The patient should be able to remember all of the items and to provide accurate responses to the information requested.**

A Memory loss

P Nervous system infection, trauma, stroke, tumor, Alzheimer's disease, seizure disorders, alcohol, and drug toxicity

Judgment

E 1. During the interview, assess whether the patient is responding appropriately to social, family, and work situations that are discussed.
2. Note whether the patient's decisions are based on sound reasoning and decision making.
3. Present hypothetical situations and ask the patient to make decisions regarding what his or her responses would be: for example, "What would you do if followed by a police car with flashing lights?" and "What would you do if you saw a house burning?"
4. Interview the patient's family or directly observe the patient to more carefully assess judgment.

N **The patient should be able to evaluate and act appropriately in situations requiring judgment.**

A Impaired judgment

P Frontal lobe damage, dementia, psychotic states, mental retardation

Insight

E 1. Ask the patient to describe personal health status, reason for seeking health care, symptoms, current life situation, and general coping behaviors.
2. If the patient describes a symptom, ask what life was like before the appearance of the symptom, what life changes the symptom has introduced, and whether the patient feels a need for help.

N **The patient should demonstrate a realistic awareness and understanding of self.**

A Unrealistic perceptions of self

P Euphoric stages of bipolar affective disorders; endogenous anxiety states; depressed states

Spatial Perception

E 1. Ask the patient to copy figures that you have previously drawn, such as a circle, a triangle, a square, a cross, and a three-dimensional cube.
2. Ask the patient to draw the face of a clock, including the numbers around the dial.
3. Ask the patient to identify a familiar sound while keeping the eyes closed: for example, a closing door, running water, or a finger snapping.
4. Have the patient identify right from left body parts.

N **The patient should be able to render the drawings without difficulty and as closely as possible to the original drawings and should be able to identify familiar sounds and left and right body parts.**

A Agnosia: inability to recognize the form, sound, and nature of objects or persons

P Lesions in the nondominant parietal lobe (impair the patient's ability to appreciate self in relation to the environment), lesions in the occipital lobe (visual agnosia), temporal lesions (auditory agnosia)

A Apraxia: inability to perform purposeful movements despite the preservation of motor ability and sensibility

P Lesions of the precentral gyrus of the frontal lobe

Calculation

The patient's ability to perform serial 7s, previously assessed as part of the attention evaluation, is also an assessment of calculation.

Abstract Reasoning

E 1. Ask the patient to describe the meaning of a familiar fable, proverb, or metaphor, for example:
- The squeaky wheel gets the grease.
- A rolling stone gathers no moss.

2. Note the degree of concreteness versus abstraction in the patient's answers.

N **The patient should be able to give the abstract meaning of proverbs, fables, or metaphors within his or her cultural understanding.**

A Conceptual concreteness: inability to describe in abstractions, to generalize from specifics, and to apply general principles

P Dementia, frontal tumor, schizophrenia

Thought Process and Content

E 1. Observe the patient's pattern of thought for relevance, consistency, coherence, logic, and organization.
2. Listen throughout the interview for flaws in content of conversation.

N **Thought processes should be logical, coherent, and goal oriented. Thought content should be based on reality.**

A Unrealistic, illogical thought processes; interruptions of the thinking processes

P Schizophrenia

A Echolalia: involuntary repetition of a word or sentence uttered by another person

P Schizophrenia, dementia

A Persecution delusions, grandiose delusions, hallucinations, illusions, obsessive-compulsiveness, paranoia

P Schizophrenia, dementia, drug use

Suicidal Ideation

E If the patient has expressed feelings of sadness, hopelessness, despair, worthlessness, or grief, explore with more specific questions.
1. Have you ever wanted to hurt yourself?
2. Do you want to hurt yourself now? Do you have a plan?

N The patient should provide a negative response.

A Suicidal ideation

P Depression, substance abuse, bipolar disorder, schizophrenia

Sensory Assessment

Exteroceptive Sensation

For the entire exteroceptive sensation assessment, expose the patient's legs, arms, and abdomen.

Light Touch

E 1. Using a wisp of cotton, apply stimulus in very light strokes. If the skin is calloused or for the thicker skin on the hands and on the soles of the feet, the stimulus may need to be intensified.
2. Begin at distal areas of the patient's limbs and move proximally.
3. Test the hand, lower arm, abdomen, foot, and leg. Assessment of sensation of the face is discussed in the cranial nerve section.
4. To prevent the patient from being able to predict the next touch, alter the rate and rhythm of stimulation. Also, vary the sites of stimulation, keeping in mind that the right and left sides must be compared.
5. Instruct the patient to respond with "now" or "yes" when the stimulus is felt and to identify the stimulated area either verbally or by pointing to it.

N/A/P Refer to Temperature.

Superficial Pain

E 1. Use a sharp object such as a sterile needle, sterile safety pin, or partially opened paper clip.

NURSING CHECKLIST

Assessing Sensation

1. Explain the procedure to the patient before starting the assessment.
2. The sensory assessment is carried out with the patient's eyes closed.
3. For a thorough sensory examination, the patient should be in a supine position.
4. The patient should be cooperative and reliable, although the pain assessment can be performed on comatose patients.
5. Note the patient's ability to perceive sensation.
6. Much of the sensory component of the neurological assessment is subjective; observe the reactions of the patient by watching for grimacing of the face or withdrawal of the stimulated extremity.
7. Compare the patient's sensations on corresponding areas bilaterally.
8. Note whether any sensory deficits follow a dermatome distribution.
9. The borders of any area exhibiting changes in sensation should be mapped.

2. Establish that the patient can identify sharp and dull by touching the patient with each stimuli and asking the patient to describe what is felt.
3. Hold the object loosely between the thumb and first finger to allow the sharp point to slide if too much pressure is applied.
4. Beginning peripherally, move distally to proximally, following the dermatomal distribution. If impaired sensation is identified, move from impaired sensation to normal sensation for comparison. Attempt to define the area of impaired sensation (map) by proceeding from the analgesic area to the normal area.
5. Alternate the sharp point with the dull end to test the patient's accuracy of superficial sensation.
6. Instruct the patient to reply "sharp," "dull," or "I don't know" as quickly as the stimulus is felt and to indicate skin areas that perceive differences in pain sensation.
7. Again, compare the two sides, taking care not to proceed too quickly or to cue the patient via regularity of stimulus presentation.

N/A/P Refer to Temperature.

Temperature

Assess temperature sensation only if abnormalities in superficial pain sensation are noted.

E **1.** Use glass vials containing warm water (40°C to 45°C or 104° to 113°F) and cold water (5°C to 10°C or 41° to 50°F). Hotter or colder temperatures will stimulate pain receptors.
2. Touch the warm or cold test tubes to the skin, distally to proximally and following dermatome distribution.
3. Instruct the patient to respond "hot," "cold," or "I can't tell" and to indicate where the sensation is felt.

N **The patient should be able to accurately perceive light touch, superficial pain, and temperature, and to accurately perceive the location of the stimulus.**

A Anesthesia: absence of touch sensation; hypoesthesia: diminished sense of touch; hyperesthesia: abnormally acute sense of touch; paresthesia: numbness, tingling, or pricking sensation; dysesthesia: inability to distinguish a stimulus such as burning or tingling from a stimulus such as touch or superficial pain

P Peripheral nerve lesions (anesthesia, hypoesthesia, hyperesthesia); lesions of the nerve roots (anesthesia, hypoesthesia)

A Analgesia: insensitivity to pain; hypoalgesia: diminished sensitivity to pain; hyperalgesia: increased sensitivity to pain

P Lesions of the thalamus and the peripheral nerves and nerve roots

A Loss of touch sensation in the hands and lower legs (glove and stocking anesthesia)

P Polyneuritis

A Unilateral loss of all sensation

P Partial lesion of thalamus, lesion situated laterally in upper brain stem, hysteria

Proprioceptive Sensation

Motion and Position

E **1.** With your thumb and index finger, grasp the patient's index finger. Hold the patient's finger at the sides and parallel to the plane of movement in order not to exert upward or downward pressure with your fingers and thus not give the patient any clues regarding direction of finger movement. The patient's fingers should be relaxed.

2. Have the patient shut his or her eyes; show the patient what "up" and "down" feel like by moving the patient's finger in those directions.

3. Use gentle, slow deliberate movements; begin with larger movements and progress to smaller and less perceptible movements.

4. Instruct the patient to respond "up," "down," or "I can't tell" after each time you raise or lower the finger.

5. With the finger of the patient's opposite hand and then with the patient's great toes, repeat steps 2 through 4.

6. If there appears to be a deficit in motion sense, repeat the test on the proximal joints such as the wrists and ankles.

N **The patient should be able to correctly identify changes in body position and motion.**

A Inability to perceive direction of movement

P Peripheral neuropathies; lesion of the posterior column, the sensory cortex, the thalamus, or the connections between them (thalamocortical connections)

Vibration Sense

E **1.** Against the ulnar surface of your hand or on your knuckles, strike the prongs of the tuning fork. Firmly place the base of the fork on the patient's skin over bony prominences.

2. Beginning with distal prominences such as a toe or finger, test each extremity.

3. Instruct the patient to say "now" when the buzzing, vibrating tuning fork is felt and to report immediately when the vibrations are no longer felt.

4. Be sure the patient is reporting the vibration sense rather than the humming sound or feeling pressure from the tuning fork handle.

5. After the patient claims to no longer be able to feel the vibrations, determine whether the vibrations can, in fact, still be felt by holding the prongs while leaving the tuning fork on the patient.

6. If you detect a deficit in vibratory sense in the peripheral bony prominences, progress toward the trunk by testing the ankles, knees, wrists, elbows, anterior superior iliac crests, ribs, sternum, and spinous processes of the vertebrae.

N **The patient should be able to perceive vibration over all bony prominences. Vibratory sensation is normally lower in patients over age 65.**

A Inability to perceive vibration sense

P Polyneuropathies (e.g., diabetic), spinal cord lesions

Cortical Sensation

Stereognosis

Stereognosis is the ability to identify objects by manipulating and touching them.

E **1.** Place a familiar object (dime, button, closed safety pin, key) into the patient's hand.
2. Ask the patient to manipulate the object and to note its size and form.
3. Ask the patient to name the object.
4. Repeat for the opposite hand and with a different object.

N **The patient should be able to identify the objects by holding them.**

A Astereognosis: inability to recognize the nature of objects via touch manipulation

P Parietal lobe dysfunction

Graphesthesia

The ability to identify numbers, letters, or shapes drawn on the skin is termed graphesthesia.

E **1.** Draw a number or letter with a blunt object on the patient's palm.
2. Ask the patient to identify what was written.
3. Repeat on the opposite side.

N The patient should be able to identify the mark made on the palm or skin surface.

A Graphanesthesia

P Parietal lobe dysfunction

Two-Point Discrimination

Two-point discrimination is tested by simultaneously and closely touching various parts of the body with two identical sharp objects.

E **1.** With two sterile pins, the tips of opened paper clips, or broken cotton-tipped applicators, simultaneously touch the tip of one of the patient's fingers, starting with the objects far apart.
2. Ask the patient whether one or two points are felt.
3. Continue to move the two points closer together until the patient is unable to distinguish two points. Note the minimum distance between the two points at which the patient reports feeling the objects separately.
4. Irregularly alternate using one or two pins throughout the test to verify that the patient is feeling two points.
5. Repeats steps 1 through 4 on the fingers of the opposite hand.
6. Other body areas that can be tested include the dorsum of the hand, the tongue, the lips, the feet, and the trunk.

N **On the fingertips, the patient should be able to identify two points at 5 mm apart. Other parts of the body vary widely with regard to distance of discrimination, such as the dorsum of the hand or foot, where a separation of as much as 20 mm may be necessary. On the tip of the tongue, the patient may be able to detect two points as close as 2 to 3 mm (1⁄16 to 1⁄8 inch) apart.**

A Distances greater than those described

P Parietal lobe lesions

Extinction

Extinction (sensory inattention) is tested by simultaneously touching opposite sides of the body at the identical site.

E **1.** Using cotton-tipped applicators or your fingers, ask the patient whether one or two points are felt and where they are felt.
2. Remove the stimulus from one side while maintaining the stimulus on opposite side.
3. Ask the patient whether one or two points are felt and to identify the area of sensation.

N **The patient should be able to feel both stimuli.**

A Inability to feel the two points simultaneously and to discriminate that one point has been removed

P Parietal lobe lesion

Cranial Nerves

Refer to Table 19-1 to assist in the review of cranial nerves.

Olfactory Nerve (CN I)

E 1. Ask the patient to close the eyes.
2. Test each side separately by asking the patient to occlude one nostril by pressing against it with a finger. Under the nostril that is not occluded, hold a vial containing an odorous substance.
3. Ask the patient to inhale deeply so that the odor surrounds the mucous membranes and thus adequately stimulates the olfactory nerve.
4. Ask the patient to identify the contents of the vial.
5. Present one odor at a time and alternate from nostril to nostril.
6. To prevent confusion of the olfactory system, allow enough time to pass between presentations of vials.
7. Note whether a difference between the right and left sides is apparent.

N **The patient should be able to distinguish and identify the odors with each nostril.**

A Anosmia: loss of the sense of smell

P Trauma to the cribriform plate, sinusitis, colds, heavy smoking

A Unilateral anosmia

P Intracranial neoplasm

Optic Nerve (CN II)

Visual acuity, and visual fields, funduscopic examination: see Chapter 12.

Oculomotor (CN III)

Cardinal fields of gaze, eyelid elevation, and pupil reactions: see Chapter 12.

Trochlear (CN IV)

Cardinal fields of gaze: see Chapter 12.

Trigeminal Nerve (CN V)

Motor Component

E 1. Instruct the patient to clench the jaw.
2. Using the finger pads of the first three fingers, palpate the contraction of the temporalis (see Figure 19-4A) and masseter (see Figure 19-4B) muscles on each side of the face.
3. Ask the patient to move the jaw from side to side against resistance from your hand. Feel for weakness on one side or the other as the patient pushes against resistance.
4. Test the muscles of mastication by having the patient bite down with the molars on each side of a tongue blade and comparing the depth of the impressions made by the teeth. If you can pull the tongue blade

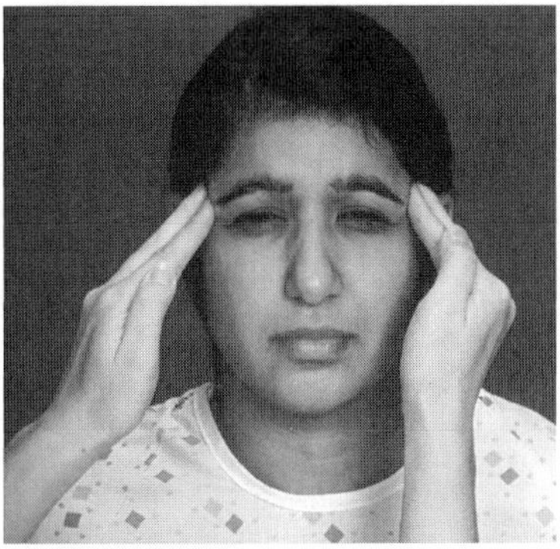

A. Temporalis Muscles

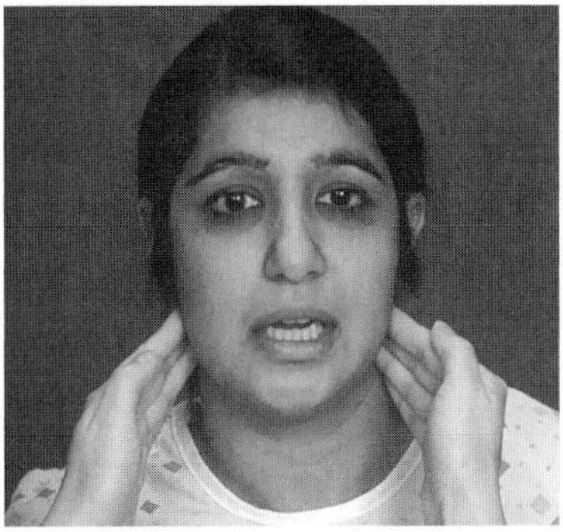

B. Masseter Muscles

Figure 19-4 Assessment of the Motor Component of CN V

out while the patient is biting on it, there is weakness in the muscles of mastication.

5. Observe for fasciculation and note the bulk, contour, and tone of the mastication muscles.

Sensory Component

E 1. Instruct the patient to close the eyes.

2. Test light touch by using a cotton wisp to lightly stroke the patient's temple and cheek on each side of the face.

3. Instruct the patient to respond by saying "now" each time the touch of the cotton wisp is felt.

4. Test and compare both sides of the face.

5. To assess superficial pain sensation, use a sterile needle or an open paperclip. Before testing, show the patient how the sharp end of the needle or paperclip feels compared with the dull, blunt end.

   a. Instruct the patient to respond with "sharp" or "dull" as each sensation is felt.

   b. Irregularly alternate the sharp and dull ends, again testing each distribution area of the trigeminal nerve on both sides of the face.

6. Test temperature sensation if other abnormalities have been detected. Use vials of hot and cold water.

   a. Alternating hot and cold, touch the vials to each dermatomal distribution area.

   b. Ask the patient to respond by saying "hot" or "cold."

7. Because sensation to the cornea is supplied by the trigeminal nerve, test the corneal reflex (the motor component is CN VII). The corneal reflex should not be routinely assessed in conscious patients, unless there is a clinical suspicion of trauma to CN V or CN VII.

   a. Ask the patient to open the eyes and look away from you.

   b. Approach the patient out of the line of vision to eliminate the blink reflex. You can stabilize the patient's chin with your hand if the chin is moving.

   c. Lightly stroke the cornea with a slightly moistened cotton wisp. Avoid stroking just the sclera or the lashes of the eye. An alternative technique is to instill normal saline eye drops instead of a light stroke of a cotton wisp.

   d. Observe for bilateral blinking of the eyes.

   e. Repeat on the opposite eye.

N **The temporalis and masseter muscles should be equally strong on palpation. The jaw should not deviate and should be equally strong on side-to-side movement against resistance. The volume and bulk of the muscles should be bilaterally equal. Sensation to light touch, superficial pain, and temperature should be present on the sensory distribution areas of the trigeminal nerve. The corneal reflex should cause bilateral blinking of eyes.**

A Reduced sensory perception, facial pain

P Aneurysms of the internal carotid artery, neoplasms that compress the gasserian ganglion or root, meningiomas, pituitary adenomas, malignant tumors of the nasopharynx, head injuries (especially basilar skull fractures)

A Trigeminal neuralgia (tic douloureux): brief, paroxysmal, unilateral facial pain along the distribution of the trigeminal nerve

P Multiple sclerosis secondary to demyelinization of CN V, posterior fossa tumor, unknown

A Postherpetic neuralgia: continuous pain, described as a constant burning ache with occasional stabbing pains unilaterally

P Herpes zoster

A Tetanus: tonic spasms interfering with the muscles that open the jaw (trismus)

P Motor root involvement of the trigeminal nerve

Abducens (CN VI)

Cardinal fields of gaze: see Chapter 12.

Facial Nerve (CN VII)

Motor Component

E **1.** Observe the patient's facial expressions for symmetry and mobility throughout the assessment.

2. Note any asymmetry of the face, such as wrinkles or lack of wrinkles on one side of the face or one-sided blinking.

3. Test muscle contraction by asking the patient to:

- **a.** Frown
- **b.** Raise the eyebrows
- **c.** Wrinkle the forehead while looking up
- **d.** Close the eyes lightly and keep them closed against your resistance
- **e.** Smile, show the teeth, purse the lips, and whistle
- **f.** Puff out the cheeks against resistance from your hands

4. Observe for symmetry of facial muscles and for weakness during the above maneuvers.

5. Note any abnormal movements such as tremors, tics, and grimaces, and note any immobility.

N **Normal findings of the motor portion of the facial nerve assessment include symmetry between the right and left sides of the face as well as between the upper and lower portions of the face, both at rest and while executing facial movements. There should be no abnormal muscle movements.**

A Bell's palsy (idiopathic facial palsy): complete flaccid paralysis of the facial muscles on the involved side

P Damage to the facial nerve

Sensory Component

E **1.** Sensory assessment of the facial nerve is limited to testing taste. The areas that are tested are as follows:

- **a.** The tip of the tongue, for sweet and salty tastes
- **b.** The tip and along the borders of the tongue, for sour taste
- **c.** The back of the tongue and the soft palate, for bitter taste

2. Test both sides of the tongue with each solution.

3. The patient's tongue should protrude during the entire assessment of taste, and talking is not allowed.

4. Cotton swabs may be used as applicators; use a different swab for each solution.

5. Dip the cotton swab into the solution being tested and place the swab on the appropriate part of the tongue.

6. Instruct the patient to state the flavor that best describes the taste perception (i.e., salty, bitter, sweet, or sour).

7. Instruct the patient to rinse the mouth with water before the next solution is tested.

8. Repeat steps 5, 6, and 7 until each solution has been tested on both sides of the tongue.

N **Normal sensation would be accurate perceptions of sweet, sour, salty, and bitter tastes.**

A Ageusia: loss of taste sensation; hypogeusia: diminution of taste sensation

P Age, excessive smoking, extreme dryness of the oral mucosa, lesions of the medulla oblongata or the parietal lobe

Acoustic Nerve (CN VIII)

Cochlear division (hearing) and Weber and Rinne tests: see Chapter 13.

Vestibular Division

The vestibular division of CN VIII assesses for vertigo.

E 1. During the history, ask the patient whether vertigo is experienced.
2. Note any evidence of equilibrium disturbances. Refer to the section on cerebellar assessment.
3. Note the presence of nystagmus.

N **Vertigo is not normally present.**

A Vertigo: an uncomfortable sensation of movement of the environment or of the self within a stationary environment

P Disorder of the labyrinth or the vestibular nerve, tumor of the cerebellopontine angle, head injury involving the labyrinth, eustachian tube blockage

A Ménière's disease: vertigo lasting for minutes or hours, low-pitched roaring tinnitus, progressive hearing loss, nausea and vomiting

P Distension of the endolymphatic system with degenerative changes in the organ of Corti

Glossopharyngeal and Vagus Nerves (CN IX and CN X)

The glossopharyngeal and vagus nerves are tested together because of their overlap in function.

E 1. Examine soft palate and uvula movement and gag reflex as described in Chapter 13.
2. Assess the patient's speech for a nasal quality or hoarseness. Ask the patient to produce guttural and palatal sounds such as *k, q, ch, b,* and *d.*
3. Assess the patient's ability to swallow a small amount of water. Observe for regurgitation of fluids through the nose. If the patient is unable to swallow, observe how oral secretions are handled.
4. The sensory portion of the glossopharyngeal and vagus nerves assessment is limited to taste on the posterior one-third of the tongue. This assessment was previously discussed with regard to CN VII.

N **Refer to Chapter 13 for normal findings on soft palate and uvula movement and gag reflex. The quality of speech is clear and without hoarseness or a nasal quality. The patient is able to swallow water or oral secretions easily. Taste (sweet, salty, sour, and bitter) is intact in the posterior one-third of the tongue.**

A Unilateral lowering and flattening of the palatine arch, weakness of the soft palate, deviation of the uvula to the normal side, some dysphagia and regurgitation of fluids and a nasal vocal quality, loss of taste sensation in the posterior one-third of the tongue, hemianesthesia of the palate and pharynx

P Unilateral glossopharyngeal and vagal paralysis (trauma or skull fractures at the base of the skull), bilateral vagus nerve paralysis (lower brain stem CN dysfunction, ALS)

Spinal Accessory Nerve (CN XI)

E 1. Place the patient in a seated or supine position. Inspect the sternocleidomastoid muscles for contour, volume, and fasciculation.
2. Place your right hand on the left side of the patient's face. Instruct the patient to turn the head sideways against resistance from your hand.
3. Use your left hand to palpate the sternocleidomastoid muscle for strength of contraction. Inspect the muscle for contraction.
4. Repeat steps 2 and 3 on the opposite side. Compare the strength of the two sides.
5. To assess the function of the trapezius muscle, stand behind the patient and inspect the shoulders and scapulae for symmetry of contour. Note any atrophy or fasciculation.
6. Place your hands on top of the patient's shoulders and instruct the patient to raise the shoulders against downward resistance from your hands.

This maneuver can be performed in front of or behind the patient.

7. Observe movement and palpate contraction of the trapezius muscles. Compare the strength of the two sides.

N **The patient should be able to turn the head in a smooth, strong, symmetric motion against resistance. The patient should also demonstrate the ability to shrug the shoulders in a strong, symmetric movement of the trapezius muscles against resistance.**

A Inability to turn the head toward the paralyzed side, a flat, noncontracting muscle on that side, and possibly a contracted contralateral sternocleidomastoid muscle; inability to elevate shoulder; asymmetric drooping of shoulder and scapula

P Unilateral paralysis of the sternocleidomastoid muscle due to trauma, tumor, or infection affecting the spinal accessory nerve

A/P For information on torticollis, see Chapter 11.

Hypoglossal Nerve (CN XII)

See Chapter 13 for assessment of tongue movement.

E Assess lingual sounds by asking the patient to say "la, la, la."

N **See Chapter 13 for normal tongue movements. Lingual speech is clear.**

A Inability to produce or difficulty in producing lingual sounds

P Hypoglossal nerve lesions

Motor System

Muscle size, tone, and strength and involuntary movements: see Chapter 18.

A Extrapyramidal rigidity evident when resistance is present during passive movement of the muscles in all directions

P Basal ganglia lesions

A Decerebrate rigidity (decerebration): Figure 19-5A.

P Diencephalic injury, midbrain dysfunction, severe metabolic disorders

A Decorticate rigidity (decortication): Figure 19-5B.

P Cerebral hemisphere lesions that interfere with the corticospinal tract

Pronator Drift

E **1.** Have the patient extend the arms forward with the palms turned up for 20 seconds.

2. Observe for downward drifting of an arm.

N **There should be no downward drifting of an arm.**

A Downward drifting of an arm

P Hemiparesis (stroke)

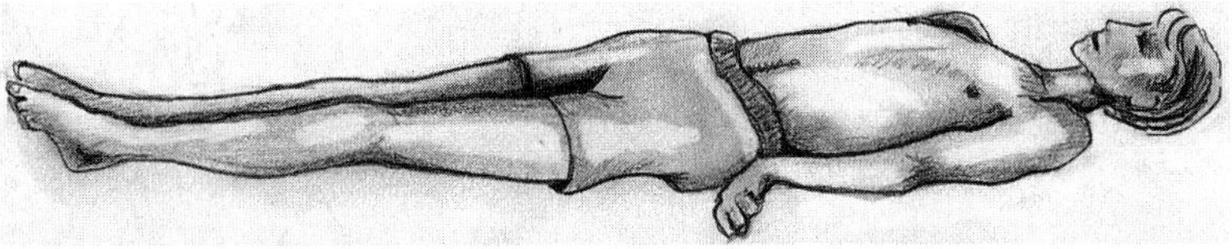

A. Decerebrate Rigidity (Abnormal Extension)

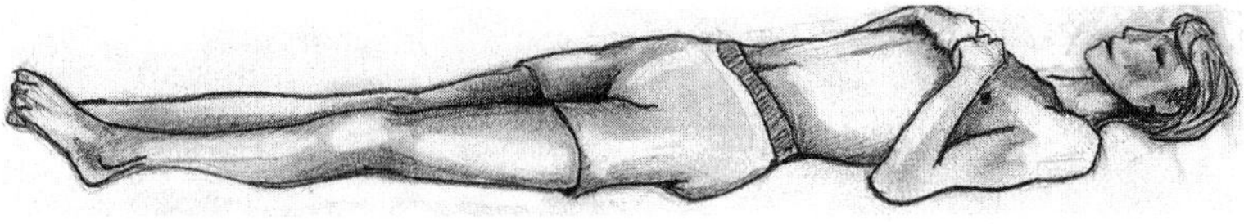

B. Decorticate Rigidity (Abnormal Flexion)

Figure 19-5 Motor System Dysfunction

Cerebellar Function (Coordination, Station, and Gait)

Coordination

E **1.** Instruct the patient to sit comfortably facing you and with the eyes open and the arms outstretched.

2. Ask the patient first to touch the index finger to nose and then to alternate rapidly with the index finger of the opposite hand.

3. Have the patient continue to rapidly touch the nose with alternate index fingers while keeping the eyes closed.

4. With the patient's eyes open, ask the patient to again touch finger to nose. Next, ask the patient to touch your index finger, which is held approximately 45 cm (18 inches) away from the patient.

5. Change the position of your finger as the patient rapidly repeats the maneuver using one finger.

6. Repeat steps 4 and 5 on the opposite hand.

7. Observe for intention tremor or

NURSING CHECKLIST

Assessing Reflexes

1. For testing reflexes, the patient should be relaxed and comfortable.
2. Position the patient so that the extremities are symmetric.
3. To elicit true reflexes, distract the patient by talking about another topic.
4. Loosely hold the reflex hammer between the thumb and index finger and use a brisk motion from the wrist to strike the tendon. The reflex hammer should make contact with the correct point on the tendon in a quick, direct manner.
5. Observe the degree and speed of response of the muscles after the reflex hammer makes contact. Grading of reflexes is as follows:

   0: absent
   + (1+): present but diminished
   ++ (2+): normal
   +++ (3+): mildly increased but not pathological
   ++++ (4+): markedly hyperactive, clonus may be present

6. Compare reflex responses of the right and left sides. Taps in the correct area should elicit a brisk (i.e., ++ or +++) contraction of the muscles involved.
7. When documenting the deep tendon reflexes (DTRs), you can use a stick figure.

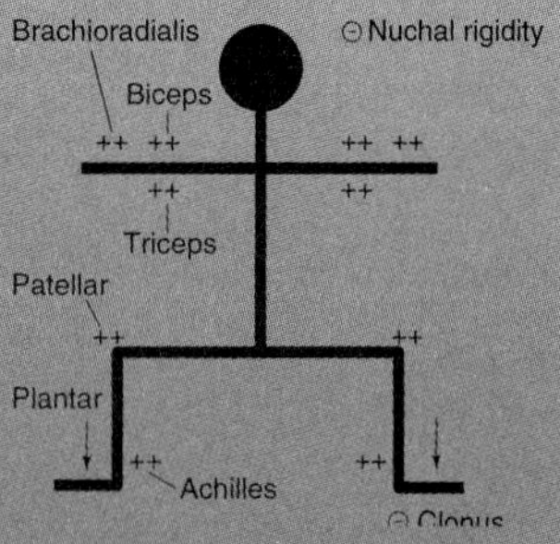

overshoot or undershoot of the patient's finger.

8. To assess rapid-alternating movements, ask the patient to rapidly alternate patting the knees first with the palms of the hands and then alternating the palms and the backs of the hands (rapid supinating and pronating of the hands).

9. Ask the patient to repeatedly touch the thumb to each of the fingers of the hand in rapid succession from index to the fifth finger and back.

10. Repeat step 9 on the opposite hand.

11. Observe coordination and the ability of the patient to perform these movements in rapid sequence.

12. With the patient in a seated or supine position, ask the patient to place the heel just below the knee on the shin of the opposite leg and to slide the heel down to the foot.

13. Repeat on the opposite foot.

14. Observe coordination of the two legs.

15. With the patient's foot either on the ground or in the air, ask the patient to use the foot to draw a circle or a figure 8.

16. Repeat on the opposite foot.

17. Observe for coordination and for regularity of the figure.

18. Test the lower extremities for rapid-alternating movement by asking the patient to rapidly extend the ankle ("tap your foot") or to rapidly flex and extend the toes of one foot.

19. Repeat on the opposite foot.

20. Note rate, rhythm, smoothness, and accuracy of the movements.

N **The patient is able to rapidly alternate touching finger to nose and moving finger from nose to your finger in a coordinated fashion. The patient is able to perform alternating movements in a purposeful, rapid, coordinated manner. The patient is able to purposefully and smoothly run heel down shin with equal coordination in both feet and to draw a figure 8 or circle with the foot.**

A Dyssynergy: lack of coordinated action of the muscle groups (movements appear jerky, irregular, and uncoordinated); dysmetria: impaired judgment of distance, range, speed, and force of movement; dysdiadochokinesia: inability to perform rapid-alternating movements

P Cerebellar disease

Station

See Chapter 18 for posture assessment techniques and findings.

Gait

See Chapter 18 for gait assessment techniques and findings.

Reflexes

Deep Tendon Reflexes

Brachioradialis

E **1.** Flex the patient's arm to 45°.
2. Support the patient's relaxed arm either on the lap or semipronated on your forearm.
3. With narrow end of reflex hammer, strike the tendon of the brachioradialis above the styloid process of the radius (several centimeters above the wrist on the thumb side Figure 19-6A).

N **Observe for flexion and supination of the forearm. An exaggerated reflex may also yield flexion of the wrist and fingers and adduction of the forearm. Innervation of this reflex is via the radial nerve, with segmental innervation of C5 and C6.**

A/P See Achilles.

Biceps

E **1.** Flex the patient's arm to between 45° and 90°.
2. Support the patient's forearm on your forearm.
3. Firmly place your thumb on the biceps tendon just above the crease of the antecubital fossa (Figure 19-6B).
4. Wrap your fingers around the patient's arm and rest them on the biceps muscle to feel it contract.
5. With the narrow end of the reflex hammer, briskly tap the thumb.

N **Observe for contraction of the biceps muscle and flexion of the elbow. Innervation of the biceps reflex is via the musculocutaneous nerve, with segmental innervation of C5 and C6.**

A/P See Achilles.

Triceps

E **1.** Flex the patient's arm to between 45° and 90°.
2. Support the patient's arm either on the lap or on your hand as shown in Figure 19-6C.
3. With the blunt end of reflex hammer, tap the triceps tendon just above its insertion above the olecranon process (elbow).

N **Observe for contraction of the triceps muscle and extension of the arm. Innervation of the triceps reflex is via the radial nerve, with segmental innervation of C7 and C8.**

A/P See Achilles.

Patellar

E **1.** Ask the patient to sit in a chair or at the edge of the examination table.
2. Place your hand over the quadriceps femoris muscle to feel contraction.
3. With the other hand and using the blunt end of the reflex hammer, tap the patellar tendon just below the patella (Figure 19-6D).
4. If the patient cannot tolerate a sitting position, use one hand to lift the flexed knee off the table and to support the leg under the knee so that the foot is hanging freely.

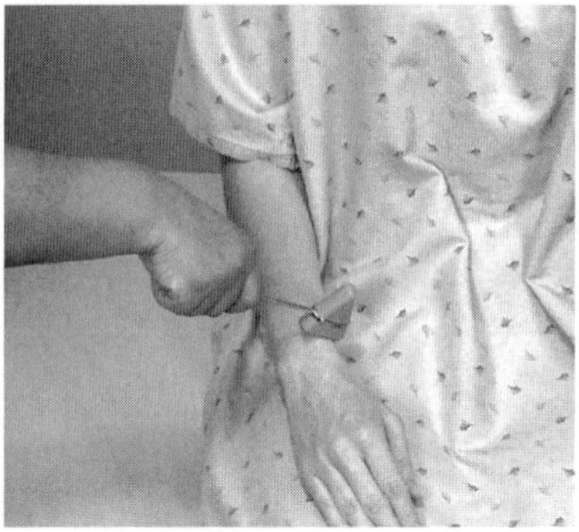

A. Brachioradialis

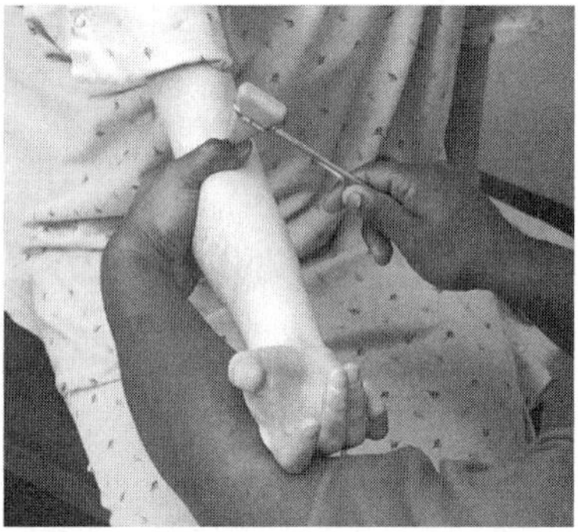

B. Biceps

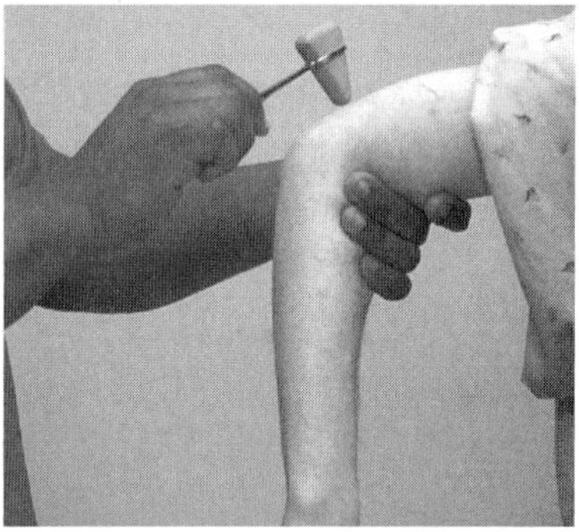

C. Triceps

Figure 19-6 Assessment of Deep Tendon Reflexes *continues*

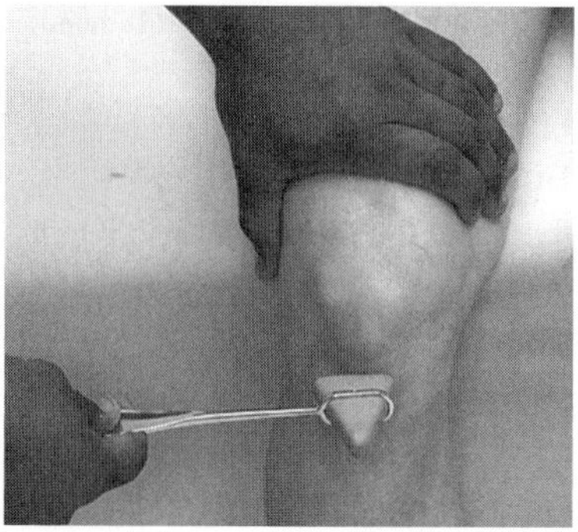

D. Patellar

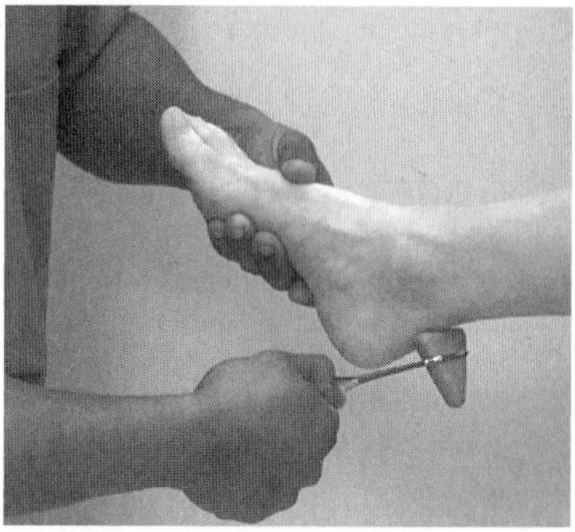

E. Achilles

Figure 19-6 Assessment of Deep Tendon Reflexes *continued*

N **There should be contraction of the quadriceps muscle and extension of the leg. Innervation of the patellar reflex is via the femoral nerve, with segmental innervation of L2, L3, and L4.**

A/P See Achilles.

Achilles

E **1.** Ask the patient to sit with the feet dangling.

2. Partially dorsiflex the patient's foot.

3. With the blunt end of the reflex hammer, tap the Achilles tendon just above its insertion at the heel.

4. If the patient is lying down, flex the leg at the knee and externally rotate the thigh. Place a hand under the foot to produce dorsiflexion. Hold the foot in your nondominant hand as shown in Figure 19-6E. Apply the stimulus as described in step 3.

N **The normal response is contraction of the calf muscles (gastrocnemius, soleus, and plantaris) and plantar flexion of the foot. Innervation of the Achilles reflex is via the tibial nerve, with segmental innervation of L5, S1, and S2.**

A Absent or decreased deep tendon reflexes

P Interference in the reflex arc, deep coma, narcosis, deep sedation, hypothyroidism, sedative-hypnotic drugs, infectious diseases, increased intracranial pressure, spinal shock

A Hyperactive deep tendon reflexes

P Loss of inhibition of the higher centers in the cortex and reticular formation, lesions of the pyramidal system, light coma, tetany, tetanus

Superficial Reflexes

Abdominal

E **1.** Drape and place the patient in a recumbent position with the arms at the sides and the knees slightly flexed. Stand to the right of the patient.

2. Use a moderately sharp object, such as a split tongue blade or the wooden tip of a cotton-tipped applicator, to stroke the skin.

3. To elicit the upper abdominal reflex, stimulate the skin of the upper abdominal quadrants. From the tip of the sternum, stroke in a diagonal (downward and inward) fashion.

4. Repeat step 3 on the opposite side.

5. To elicit the lower abdominal reflex, stimulate the skin of the lower abdominal quadrants. From the area below the umbilicus, stroke in a diagonal (downward and inward) fashion toward the symphysis pubis.

6. Repeat step 5 on the opposite side.

N **Observe for contraction of the upper abdominal muscles upward and outward and deviation of the umbilicus toward the stimulus. The upper abdominal reflex is innervated via the intercostal nerves through segments T7, T8, and T9. Observe for contraction of the lower abdominal muscles and contraction of the umbilicus toward the stimulus. The lower abdominal reflex is innervated via the lower intercostal, iliohypogastric, and ilioinguinal nerves through segments T10, T11, and T12.**

A/P See Bulbocavernosus.

Plantar

E 1. With the handle of the reflex hammer, stroke the outer aspect of the sole of the foot from the heel across the ball of the foot to just below the great toe.

2. Repeat on the opposite foot.

N **Observe for plantar flexion of the toes. The plantar reflex is innervated via the tibial nerve, with segmental innervation of L5, S1, and S2.**

A/P See Bulbocavernosus.

Cremasteric

E 1. The male patient should be lying down with the thighs exposed and the testicles visible.

2. Stroke the skin of the inner aspect of the thigh near the groin from above downward.

3. Repeat step 2 on the opposite side.

N **Observe for contraction of the cremasteric muscle with corresponding elevation of the ipsilateral testicle. Innervation of the cremasteric reflex is via the ilioinguinal and genitofemoral nerves, with segmental innervation of T12, L1, and L2.**

A/P See Bulbocavernosus.

Bulbocavernosus

E Pinch the skin of the foreskin or the glans penis.

N **Observe for contraction of the bulbocavernosus muscle in the perineum at the base of the penis. The presence of this reflex in a paraplegic patient after acute spinal cord injury indicates that the initial stage of spinal shock has passed. The bulbocavernosus reflex is innervated via segments S3 and S4.**

A Decreased or absent superficial reflexes

P Dysfunction of the reflex arc, lesions in the pyramidal tracts, deep sleep, coma

Pathological Reflexes

All the reflexes described in this section are abnormal findings in adults and are not usually assessed unless the patient's clinical presentation warrants assessment.

Glabellar

E 1. With your finger, tap the patient on the forehead between the eyebrows.

2. Observe for a hyperactive blinking response.

A Reflex is abnormal.

P Lesions of the corticobulbar pathways from the cortex to the pons, Parkinson's disease, glioblastoma of the corpus callosum

Clonus

E 1. Have the patient assume a recumbent position. Stand to the side.

2. Support the patient's knee in a slightly flexed position.

3. Quickly dorsiflex the foot and maintain it in that position.

4. Assess for clonus (a rhythmic oscillation of involuntary muscle contraction).

A Sustained clonus

P Sustained clonus, in combination with muscle spasticity and hyperreflexia, indicates upper motor neuron disease; Women with preeclampsia and eclampsia

Babinski

E With the handle of the reflex hammer, stroke the patient's sole as you did for the plantar reflex. Use a slow and deliberate motion.

N **A Babinski reflex is normal in infants and toddlers until 15 to 18 months of age.**

A Positive Babinski's reflex, the patient's toes abduct (fan) and the great toe dorsiflexes

P Lesions in the pyramidal system, stroke or trauma

20

Female Genitalia

Anatomy and Physiology

The components of the external female genitalia are collectively referred to as the vulva. They consist of the mons pubis, the labia majora, the labia minora, the clitoris, the vulval vestibule and its glands, the urethral meatus, and the vaginal introitus (Figure 20-1).

The vestibule is the area between the two skin folds of the labia minora that contains the urethral meatus, the openings of the Skene's glands, the hymen, the openings of the Bartholin's glands, and the vaginal introitus.

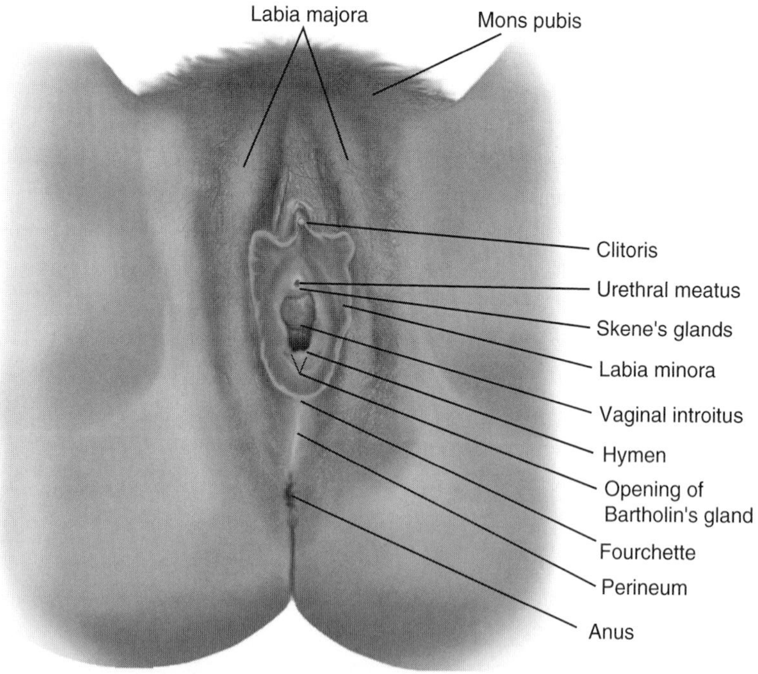

Figure 20-1 External Female Genitalia

The perineum is located between the fourchette and the anus. Its composition of muscle, elastic fibers, fascia, and connective tissue gives it an exceptional capacity for stretching during childbirth.

The anal orifice is located at the seam of the gluteal folds and serves as the exit of the gastrointestinal tract.

The components of the internal female genitalia are the vagina, the cervix, the uterus, the fallopian tubes, and the ovaries (Figure 20-2).

The vagina is a pink, hollow, muscular tube extending from the cervix to the vulva.

The uterus is an inverted pear-shaped, hollow, muscular organ in which an impregnated ovum develops into a fetus. The inferior aspect is the cervix; the superior aspect is the fundus.

The adnexa of the uterus consists of the fallopian tubes, the ovaries, and their supporting ligaments. The fallopian tubes extend from the cornu of the uterus to the ovaries and are supported by the broad ligaments. Fertilization of the ova takes place in the fallopian tubles. The ovaries are a pair of almond-shaped glands where development and formation of an ovum and hormonal production occur.

The female reproductive cycle consists of two interrelated cycles called the ovarian and menstrual cycles. Ovulation, or release of an egg, occurs during the ovarian cycle.

The menstrual cycle begins if implantation does not occur. The menstrual flow lasts from 2 to 7 days, and the cycles occur every 25 to 34 days, with the average being 28 days.

If conception and implantation of the fertilized ovum occur, the corpus luteum is maintained by the presence of human chorionic gonadotropin (HCG), which is secreted by the implanting blastocyst. Human chorionic gonadotropin is the hormone tested in at-home pregnancy kits.

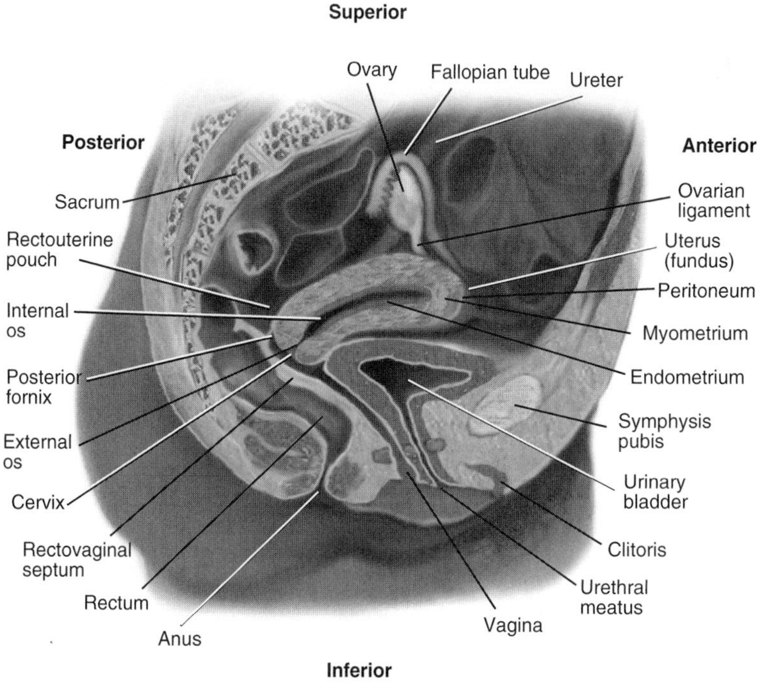

Figure 20-2 Left-Sided Sagittal Section at Midline of Internal Pelvic Organs

HEALTH HISTORY

Medical History
See Table 20–1.

Surgical History
Hysterectomy, myomectomy, salpingectomy, oophorectomy, dilatation and curettage, laparoscopy, vulvectomy, tubal ligation, colpotomy, cesarean section, colposcopy, cryotherapy, uterine cryoablation

Communicable Diseases
Sexually transmitted diseases: gonorrhea, syphilis, herpes, HIV/AIDS, hepatitis B or C, *Chlamydia*, pelvic inflammatory disease, human papillomavirus, trichomoniasis, chancroid, molluscum contagiosum

Injuries and Accidents
Abdominal trauma, rape, sexual abuse, vaginal trauma or injury, pelvic fractures, lumbar spine, sacral coccyx injuries

Childhood Illnesses
Fetal DES exposure

Family Health History
Cancers of the reproductive organs, maternal use of diethylstibestrol (DES) while pregnant with patient, STDs, HIV/AIDS, multiple pregnancies, congenital anomalies, hepatits B or C

TABLE 20-1 Female Reproductive Health History

MENSTRUAL HISTORY
Age of menarche, last menstrual period (LMP), length of cycle, regularity of cycle, duration of menses, amenorrhea, menorrhagia, presence of clots or vaginal pooling, number and type of tampons or pads used during menses, dysmenorrhea, spotting between menses, missed menses

PREMENSTRUAL SYNDROME (PMS)
Symptoms occur from 3 to 7 days before the onset of menses with cessation of symptoms after second day of cycle. Symptoms include: breast tenderness, bloating, moodiness, cravings (salt, sugar, or chocolate), fatigue, weight gain, headaches, joint pain, nausea, and vomiting.

OBSTETRIC HISTORY
See Chapter 23.

MENOPAUSE HISTORY
Menopause (cessation of menstruation), spotting, associated symptoms of menopause (such as hot flashes, palpitations, numbness, tingling, drenching sweats, mood swings, vaginal dryness, itching), treatment for symptoms (including hormone replacement therapy), feelings about menopause

VAGINAL DISCHARGE
Color, consistency, odor, pruritis (itching), amount

ASSOCIATED SYMPTOMS
Dyspareunia (painful intercourse), dysuria, abdominal/pelvic pain, cramping symptoms in partner(s)

continues

TABLE 20-1 Female Reproductive Health History *continued*

HISTORY OF UTERINE BLEEDING
Consistency, color, number of pads or tampons used in 24 hours, duration, frequency of flow, abdominal pain/cramping, passage of clots or tissue, relationship to menses, IUD

SEXUAL FUNCTIONING
Sexual preference, number of partners, interest, satisfaction, dyspareunia, inorgasmia

REPRODUCTIVE MEDICAL HISTORY
Vaginal infections, salpingitis, endometritis, endometriosis, cervicitis, fibroids, ovarian cysts, cancer of the reproductive organs, infertility, Pap smear records

METHOD OF BIRTH CONTROL
Type, frequency of use, methods to prevent STDs, any associated problems with birth control or STD prevention methods, such as a reaction to the spermicides used with vaginal sponges, diaphragms, and condoms

Equipment

- Examination table with stirrups
- Stool (preferably mounted on wheels)
- Large hand mirror
- Gooseneck lamp
- Clean gloves
- Linens for draping
- Vaginal speculum:
  - Graves' bivalve speculum, sizes medium and large; useful for most adult, sexually active women
  - Pederson bivalve speculum, sizes small and medium; useful for non-sexually active women, for children, and for menopausal women
- Cytological materials:
  - Ayre spatulas
  - Cytobrushes
  - Cervical broom
  - Cotton-tipped applicators
  - Liquid-based preparation vial
  - Microscope slides, cover slips, Thayer-Martin culture plates (labeled with the patient's name and identification number and the date of specimen collection)
  - Cytology fixative spray
  - Reagents: normal saline, potassium hydroxide (KOH), acetic acid (white vinegar)
- Thin-Prep supplies
- Warm water
- Water-soluble lubricant

NURSING CHECKLIST

General Approach to Female Genitalia Assessment

Before the assessment:

1. Ensure the patient will not be menstruating at the time of the examination.
2. Instruct the patient not to use vaginal sprays, to douche, to have coitus, or to place tampons in the vagina for 24 to 48 hours before the scheduled physical assessment. The products of coitus and commercial sprays, douches, and tampons may affect the Pap smear and other vaginal cultures.
3. Encourage the patient to express any anxieties and concerns about the physical assessment. Reassure the patient by acknowledging anxieties and validating concerns. Virgins may desire reassurance that the pelvic assessment will not affect the hymen.

continues

General Approach to Female Genitalia Assessment *continued*

4. Show the speculum and other equipment to the patient and allow her to touch and explore any items that do not have to remain sterile.
5. Inform the patient that the assessment should not be painful but may be uncomfortable at times and that she should inform you if she experiences any pain.
6. Instruct the patient to empty her bladder and to then undress from the waist to the ankles.
7. Ensure that the room is warm enough to prevent chilling; provide additional draping material as necessary.
8. Place drapes or sheep skin over the stirrups to increase patient comfort.
9. Use warm water to warm your hands before gloving.
10. Ensure that privacy will be maintained during the assessment. Provide screens and a closed door.
11. Warm the speculum with water or a warming device before insertion.

During the assessment:

1. Inform the patient of what you are going to do before you do it. Tell her she may feel pressure when the speculum is opened and a pinching sensation during the Pap smear.
2. Adopt a nonjudgmental and supportive attitude.
3. Maintain eye contact with the patient as much as possible to reinforce a caring relationship.
4. Use a mirror to show the patient what you are doing and to educate her about her body. Help her in positioning the mirror during the examination so she will feel comfortable when using this technique at home to assess her genitalia.
5. Offer the patient the opportunity to ask questions about her body and sexuality.
6. Encourage the patient to use relaxation techniques, such as deep breathing or guided imagery, to prevent muscle tension during the assessment.

After the assessment:

1. Assess whether the patient needs assistance in dressing.
2. Offer tissues with which to wipe excess lubrication.
3. After the patient is dressed, discuss the experience with her, invite questions and comments, listen carefully, and provide information regarding the assessment and any available laboratory information.
4. Tell the patient she may experience a small amount of spotting after the Pap smear.

Assessment of the Female Genitalia

Inspection of the External Genitalia

E 1. With the patient seated, place a drape over the patient's torso and thighs until positioning is completed.

2. Instruct the patient to sit between the stirrups on the examination table and facing away from the head of the table.

3. Assist the patient in assuming a dorsal recumbent or lithotomy position on the examination table. Help the patient place her heels in the stirrups, thus abducting her legs and

flexing her hips (see Chapter 8 for positioning).

4. Don clean gloves.

5. Assist the patient as she moves her buttocks down to the lower end of the examination table so that the buttocks are flush with the edge of the table. If the patient desires, raise the head of the examination table slightly to elevate her head and shoulders. This position allows you to maintain eye contact with the patient and prevents abdominal muscle tensing.

6. Readjust the drape to cover the abdomen, thighs, and knees; adjust the stirrups as necessary for patient comfort. Push the drape down between the patient's knees so you can see the patient's face.

7. Sit on a stool at the foot of the examination table and facing the patient's external genitalia.

8. Adjust your lighting source and provide the patient with a mirror. Before touching the patient's genitalia, show her how to hold the mirror to view the examination.

Pubic Hair

E 1. Observe the pattern of pubic hair distribution.

2. Note the presence of nits or lice.

N **Female pubic hair distribution should resemble an inverse triangle. There may be some growth on the abdomen and upper inner thighs. Sexual maturity ratings can be determined at this time for adolescent patients. A diamond-shaped pattern from the umbilicus may be due to cultural or familial differences.**

A Diamond-shaped pattern from the umbilicus

P Hirsutism secondary to an endocrine disorder

P Alopecia, age, obesity, systemic disease

A Pubic lice or nits in the pubic hair, flecks of residual blood on the external genitalia

P Pediculosis pubis: infestation of the hairy regions of the body, usually the pubic area

Skin Color and Condition

Mons Pubis and Vulva

E 1. Observe skin color and skin condition at the mons pubis and vulva.

2. With gloved hands, using the thumb and index finger of the dominant hand, separate the labia majora.

3. Observe the labia majora and labia minora for color, lesions, and trauma.

N **The skin over the mons pubis should be clear except for nevi and normal hair distribution. The labia majora and labia minora should appear symmetric and should have a smooth to somewhat wrinkled, unbroken, slightly pigmented skin surface. There should be no ecchymosis, excoriation, nodules, swelling, rash, or lesions. An occasional sebaceous cyst is within normal limits. These cysts are nontender, yellow nodules less than 1 cm in diameter.**

A Edema or swelling of the labia

P Hematoma formation, Bartholin's cyst, obstruction of the lymphatic system

A Broken areas in the skin surface

P Ulcerations or abrasions secondary to infection or trauma

A Rashes over the mons pubis and labia

P Contact dermatitis, infestations

A Chancre: reddish, nontenter, round ulcer with a depressed center and raised, indurated edges

P Primary stages of syphilis at the site where the treponema enters the body

A Condylomata lata: raised, round, wartlike plaques that have moist surfaces and are covered with gray exudate

P Secondary stage of syphilis

A Condyloma acuminatum: white, dry, cauliflowerlike, painless growths that have narrow bases

P Human papillomavirus

A Small, shallow, red vesicles that fuse together to form a large, possibly painful and itchy ulcer

P Herpes simplex lesions

A A painless mass possibly accompanied by pruritus; a mass that develops into a cauliflowerlike growth

P Suggestive of malignancy

A Varicose veins: venous prominences of the labia

P Congenital predisposition, prolonged standing, pregnancy, aging

A Ecchymosis

P Accident, trauma, or abuse

Clitoris

E 1. Using the dominant thumb and index finger, separate the labia minora laterally to expose the prepuce of the clitoris.
2. Observe the clitoris for size and condition.

N **The clitoris is approximately 2.0 cm in length and 0.5 cm in diameter and is without lesions.**

A Hypertrophy of the clitoris

P Female pseudohermaphroditism due to androgen excess

A Chancre: a reddish, round ulcer with a depressed center and raised, indurated edges

P The primary lesion of syphilis

Urethral Meatus

E 1. With a gloved hand, using the dominant thumb and index finger, separate the labia minora laterally to expose the urethral meatus. Do not touch the urethral meatus because doing so may cause pain and urethral spasm.
2. Observe the shape, color, and size of the urethral meatus.

N **The urethral opening is slitlike in appearance and is midline; it is free of discharge, swelling, and redness and is approximately the size of a pea.**

A Meatus discharge of any color

P Urinary tract infection

A Swelling or redness around the urethral meatus

P Skene's gland infection, urethral caruncle (small, red growth that protrudes from the meatus), urethral carcinoma, prolapse of the urethral mucosa

Vaginal Introitus

E 1. Keep the labia minora retracted laterally to inspect the vaginal introitus.
2. Ask the patient to bear down.
3. Observe for patency and bulging.

N **The introitus mucosa should be pink and moist. Normal vaginal discharge is clear to white in color and is free of foul odor. It may contain some white clumps, which are mass numbers of epithelial cells. The introitus should be patent and without bulging.**

A Pale color and dryness

P Atrophy from topical steroids, aging process, and estrogen deficiency

A Malodorous white, yellow, green, or gray discharge

P Gonorrhea, *Chlamydia*, *Candida* vaginosis, *Trichomonas* vaginitis, bacterial vaginosis, atrophic vaginitis, cervicitis (Table 20-2)

A An external tear or impatency of the vaginal introitus

P Trauma, fissure of the introitus

A Cystocele: bulging of the anterior vaginal wall

P Weakened supporting tissues and ligaments cause the upper two-thirds of the anterior vaginal wall along with the bladder to push forward into the introitus

A Cystourethrocele: bulging of the anterior vaginal wall, the bladder, and the urethra into the vaginal introitus

P Weakening of the entire anterior vaginal wall, fissure

TABLE 20-2 Description of Vaginal Discharges

DISCHARGE	NORMAL PHYSIOLOGICAL DISCHARGE	BACTERIAL VAGINOSIS (BV)	TRICHOMONAS	CANDIDA	GONOCOCCAL
Color	White	Gray	Grayish yellow	White	Greenish yellow
Odor	Absent	Fishy	Fishy	Absent	Absent
Consistency	Nonhomogenous	Homogenous	Purulent, often with bubbles	Cottage cheeselike	Mucopurulent
Location	Dependent	Adherent to walls	Often pooled in fornix	Adherent to walls	Adherent to walls
Vaginal pH	4	5–6	5–6	4–4.5	—
Anatomic Appearance					
Vulva	Normal	Normal	Edematous	Erythematous	Erythematous
Vaginal mucosa	Normal	Normal	Usually normal	Erythematous	Normal
Cervix	Normal	Normal	May show red spots	Patches of discharge	Pus in os

A Rectocele: bulging of the posterior vaginal wall and a portion of the rectum

P Weakening of the entire posterior vaginal wall

Perineum and Anus

E 1. Observe color and shape of the anus.
2. Observe texture and color of the perineum.

N **The perineum should be smooth and slightly darkened. A well-healed episiotomy scar is normal after vaginal delivery. The anus should be dark pink to brown and puckered. Skin tags are not uncommon around the anal area.**

A A fissure or tear of the perineum

P Trauma, abscess, unhealed episiotomy, herpes simplex

A External hemorrhoids: venous prominences of the anal area

P Varicose dilatation of a vein of the inferior hemorrhoidal plexus covered with modified anal skin

Palpation of the External Genitalia

Labia

E 1. Between the thumb and the index finger of your dominant hand, palpate each labium.
2. Observe for swelling, induration, pain, and discharge from the Bartholin's gland ducts.

N **The labium should feel soft, be uniform in structure, and exhibit no swelling, pain, or induration.**

A Bartholin's gland infection: swelling, redness, induration, or purulent discharge from the labial folds along with hot, tender areas

P Gonococci, *Chlamydia trachomatis*

Urethral Meatus and Skene's Glands

E 1. Insert your dominant index finger into the vagina.

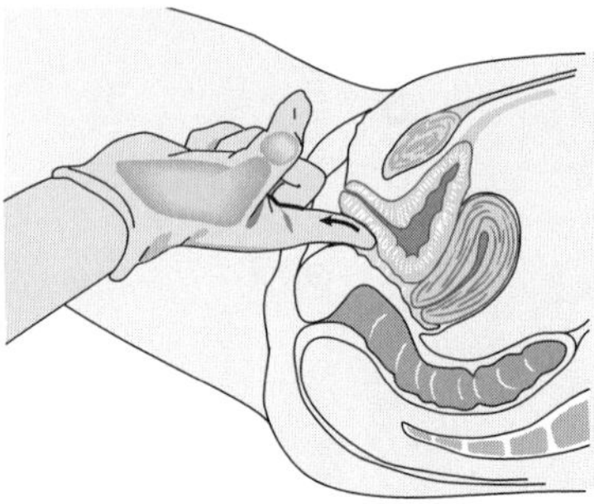

Figure 20-3 Milking the Urethra

2. Apply pressure to the anterior aspect of the vaginal wall and milk the urethra (Figure 20-3).
3. Observe for discharge and patient discomfort.

N **Milking the urethra should not cause pain or urethral discharge.**

A Urethral discharge and pain on contact

P Skene's gland infection, urinary tract infection

Vaginal Introitus

E 1. While your finger remains in the vagina, ask the patient to squeeze the vaginal muscles around your finger.
2. Evaluate muscle strength and tone.

N **In a nulliparous woman, vaginal muscle tone should be tight and strong, whereas in a parous woman, it will be diminished.**

A Significantly diminished or absent vaginal muscle tone, bulging of vaginal or pelvic contents (cystocele, rectocele, uterine prolapse)

P Weakened muscle tone secondary to injury, age, childbirth, or medication

Perineum

E 1. Withdraw your finger from the introitus until you can place only your dominant index finger posterior to the perineum and place your dominant thumb anterior to the perineum.

2. Between the dominant thumb and index finger, assess the perineum for muscle tone and texture.

N **The perineum should be smooth, firm, and homogenous in the nulliparous woman and thinner in the parous woman. A well-healed episiotomy scar is within normal limits for a parous woman.**

A Thin, tissuelike perineum; fissures; tears

P Atrophy, trauma, unhealed episiotomy

Speculum Examination of the Internal Genitalia

Cervix

E 1. Select the appropriately sized speculum. Base your selection on the patient's history, size of the vaginal introitus, and vaginal muscle tone.

2. Lubricate and warm the speculum by rinsing it under warm water. Do not use other lubricants because they may interfere with the accuracy of cytologic samples and cultures.

3. Between your dominant index and middle fingers, hold the speculum with the blades closed The index finger should rest at the proximal end of the superior blade. Wrap the other fingers around the handle, with the thumbscrew over the thumb.

4. Insert your nondominant index and middle fingers, ventral sides down, just inside the vagina and apply pressure to the posterior vaginal wall. Encourage the patient to bear down to help relax the perineal muscles.

5. Encourage the patient to take deep breaths to relax. Be careful not to pull on pubic hair or to pinch the labia.

6. When you feel the muscles relax, insert the speculum at an oblique angle and in a plane parallel to the examination table until the speculum reaches the end of the fingers in the vagina (see Figure 20-4A).

7. Withdraw the fingers of your nondominant hand.

8. Gently rotate the speculum blades to a horizontal angle and advance the speculum at a 45° downward angle against the posterior vaginal wall until the speculum reaches the end of the vagina.

9. Using your dominant thumb, depress the lever to open the blades and visualize the cervix (Figure 20-4B).

10. If the cervix is not visualized, close the blades, withdraw the speculum 2 to 3 cm, and reinsert the speculum at a slightly different angle to ensure that it is inserted far enough into the vagina.

11. Once the cervix is fully visualized, lock the speculum blades in place. (This procedure varies with the type of speculum being used.)

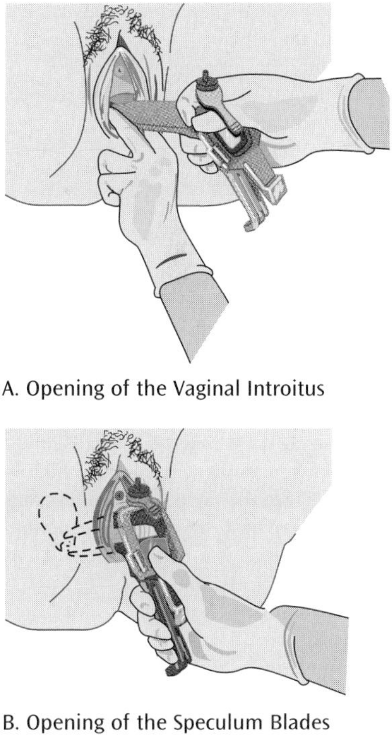

A. Opening of the Vaginal Introitus

B. Opening of the Speculum Blades

Figure 20-4 Speculum Examination

12. Adjust your light source so that it shines through the speculum.

13. If any discharge obstructs the visualization of the cervix, clean it away with a cotton-tipped applicator.

14. Inspect the cervix and the cervical os for color, position, size, surface characteristics such as polyps and lesions, discharge, and shape.

Color

N **The normal cervix is a glistening pink; it may be pale after menopause or blue (Chadwick's sign) during pregnancy.**

A Redness or a friable appearance

P Inflammation from infection such as *Chlamydia* or gonorrhea

Position

N **The cervix is located midline in the vagina with an anterior or posterior position relative to the vaginal vault and projecting approximately 2.5 cm into the vagina.**

A Lateral positioning of the cervix

P Tumor, adhesions, a normal variant

A Projection of the cervix into the vaginal vault greater than normal limits

P Uterine prolapse

Size

N **Normal size is 2.5 cm.**

A Cervical size greater than 4 cm (hypertrophy)

P Inflammation, tumor, multiparous

Surface Characteristics

N **The cervix is covered by a glistening pink squamous epithelium, which is similar to the vaginal epithelium, and a deep-pink to red columnar epithelium, which is a continuation of the endocervical lining.**

A Ectropion, or eversion: reddish circle around the cervical os

P Appearance of the squamocolumnar junction on the ectocervix as a result of lacerations during childbirth or congenital variation

A Nabothian cysts: small, cystic, yellow, benign lesions on the cervical surface

P Obstruction of the cervical glands

A Cervical polyp: bright-red, soft protrusion through the cervical os

Nursing Alert

Risk Factors for Female Genitalia Cancer

Cervical Cancer
- Early age at first intercourse
- Multiple sex partners
- Prior history of human papillomavirus (HPV), herpes simplex virus (HSV)
- Tobacco use
- Family history
- African American
- Immunosuppressed
- Drug use
- Women of lower socioeconomic status
- HIV
- History of STDs
- Cervical cancer of dysplasia

Endometrial Cancer
- Early or late menarche (before age 11 or after age 16)
- History of infertility
- Failure to ovulate
- Unopposed estrogen therapy
- Use of tamoxifen
- Obesity
- Family history

Ovarian Cancer
- Advancing age
- Nulliparity
- History of breast cancer
- Family history of ovarian cancer
- Infertility treatment

Vaginal Cancer
- Daughters of women who ingested DES during pregnancy
- HPV

P Originate from the endocervical canal; usually benign, but tend to bleed if abraded

A Strawberry spots: hemorrhages dispersed over the surface of the cervix

P Trichomonal infection

A Irregularities of the cervical surface that may be cauliflowerlike in appearance

P Carcinoma of the cervix

A Columnar epithelium covering most of the cervix and extending to the vaginal wall (vaginal adenosis) and a collar-type ridge between the cervix and the vagina

P Fetal exposure to DES

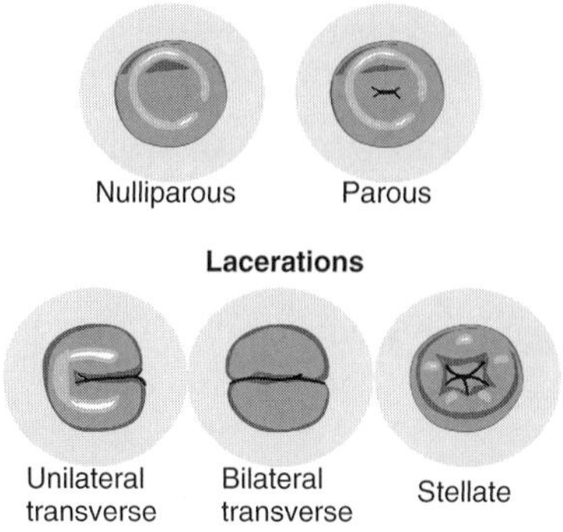

Figure 20-5 Shapes of the Cervical Os

Discharge

See Table 20-2.

Shape of the Cervical Os

N **In the nulliparous woman, the os is small and either round or oval. In the parous woman who has had a vaginal delivery, the os is a horizontal slit.**

A A unilateral transverse, bilateral transverse, irregular, or stellate cervical os (Figure 20-5)

P Rapid second-stage childbirth delivery, forceps delivery, trauma

Collecting Specimens for Cytological Smears and Cultures

Collect the Papanicolaou (Pap) smear first, followed by the chlamydial, the gonococcal, and any other vaginal smears or cultures.

Pap Smear

If the patient has three or more consecutive normal Pap smears, the Pap may be done every 2 to 3 years. If the patient had a hysterectomy for benign disease, discontinue routine screening. If the patient had CIN II or III or in situ, screen three times then discontinue. This screen is for vaginal cancer. Though Pap smears can be spaced every 3 years, a woman should have an annual pelvic examination at least until age 80 to 85. Many providers now use liquid-based cytology systems such as ThinPrep and PapSure.

Endocervical Smear

E **1.** Using your dominant hand, insert the cytobrush or cervical broom through the speculum and into the cervical os approximately 1 cm. This procedure causes a cramping sensation in many patients, so forewarn your patient that she may feel discomfort during this portion of the assessment.

2. Rotate the cytobrush between your index finger and thumb 360° first clockwise and then counterclockwise. Keep the cytobrush in contact with the cervical tissue. *Note:* If you must use a cotton-tipped applicator instead of a cytobrush, leave the applicator in the cervical os for 30 seconds to ensure saturation. If you use a cervical broom, rotate the broom six times clockwise.

3. Remove the cytobrush. Using a rolling motion, spread the cells on the section of the slide marked *E*, if a sectional slide is being used. Do not press down hard or wipe the cytobrush back and forth because doing either will destroy the cells. If using

a cervical broom, place the broom in the liquid-based preparation container.
4. Discard the brush.
5. If using the ThinPrep method, follow the manufacturer's directions.

N/A/P See Vaginal Pool Smear.

Cervical Smear

E 1. Insert the bifurcated end of the Ayre spatula through the speculum base. Place the longer projection of the bifurcation into the cervical os. The shorter projection should be snug against the ectocervix.
2. Rotate the spatula 360° one time only. Make sure the transformation zone is well sampled.
3. Remove the spatula and gently spread the specimen on the section of the slide labeled *C*, if a sectional slide is being used.

N/A/P See Vaginal Pool Smear.

Vaginal Pool Smear

E 1. Reverse the Ayre spatula, insert the rounded end into the posterior vaginal fornix, and gently scrape the area. *Note*: A cotton-tipped applicator can also be used to obtain the smear and may be the preferred vehicle for obtaining the specimen if vaginal secretions are viscous or dry. By moistening the cotton-tipped applicator with normal saline, viscous secretions can be removed with less trauma to the surrounding membranes.
2. Remove the spatula and gently spread the specimen on the section of the slide marked *V*, if a sectional slide is being used.
3. Dispose of the spatula or cotton-tipped applicator.
4. Spray the entire slide or slides with cytological fixative.
5. Submit the specimens to the appropriate laboratory per your institution's guidelines for cytology specimens.

N **Using the Bethesda System 2001, cervicovaginal cytology should read "Specimen Adequacy—adequate for evaluation," and "General Categorization—negative for intraepithelial lesion or malignancy," which denotes a lack of pathogenesis.**

A Report finding of "benign cellular changes"

P Fungal, bacterial, protozoan, or viral infections

A Report finding of "atypical squamous cells of undetermined significance"

P Inflammatory or infectious processes, preliminary lesion, unknown phenomenon

A Report finding of "epithelial cell abnormalities"

P Transient or intransient squamous intraepithelial lesion; squamous cell carcinoma; glandular cell abnormalities (seen in postmenopausal women who are not on hormone replacement therapy)

Gonococcal Culture Specimen

E 1. Insert a sterile cotton swab applicator 1 cm into the cervical os.
2. Hold the applicator in place for 20 to 30 seconds.
3. Remove the swab.
4. Roll the swab in a large Z pattern over a Thayer-Martin culture plate. Simultaneously rotate the swab as you roll it to ensure that all of the specimen is used.
5. Dispose of the swab.
6. Submit the specimen to the appropriate laboratory per your institution's guidelines for culture specimens.

N **Cervicovaginal tissues are normally free of *Neisseria gonorrhoeae*.**

A Large number of gram-negative diplococci present in cervicovaginal secretions

P *N. gonorrhoeae* organism invasion of columnar and stratified epithelium

Saline Mount or "Wet Prep"

E Spread a sample of the cervicovaginal specimen onto a microscope slide, add one drop of normal saline, and apply a cover slip.

N **The sample should have fewer than 10 WBCs per field.**

A A sample with more than 10 WBCs per field, protozoa, or clue cells (bacteria-covered epithelium)

P Large number of WBCs: inflammatory response, *Chlamydia trachomatis*, bacterial infection; protozoa: trichomoniasis; clue cells: bacterial vaginosis

KOH Prep

E Spread a sample of the cervicovaginal specimen onto a microscope slide, add one drop of potassium hydroxide, and apply a cover slip; note any odor, and examine under a microscope.

N **Cervicovaginal tissues are normally free of *Candida albicans* except in a small percentage of women.**

A The presence of yeast and pseudohyphae forms (chains of budding yeast)

P Overgrowth of *Candida*

A Fishy odor (positive whiff test)

P Bacterial vaginosis

Five Percent Acetic Acid Wash

E After completing all other vaginal specimens, swab the cervix using a cotton-tipped applicator that has been soaked in 5% acetic acid.

N **The normal response is no change in the appearance of the cervix.**

A A rapid acetowhitening or blanching with jagged borders

P Human papillomavirus (causative agent of genital warts)

Anal Culture

E **1.** Insert a sterile cotton swab applicator 1 cm into the anal canal.
2. Hold the applicator in place for 20 to 30 seconds.
3. Remove the swab. If fecal material is collected, discard the applicator and start again.
4. Roll and rotate the swab in a large Z pattern over a Thayer-Martin culture plate.
5. Dispose of the swab.

N **Anal tissues are normally free of *Neisseria gonorrhoeae*.**

A A large number of gram-negative diplococci

P *N. gonorrhoeae*

Inspection of the Vaginal Wall

E **1.** Disengage the locking device of the speculum.
2. Slowly withdraw the speculum without closing the blades.
3. To allow full inspection of the vaginal walls, rotate the speculum into an oblique position as you retract it. Observe vaginal wall color and texture.

N **The vaginal walls should be pink, moist, deeply rugated, and without lesions and redness.**

A Spots that look like white paint on the walls

P Leukoplakia: secondary to *Candida*, HIV disease

A Pallor of vaginal wall

P Anemia, menopause

A Redness of vaginal walls

P Inflammation, hyperemia, trauma from tampon insertion or removal

A Vaginal lesions or masses

P Carcinoma, tumors, DES exposure

Bimanual Examination

E **1.** Observe the patient's face for signs of discomfort during the assessment process.
2. Inform the patient of the steps of the bimanual assessment, and warn her that the lubricant gel may be cold.

3. Squeeze water-soluble lubricant onto the fingertips of your dominant hand.
4. Stand between the legs of the patient as she remains in the lithotomy position, and place your nondominant hand on her abdomen and below the umbilicus.
5. Insert your dominant index and middle fingers 1 cm into the vagina. The fingers should be extended with the lateral sides up. Exert gentle posterior pressure.
6. Inform the patient that pressure from palpation may be uncomfortable. Instruct the patient to relax the abdominal muscles by taking deep breaths.
7. When you feel the patient's muscles relax, insert your fingers their full length into the vagina. Insert your fingers slowly so that you can simultaneously palpate the vaginal walls.
8. In order to prevent pain and spasm, remember to keep your thumb widely abducted and away from the urethral meatus and clitoris throughout the palpation.

Vagina

N **The vaginal wall is nontender and has a smooth or rugated surface and no lesions, masses, or cysts.**

A Lesions, masses, scarring, cysts

P Benign lesions (inclusion cysts, myomas, fibromas), malignant lesions (most commonly found on the upper one-third of the posterior vaginal wall)

Cervix

E 1. Rotate your dominant hand 90° so that the palmar surface faces upward.
2. Place your nondominant hand on the abdomen approximately one-third of the way down between the umbilicus and symphysis pubis.
3. Use the palmar surfaces of the dominant hand's fingertips, which

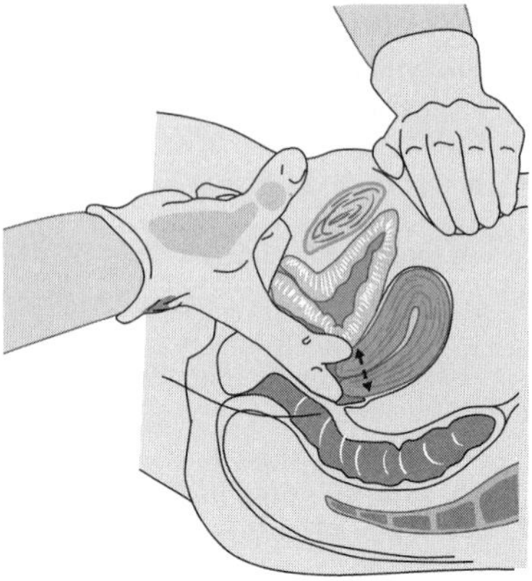

Figure 20-6 Assessment of Cervical Mobility

are in the vagina, to assess the cervix for consistency, position, shape, tenderness, and mobility.
4. Between your fingertips, grasp the cervix and move it from side to side to assess mobility (Figure 20-6).

N **The normal cervix is mobile, without pain, smooth and firm, symmetrically rounded, and midline.**

A Positive Chandelier's sign: pain on palpation or on assessment of mobility

P Pelvic inflammatory disease, ectopic pregnancy

A Positive Goodell's sign: softening of the cervix

P Fifth to sixth week of pregnancy

A Irregular surface, immobility, nodular surface

P Malignancy, nabothian cysts, polyps, and fibroids

Fornices

E 1. Using the fingertips and palmar surfaces of the fingers, palpate around the fornices.
2. Note any nodules and irregularities.

N **The walls should be smooth and without nodules.**

A Nodules, irregularities

P Malignancy, polyps, herniations (if fornices' walls are inpatent)

Uterus

E **1.** With the dominant hand, which is in the vagina, push the pelvic organs out of the pelvic cavity and provide stabilization while using the nondominant hand, which is on the abdomen, to perform palpation (Figure 20-7).

2. Press the hand that is on the abdomen inward and downward toward the vagina and try to grasp the uterus between your hands.

3. Evaluate the uterus for size, shape, consistency, mobility, tenderness, masses, and position (e.g., anteflexed, anteverted, naid position, retroverted, retroflexed).

4. Place the fingers of the dominant hand, which is in the vagina, into the anterior fornix and palpate the uterine surface.

N **The size of the uterus varies on the basis of parity; it should be pear shaped in the nongravid patient and more rounded in the parous patient. The uterus should be smooth, firm, mobile, nontender, and without masses. A nonpalpable uterus in the older woman may be a normal finding secondary to uterine atrophy. See Figure 20-8 for position of the uterus.**

A Significant exterior enlargement and changes in the shape of the uterus

P Intrauterine pregnancy or tumor

A Nodules, irregularities

P Leiomyomas: tumors composed of muscle tissue

A Inability to assess uterus

P A retroverted and retroflexed uterus (can best be assessed via rectovaginal assessment), hysterectomy

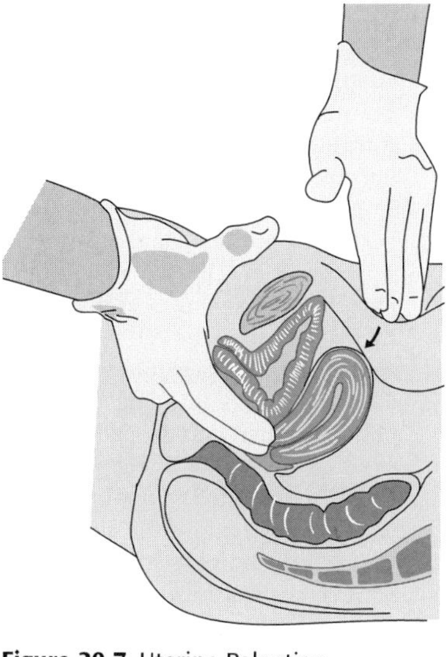

Figure 20-7 Uterine Palpation

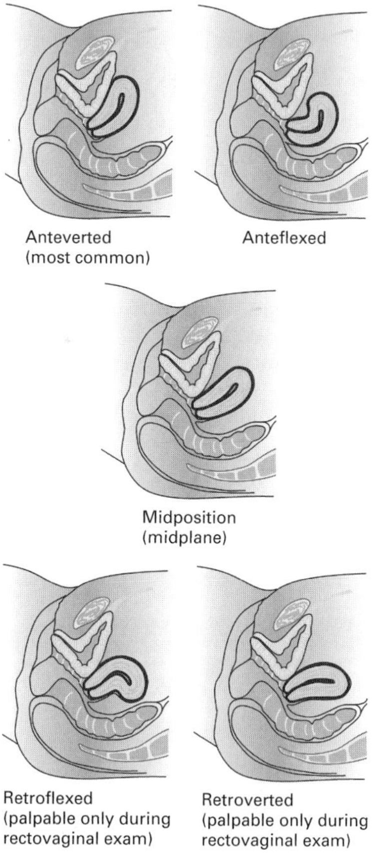

Figure 20-8 Positions of the Uterus

Adnexa

The fallopian tubes are rarely palpable, and palpation of the ovaries depends on patient age and size. The ovaries often are not palpable, and this procedure can be painful for the patient either during the luteal phase of the menstrual cycle (postovulation) or because of normal visceral tenderness.

E 1. Move your dominant hand, which is in the vagina, to the right lateral fornix, and move your nondominant hand, which is on the abdomen, to the right lower quadrant just inside the anterior iliac spine. Press deeply inward and upward toward the hand on the abdomen.

2. Push inward and downward with the hand on the abdomen and try to catch the ovary between your fingertips.

3. Palpate for size, shape, consistency, and mobility of adnexa.

4. Repeat the above maneuvers on the left side (Figure 20-9).

N **The ovaries are normally almond shaped, firm, smooth, mobile, and without tenderness.**

A Enlarged, irregular, nodular, painful, pulsatile ovaries with decreased mobility

P Ectopic pregnancy, ovarian cyst, pelvic inflammatory disease, malignancy

> **Nursing Alert**
>
> **Warning Signs of Ectopic Pregnancy**
>
> Any signs or symptoms of an ectopic pregnancy (such as late menstruation followed by spotting and abdominal soreness or pain on the affected side) constitute a medical emergency and thus require immediate medical attention.

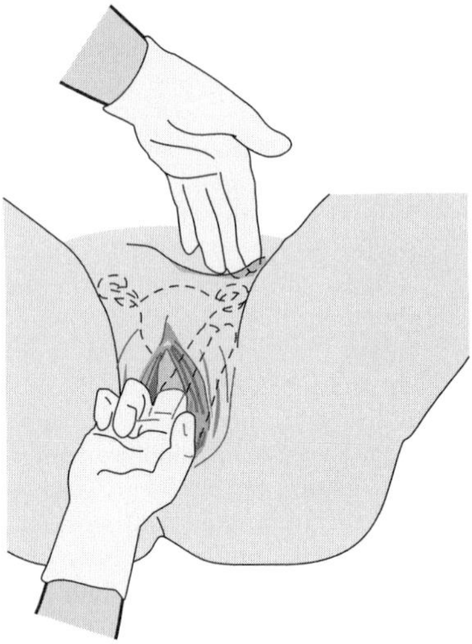

Figure 20-9 Palpation of the Left Adnexa

Rectovaginal Examination

E 1. Withdraw your dominant hand from the vagina and change gloves. Apply additional lubricant to the fingertips of your dominant hand.

2. Tell the patient you will be inserting one finger into her vagina and one finger into her rectum. Remind her that the lubricant jelly will feel cold and that the rectal exam will be uncomfortable.

3. Insert your dominant index finger back into the vagina.

4. In order to relax the anal sphincter, ask the patient to bear down as if she is having a bowel movement. Assess anal sphincter tone.

5. Insert the middle finger of your dominant hand into the patient's rectum as she bears down (Figure 20-10). If the rectum is full of stool, carefully and digitally remove the stool from the rectum.

6. Advance the finger in the rectum forward while using the nondominant hand to depress the abdomen.

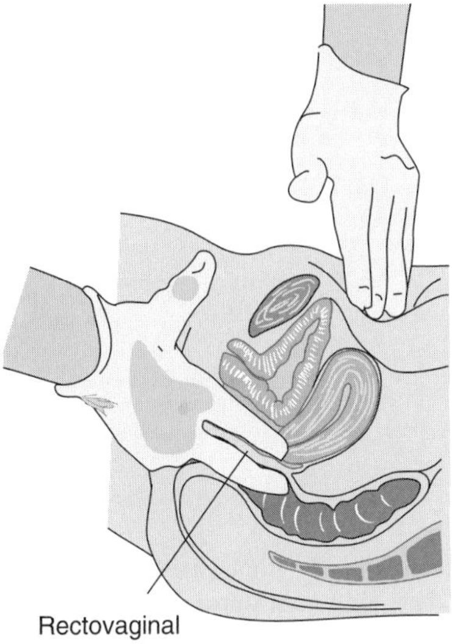

Figure 20-10 Rectovaginal Examination

Assess the rectovaginal septum for patency, the cervix and uterus for anomalies such as posterior lesions, and the rectouterine pouch for contour lesions.

7. On completion of the assessment, withdraw the fingers from the vagina and rectum. If any stool is present on the glove, test for occult blood.

8. Use a tissue to clean the patient's genitalia and anal area or allow the patient to do so. Assist the patient back to a sitting position.

N **The rectal walls are normally smooth and free of lesions. The rectal pouch is rugated and free of masses. Anal sphincter tone is strong. The cervix and uterus, if palpable, are smooth. The rectovaginal septum is smooth and intact. See Chapter 22 for further information on the complete rectal examination.**

A Masses or lesions

P Malignancy, internal hemorrhoids

A Lax sphincter tone

P Perineal trauma from childbirth or anal intercourse; neurological disorders

Nursing Tip

Examining the Patient with a Hysterectomy

If the patient has had a hysterectomy, follow the same assessment sequence but omit the following: cervical inspection and palpation, uterine inspection and palpation, endocervical and cervical smears. The vaginal walls are evaluated and the adnexa are evaluated if they were not surgically removed during the hysterectomy.

BIBLIOGRAPHY

Apgar, B., Zoschnick, L., & Wright, T. (2003). The 2001 Bethesda System terminology. *American Family Physician, 68*(10). Retrieved May 9, 2005, from http://www.aafp.org/afp/2003115/1992.html

21

Male Genitalia

Anatomy and Physiology

The male reproductive system includes essential and accessory organs, ducts, and supporting structures (Figure 21-1). The essential organs are the testes, or male gonads. The accessory organs include the seminal vesicles and bulbourethral glands. There are several ducts including the epididymis, ductus (vas) deferens, ejaculatory ducts, and urethra. The supporting structures include the scrotum, penis, and spermatic cords. The prostate is discussed in Chapter 22.

The testes, or testicles, are two oval glands located in the scrotum. The seminal vesicles are two pouches located posteriorly to and at the base of the bladder. They contribute approximately 60% of the volume of semen. The bulbourethral glands, or Cowper's glands, are pea-sized glands located just below the prostate. The bulbourethral glands secrete an alkaline substance that protects sperm by neutralizing the acidic environment of the vagina. These glands also provide lubrication at the end of the penis during sexual intercourse.

The epididymis is a comma-shaped, tightly coiled tube that is located on the top and behind the testis and inside the scrotum. Sperm mature and develop the power of motility as they pass through the epididymis. The ductus (vas) deferens is

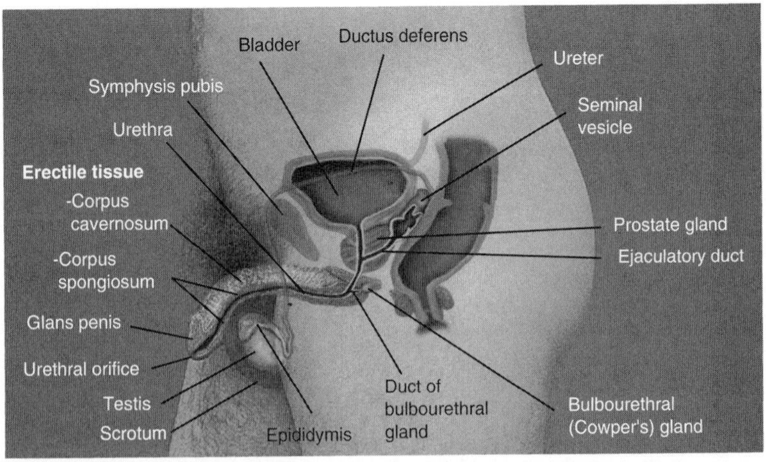

Figure 21-1 Male Genitalia

an extension of the tail of the epididymis. The ejaculatory ducts are two short tubes located posterior to the bladder that eject spermatozoa into the prostatic urethra just before ejaculation. The urethra is the terminal duct of the seminal fluid passageway, and passes through the prostate gland and penis.

The scrotum is a pouchlike supporting structure for the testes and consists of rugated, deeply pigmented, loose skin.

The penis, or male organ of copulation, is hairless, slightly pigmented, and cylindrical. The penis contains the urethra, a slitlike opening on the tip of the glans. The urethra terminates at the urethral meatus and is the passageway for urine.

The spermatic cord is made up of testicular arteries, autonomic nerves, veins that drain the testicle, lymphatic vessels, and the cremaster muscle. The testicles are suspended by the spermatic cord. The left side of the spermatic cord is longer than the right side, causing the left testicle to be lower in the scrotal sac.

The primary function of the male reproductive system is to produce sperm to fertilize eggs. The male sexual act consists of four stages: erection, lubrication, emission, and ejaculation.

HEALTH HISTORY

Medical History

Prior history of sexually transmitted disease (STD), prostatitis, epididymitis, urinary tract infection, nephrolithiasis, cryptorchidism, trauma, cancer, benign prostatic hypertrophy (BPH), congenital or acquired deformity (epispadias, hypospadias), premature ejaculation, impotence, infertility, erectile dysfunction (ED)

Nonmale Genitalia Specific

Mumps, rashes, joint pain, renal disease, CHF, spinal cord injury, pelvic fracture, diabetes mellitus, hypertension, TB, depression, anxiety, MS

Surgical History

Prostatectomy, transurethral prostatectomy, circumcision, orchidectomy, correction of testicular malpositioning, vasectomy, lesion or nodule removal, epispadias repair, hypospadias repair, hernia repair

Medications

Antibiotics, hormone replacement, antihypertensives, psychotropic agents, 5-alpha reductase inhibitors

Injuries and Accidents

Trauma, testicular torsion

Family Health History

Varicocele, testicular cancer, infertility, hypospadias, mother's use of hormones (diethylstilbestrol [DES]) during pregnancy

Social History

Drug use: cocaine (priapism with chronic abuse, impotence, increased sexual excitability), barbiturates (impotence), amphetamines (increased libido and delayed orgasm in moderate users, impotence in chronic users)

Sexual practice: multiple partners, partner with multiple partners, new sexual partner, condom use (frequency and accuracy of use), sexual orientation, anal or oral intercourse

Equipment

- Nonsterile gloves
- Penlight
- Stethoscope
- Culturette tube
- Sterile cotton swabs
- Chux
- 1½" to 2" gauze wrap
- Five percent acetic acid solution in spray bottle
- Thayer-Martin culture plate
- Male gen probe
- 10× power magnifying lens

NURSING CHECKLIST

General Approach to Male Genitalia Assessment

1. Greet the patient and explain the assessment techniques that you will be using.
2. Ensure that the examination room is at a warm, comfortable temperature to prevent patient chilling and shivering.
3. Ensure that the light in the room provides sufficient brightness to adequately observe the patient.
4. Instruct the patient to remove his pants and underpants.
5. Place the patient in a supine position on the examination table (with the patient's legs spread slightly), drape the patient, and stand to the patient's right side, *or*
6. Sit and have the patient stand in front of you.
7. Don clean gloves.
8. Expose the genitalia and the entire groin area.

Assessment of the Male Genitalia

Inspection

Sexual Maturity Rating

E 1. Assess the developmental stage of the pubic hair, penis, and scrotum.
2. Determine the sexual maturity rating (SMR).

N **Males usually begin puberty between the ages of 9½ and 13½. The average male proceeds through puberty in about 3 years, with a possible range of 2 to 5 years.**

A SMR less than expected for the patient's age.

P Familial, chronic illnesses

Hair Distribution

E 1. Note hair distribution pattern.
2. Note the presence of nits or lice.

N **Pubic hair is distributed in an inverse triangular formation, is sparsely distributed on the scrotum and inner thigh, and is absent on the penis. Genital hair is coarser than scalp hair. There are no nits or lice.**

A Alopecia: sparse or absent hair distribution in the genital area

P Genetic factors, aging, local or systemic disease

A Nits or lice

P Pediculosis

Penis

E 1. Inspect the glans, foreskin, and shaft for lesions, swelling, and inflammation. If the patient is uncircumcised, ask him to retract the foreskin so that the underlying area can be inspected. After the assessment, replace the foreskin.

2. Inspect the dorsal surface of the penis first, then lift the penis to inspect the ventral surface.
3. Note the size and shape of the penis.

N **The skin is free of lesions and inflammation. The shaft skin appears loose and wrinkled in the patient without an erection. The glans is smooth and without lesions, swelling, and inflammation. The foreskin retracts easily, and there is no discharge (although there may be a small amount of smegma, a white, cottage cheeselike substance). The dorsal vein is sometimes visible. The penis is cylindrical. Penises vary greatly in size. Glans penises also vary in size and shape and may appear rounded or broad.**

A Chancre: small, papular lesion that enlarges and undergoes superficial necrosis to produce a sharply marginated ulcer on a clean base

P Primary syphilis (*Treponema pallidum*)

A Chancroid: tender, ulcerated, exudative, papular lesion with an erythematous halo, surrounding edema, and a friable base

P *Haemophilus ducreyi*

A Condyloma acuminatum (genital warts): pinhead papules to cauliflowerlike groupings of filiform skin-colored lesions that are pink or red

P Human papillomavirus

A Penile lesion (small induration to a small papule)

P Penile carcinoma

Nursing Alert

Warning Signs of STDs in the Male Patient

- Bloody or purulent urethral discharge
- Scrotal or testicular pain
- Burning or pain on urination
- Penile lesion

A Multifocal, maculopapular lesions that are tan, brown, pink, violet, or white

P Intraepithelial neoplasia

A Erythematous plaque developing into vesicular lesions that may become pustular

P Herpes simplex virus

A *Candida*: multiple, discrete, flat pustules with slight scaling and surrounding edema

P Superficial mycotic infection of moist cutaneous sites

A Tinea cruris: erythematous plaques with scaling, papular lesions with sharp margins, occasionally with clear centers and pustules

P Fungal infection of the groin caused by *Epidermophyton floccosum* or *Trichophyton rubrum*

A Phimosis: unusually narrow foreskin that cannot be retracted over the glans penis

P Normal in infancy; in later years, possibly an acquired constricting circumferential scar that follows healing of a split foreskin

A Paraphimosis: fixed constriction proximal to the glans

P Retracted foreskin that is not returned to its original position

A Microphallus: normally formed but diminutive penis

P Disorder in the hypothalamus or pituitary gland; idiopathic

A Abnormally large penis before the age of normal puberty

P Hormonal influence of tumors of the pineal gland or hypothalamus; tumors from the Leydig cells of the testes; tumors of the adrenal gland; precocious genital maturity

A Priapism: continuous and pathological erection of the penis

P Leukemia, metastatic carcinoma, created by a positive imbalance between arterial blood supply and its return

A Ventral or dorsal penile curvature (chordee)

P Congenital: caused by a fibrous band along the usual course of the corpus spongiosum; Peyronie's disease: cause unknown

A Inflammation of the glans penis

P Balanitis, a bacterial infection associated with phimosis and in diabetic men

Scrotum

E 1. Displace the penis to one side in order to inspect the scrotal skin.
2. Lift up the scrotum to inspect the posterior side.
3. Observe for lesions, inflammation, swelling, and nodules.
4. Note size and shape.
5. The patient should then stand with legs slightly spread apart.
6. Have the patient perform the Valsalva maneuver.
7. Observe for a mass of dilated testicular veins in the spermatic cord above and behind the testes.

N **Scrotal skin appears rugated, thin, and more deeply pigmented than body color. The skin should hug the testicles firmly in the young patient and should be elongated and flaccid in the elderly patient. All skin areas should be free of lesions, nodules, swelling, and inflammation. Scrotal size and shape vary greatly from one individual to another. The left scrotal sac is lower than the right. There should be no dilated veins.**

A Condyloma acuminatum, tinea cruris, and *Candida*

P See page 299

A Enlargement of or masses within the scrotum

P Inguinal hernia, hydrocele, varicocele, spermatocele, tumor, edema

A Hydrocele: a large pear-sized mass in the scrotum

P Accumulation of fluid between the two layers of the tunica vaginalis (idiopathic or resulting from trauma, inguinal surgery, epididymitis, or testicular tumor)

A Spermatocele: well-defined, cystic mass on the superior testis or in the epididymis

P Blockage of the efferent ductules of the rete testis resulting in formation of sperm-filled cysts

A Varicocele: in light-skinned individuals, a scrotal mass (most often in the left hemiscrotum) with a bluish discoloration

P Dilated veins in the pampiniform plexus of the spermatic cord

A Sebaceous cysts: round, firm, cystic nodules confined within the scrotal skin

P Decrease in localized circulation and closure of sebaceous glands or ducts

Urethral Meatus

E 1. Note the location of the urethral meatus.
2. Observe for discharge.
3. Culture any discharge.
4. If the patient complains of penile discharge, but none is present, ask the patient to milk the penis from the shaft to the glans.

N **The urethral meatus is located centrally. It is pink and without discharge.**

A Urethritis: erythema and swelling at the urethral meatus

P Localized tissue inflammation resulting from bacterial, viral, or fungal infection or from urethral trauma

A Epispadias: dorsally displaced urethral meatus

P Congenital abnormality caused by a complete or partial dorsal fusion defect of the urethra

A Hypospadias: urethral meatus opens on the ventral aspect of the glans penis or on the perineum

P Congenital abnormality usually associated with chordee

Inguinal Area

E 1. If the patient is supine, ask the patient to stand.
2. Stand facing the patient.
3. Observe for swelling and bulges.
4. Ask the patient to bear down.
5. Observe for swelling and bulges.

N **The inguinal area is free of swelling and bulges.**

A Bulge in the inguinal area
P Hernia (see Chapter 17)

Palpation

Penis

E 1. Stand in front of the patient's genital area.
2. Don clean gloves.
3. Between the thumb and first two fingers, palpate the entire length of the penis.
4. Note any pulsations, tenderness, masses, and plaques.

N **Pulsations are present on the dorsal sides of the penis. The penis is nontender. No masses or firm plaques are palpated.**

A Vascular insufficiency: diminished or absent palpable pulse or pulsations
P Systemic disease, localized trauma, localized disease
A Generalized penile swelling
P Anasarcic states, trauma, obstruction of the penile veins, or inflammation of the penis resulting in local edema
A Fibrotic plaques or ridges along the dorsal shaft
P Perivascular inflammation between the tunica albuginea and the underlying spongy erectile tissue

Urethral Meatus

E 1. Stand in front of the patient's genital area.
2. Between the thumb and forefinger, grasp the glans penis and gently squeeze to expose the urethral meatus (Figure 21-2).
3. If the patient complains of a urethral discharge, a culture should be taken.

N **The urethral meatus is free of discharge and drainage.**

A Urethral discharge of pus and mucus shreds
P Bacterial infection

Scrotum

E 1. Between the thumb and first two fingers, gently palpate the right testicle.
2. Note size, shape, consistency, and presence of masses.
3. Palpate the epididymis.
4. Note consistency and the presence of tenderness and masses.
5. Between the thumb and the first two fingers, palpate the spermatic cord from the epididymis to the external ring.
6. Note consistency and the presence of tenderness and masses.
7. Repeat on the left side (Figure 21-3).

N **The scrotum contains on each side a testis (testicle) and epididymis. The testicles should be firm but not hard, ovoid, smooth, and equal in size**

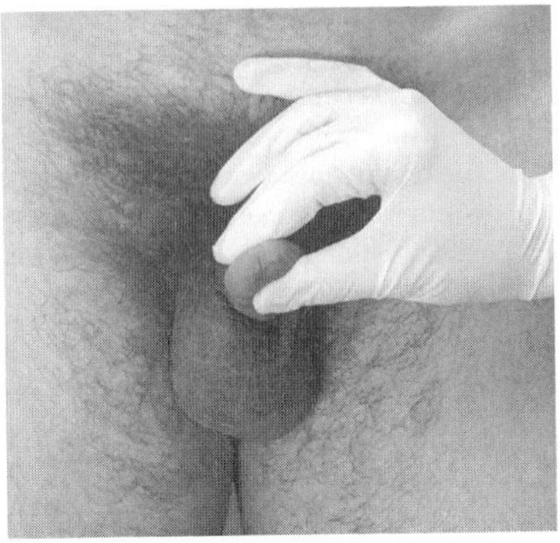

Figure 21-2 Palpation of the Urethral Meatus

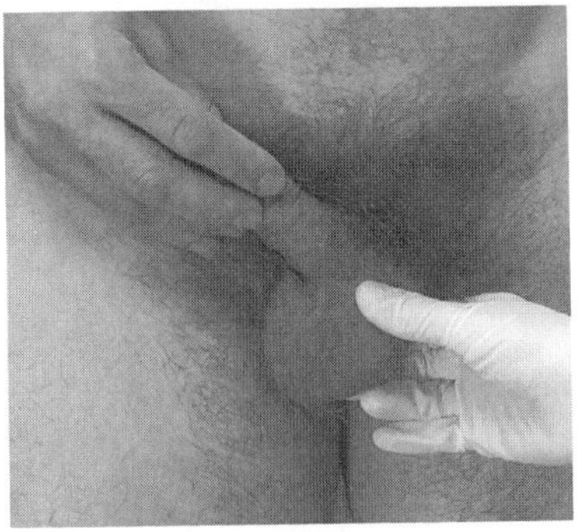

Figure 21-3 Palpation of the Testicle

bilaterally. They should be sensitive to pressure but not tender. The epididymis is comma-shaped and should be distinguishable from the testicle. The epididymis should be insensitive to normal pressure. The spermatic cord should feel smooth and round.

A A unilateral mass palpated within or near the testicle

P Intratesticular masses: consider malignant until proven otherwise, usually nodular and associated with painless swelling, usually benign; inguinal hernia

A/P Hydrocele, spermatocele: see page 300

A Scrotal mass that is superior to the testis and feels like a "bag of worms"

P Varicocele

A Testicular torsion: enlarged, retracted, laterally positioned, extremely sensitive testicle (Figure 21-4)

P Twisting or torsion of the testis resulting in venous obstruction, edema, and eventual arterial obstruction and lack of perfusion to the testicle

A Epididymitis: indurated, swollen, tender epididymis

P Bacterial pathogens (e.g., *Chlamydia trachomatis* and *Neisseria gonorrhoeae*)

A Cryptorchidism: one or both testes undescended (Figure 21-5)

P Testicular failure, deficient gonadotrophic stimulation, mechanical obstruction, gubernacular defects

A Orchitis: acute, painful onset of testicular swelling and warm scrotal skin

P Mumps, coxsackievirus B, infectious mononucleosis, varicella

A Testicle that is smaller and softer than normal

P Atrophic testicle (Klinefelter's syndrome [hypogonadism], hypopituitarism, estrogen therapy, orchitis)

A In light-skinned individuals, enlarged, taut, reddened scrotum with pitting edema

P Scrotal edema associated with edema of the lower half of the body, such as in congestive heart failure (CHF), renal failure, and portal vein obstruction

A Acute, painful, scrotal swelling occurring in conjunction with a history of trauma

P Scrotal or testicular hematoma formation, testicular rupture

A Soft testes

P Hypogonadism

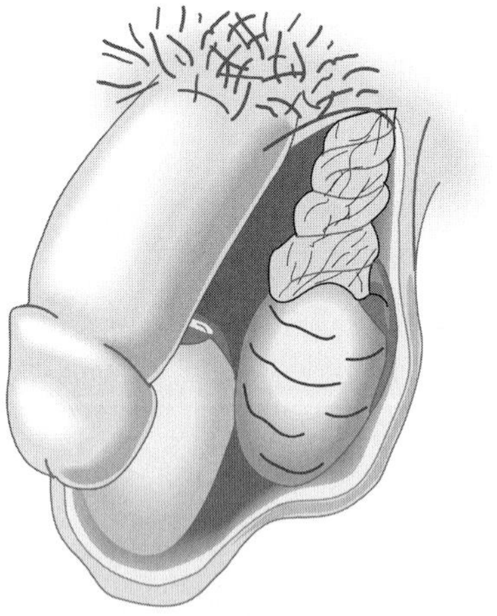

Figure 21-4 Testicular Torsion

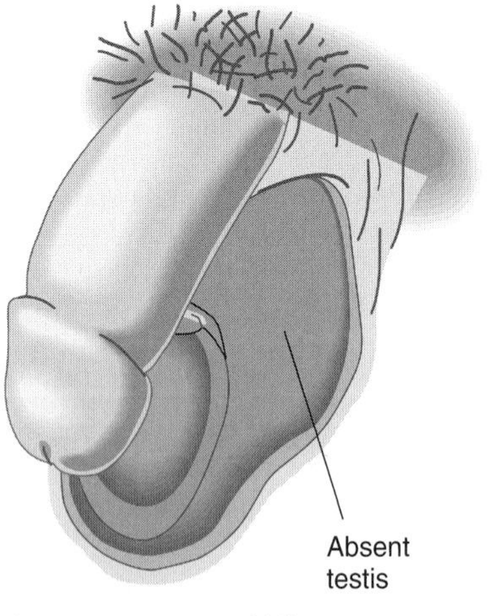

Figure 21-5 Cryptorchidism

Nursing Tip

Teaching Testicular Self-Examination

Testicular self-examination (TSE) should be taught to the patient during the scrotal examination.

- Ask the patient whether monthly TSE is performed.
- Explain the rationale for the examination (i.e., monthly testicular examination allows for earlier detection of testicular cancer, which occurs most often in 16 to 35 year olds).
- Pick a date to perform TSE every month. The best time to perform the examination is after a warm shower, when both hands and scrotum are warm.
- Instruct the patient to gently feel each testicle, using the thumb and first two fingers (Figure 21-6A).
- Remind the patient that the testicles are ovoid and movable and feel firm and rubbery. The epididymis is located on top and behind the testis, is softer, and feels ropelike.
- Instruct the patient to report any variations from normal findings, including any lumps and nodules, especially if they are nonmobile.
- Instruct the patient to squeeze the tip of the penis and to observe for any discharge (Figure 21-6B).

Nursing Alert

Risk Factors for Testicular Cancer

- Caucasian race, especially Scandinavian background
- Higher socioeconomic status
- Unmarried
- Rural resident
- History of cryptorchidism (even if previously repaired)

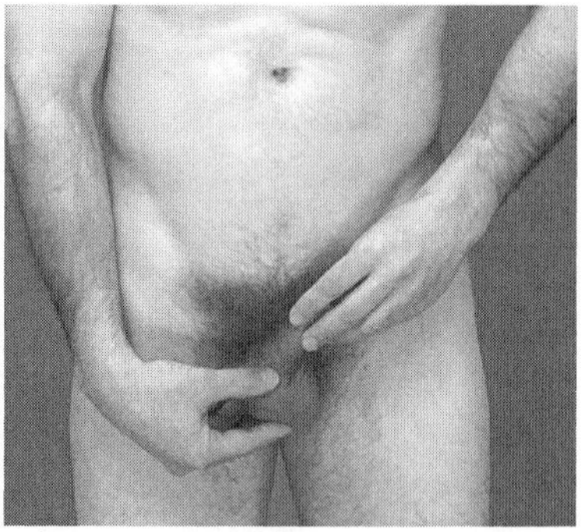

A. Palpating the Testis

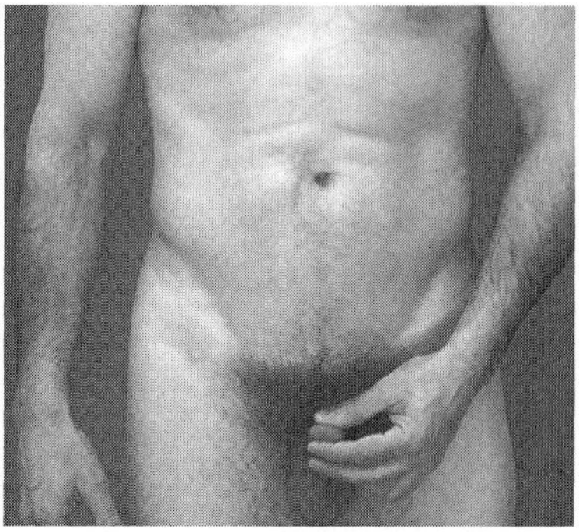

B. Assessing for Penile Discharge

Figure 21-6 Testicular Self-Examination

Inguinal Area

E **1.** With the index and middle fingers of your right hand, palpate the skin overlying the inguinal and femoral areas for lymph nodes.

2. Note size, consistency, tenderness, and mobility.

3. Ask the patient to bear down while you palpate the inguinal area.

4. Place your right index finger in the patient's right scrotal sac above the right testicle and invaginate the scrotal skin. Follow the spermatic cord until you reach a triangular, slit-like opening (the external inguinal ring).

5. Place your finger with the nail facing inward and the finger pad facing outward (Figure 21-7).

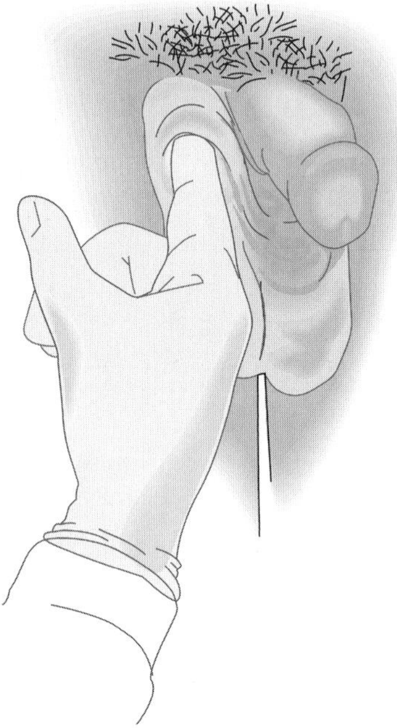

Figure 21-7 Inguinal Palpation

6. If the inguinal ring is large enough, continue to advance your finger along the inguinal canal and ask the patient to cough.

7. Note any masses felt against the finger.

8. Repeat on the left side, using the left hand to perform the palpation.

9. Palpate the femoral canal. Ask the patient to bear down.

N **It is normal for there to be small (1.0 cm), freely mobile lymph nodes present in the inguinal area. However, no bulges should be present in the inguinal area, and no palpable masses should be present in the inguinal canal. No portion of the bowel should enter the scrotum.**

A Unilaterally enlarged lymph nodes with erythematous overlying skin

P Possible lymphogranulam venereum (LGV)

A Lymphadenopathy: unilateral or bilateral enlargement of the inguinal lymph nodes, which may be tender or painless

P Immune system response to bacterial infection, trauma, carcinoma, or herpes simplex

A/P Table 21-1 compares the different types of hernias. Refer to Figures 21-8, 21-9, and 21-10.

TABLE 21-1 Comparison of Inguinal and Femoral Hernias

FEATURE	INDIRECT INGUINAL HERNIA	DIRECT INGUINAL HERNIA	FEMORAL HERNIA
Occurrence	More common in infants <1 year and males 16 to 25 years of age	Middle-aged and elderly men	More frequent in women
Origin of swelling	Above inguinal ligament. Hernia sac enters canal at internal ring and exits at external ring Can be found in the scrotum	Above inguinal ligament Directly behind and through external ring	Below inguinal ligament

continues

TABLE 21-1 Comparison of Inguinal and Femoral Hernias *continued*

FEATURE	INDIRECT INGUINAL HERNIA	DIRECT INGUINAL HERNIA	FEMORAL HERNIA
Cause	Congenital or acquired	Acquired weakness brought on by heavy lifting, obesity, COPD	Acquired, due to increased abdominal pressure and muscle weakness
Signs and symptoms	Lump or fullness in the groin, which may be associated with a cough or crying	Lump or fullness in the groin area; it may cause an aching or dragging sensation	Firm or rubbery lump in the groin; pain may be severe

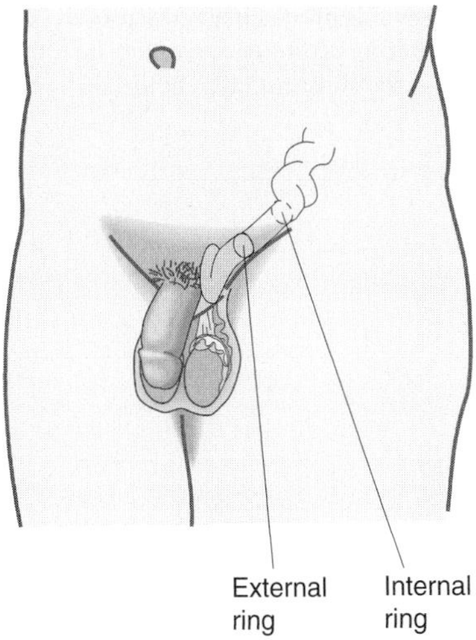

Figure 21-8 Indirect Inguinal Hernia

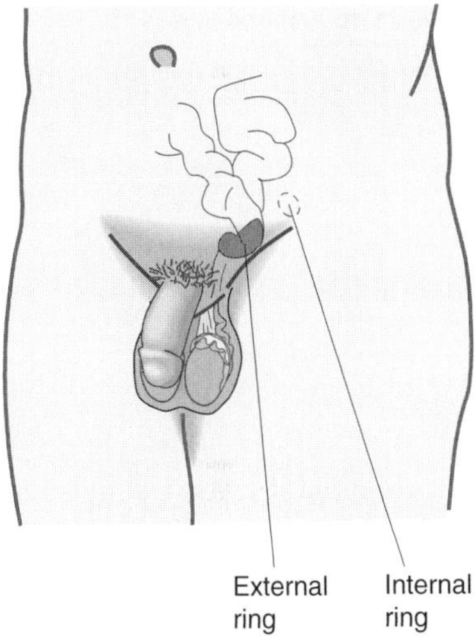

Figure 21-9 Direct Inguinal Hernia

Nursing Tip

Warning Signs of a Hernia

- Scrotal or inguinal mass
- Mild aching or discomfort in the scrotal or inguinal area, or both
- Bulging in the groin area upon coughing and heavy lifting

If any of the above are present, refer the patient for further treatment.

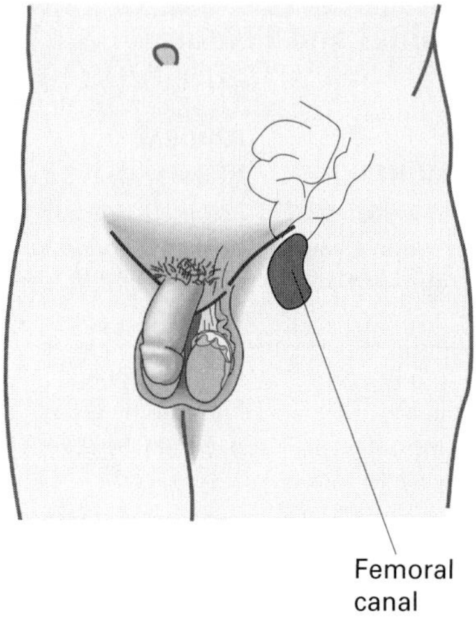

Figure 21-10 Femoral Hernia

Auscultation

Auscultation is performed if a scrotal mass is found on inspection or palpation.

Scrotum

E **1.** Place the patient in a supine position.

2. Stand at the patient's right side at the genital area.

3. Place your stethoscope over the scrotal mass.

4. Listen for the presence of bowel sounds.

5. Clean the stethoscope with alcohol after auscultation.

N **No bowel sounds are present in the scrotum.**

A Indirect inguinal hernia: bowel sounds in the enlarged scrotum

P Loops of bowel extending into the scrotum via an indirect hernia

22

Anus, Rectum, and Prostate

Anatomy and Physiology

Rectum

The large intestine is composed of the cecum, the colon, the rectum, and the anal canal. The cecum and colon are discussed in Chapter 17. The sigmoid colon begins at the pelvic brim. Beyond the sigmoid colon, the large intestine passes downward in front of the sacrum. This portion is called the rectum (Figure 22-1). The rectum contains three transverse folds, or valves of Houston. These valves work to retain fecal material so that it is not passed along with flatus.

Anus

The terminal 3 to 4 cm of the large intestine is called the anal canal. The anal canal fuses with the rectum at the anorectal junction, or the dentate line, and together these structures form the anorectum.

In the superior half of the anal canal are anal columns, which are longitudinal folds of mucosa (also called columns of Morgagni). The anal valves are formed by inferior joining anal columns. Pockets located superior to the valves and called the anal sinuses secrete mucus when they are compressed by feces, providing lubrication that eases fecal passage during defecation (Figure 22-2).

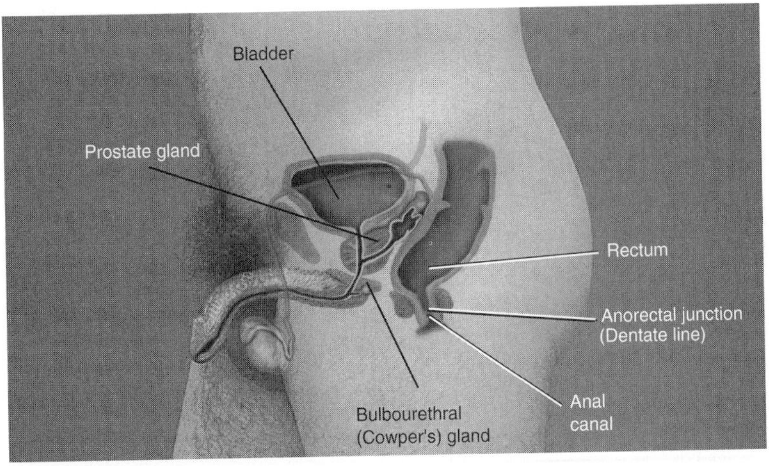

Figure 22-1 The Anorectum and Prostate

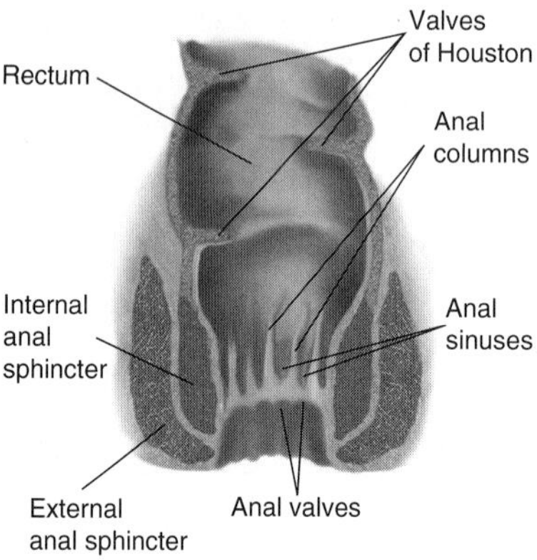

Figure 22-2 Anal Canal

The anal canal opens to the exterior through the anus. Internal and external anal sphincter muscles surround the anus. Smooth muscle, which is under involuntary control, forms the internal sphincter. Skeletal muscle forms the external sphincter and is under voluntary control, allowing a person to control bowel movements.

Prostate

Contiguous with part of the anterior rectal wall in the male is the prostate gland. The prostate is an accessory male sex organ approximately the size and shape of a chestnut (approximately 3.5 cm long by 3.0 cm wide). It consists of glandular tissue and muscle, and its small ducts drain into the urethra.

The prostate can be divided into five lobes: anterior, posterior, median, and (two) lateral. The median sulcus is the groove between the lateral lobes. The right and left lateral lobes are accessible to examination.

HEALTH HISTORY

Medical History
Trauma, inflammatory bowel disease, prior history of STD, polyps, rectal cancer, prostate cancer, prostatitis, benign prostatic hypertrophy (BPH), hemorrhoids, pruritus ani, constipation, diarrhea, incontinence

Surgical History
Sigmoidoscopy, colonoscopy, rubber band ligation, injection sclerotherapy, hemorrhoidectomy, drainage of fistula or abscess, prostatectomy, transurethral resection of the prostate (TURP)

Medications
Laxatives, constipating agents, alpha blockers, 5–alpha-reductase inhibitors, antifungals, astringent ointments, suppositories

Communicable Diseases
HIV, *Neisseria gonorrhoeae, Treponema pallidum, Chlamydia trachomatis*, human papillomavirus (HPV), herpes simplex virus (HSV)

Family Health History
Rectal polyps, rectal cancer, prostate cancer, pilonidal cyst

Social History
Sexual practice: rectal penetration increases the risk of anal carcinoma and anorectal STDs; use of foreign objects in the rectum can lead to anal valve incompetence.

Diet: prostate and rectal cancers: increased amounts of dietary fat, cured and smoked meats, and charcoal-broiled foods and decreased amounts of fiber, fruits, and vegetables; with pruritus ani: excessive intake of milk, coffee, tea, cola, and spices; vitamins A, C, E and folate may protect against developing rectal cancer.

NURSING CHECKLIST

General Approach to Anus, Rectum, and Prostate Assessment

1. Greet the patient and explain the assessment techniques that you will be using.
2. Ensure that the examination room is at a warm, comfortable temperature to prevent patient chilling and shivering.
3. Ensure that the light in the room provides sufficient brightness to adequately observe the patient. It may be helpful to have a gooseneck lamp available for additional lighting when lesions are observed.
4. Instruct the patient to void and, if possible, to defecate before the assessment.
5. Instruct the patient to remove pants and underpants and to cover up with a drape sheet.
6. For inspection, place the patient in the left lateral decubitus position and visualize the perianal skin (Figure 22-3A). This position can also be used for palpation.
7. For palpation, have the patient stand at the end of the examination table, bend over the end of the table, rest the elbows on the table, and spread the legs slightly apart (Figure 22-3B), *or*

7A. For the patient who cannot stand, have the patient assume the knee-chest position (Figure 22-3C).

7B. Have the female who is undergoing a rectovaginal examination assume the lithotomy position (see Chapter 20).

8. Don nonsterile gloves.
9. In the female patient, proceed from the anus to the rectum; in the male patient, proceed from the anus to the prostate.

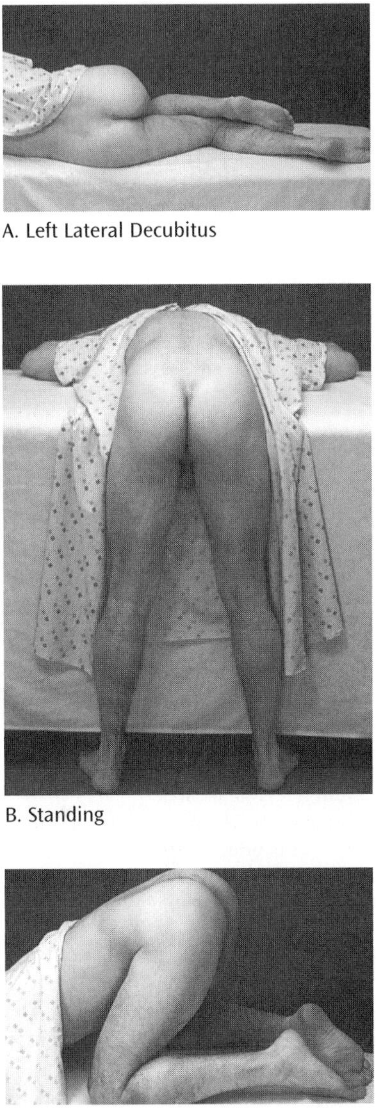

A. Left Lateral Decubitus

B. Standing

C. Knee-Chest

Figure 22-3 Patient Positions for the Anus, Rectum, and Prostate Examination

Equipment

- Nonsterile gloves
- Water-soluble lubricant
- Hemoccult cards
- Gooseneck lamp

Assessment of the Anus, Rectum, and Prostate

Inspection

Perineum and Sacrococcygeal Area

E Inspect the buttocks and the sacral region for lesions, swelling, inflammation, and tenderness.

N **These areas should be smooth and free of lesions, swelling, inflammation, and tenderness. There should be no evidence of feces or mucus on the perianal skin.**

A Pilonidal disease: one or several tiny openings (often with hair protruding from them) in the midline over the sacral region

P Acquired condition of the midline coccygeal skin region induced by local stretching forces; small skin pits representing enlarged hair follicles precede development of draining sinuses or abscesses

A Pruritus ani: possibly intensely pruritic areas of hyperpigmentation coupled with excoriation and thickened skin in the perianal area

P Pinworms in children, fungal infections in adults

A Psoriasis: dry, well-circumscribed, silvery, scaly papules and plaques of various sizes

P Increased epidermal cell proliferation, family history of psoriasis

A *Candida albicans:* well-demarcated, erythematous, sometimes itchy, exudative patches of varying size and shape and rimmed with small, red-based pustules

P Systemic antibacterial, corticosteroid, or antimetabolic therapy, pregnancy, obesity, diabetes mellitus, blood dyscrasias, immunologic defects

Anal Mucosa

E 1. To expose the anus, spread the patient's buttocks apart with both hands.

2. Instruct the patient to bear down as though moving the bowels.

3. Examine the anus for color, appearance, lesions, inflammation, rashes, and masses.

N **The anal mucosa is deeply pigmented, coarse, moist, and hairless. It should be free of lesions, inflammation, rashes, masses, and additional openings. The anal opening should be closed. There should be no leakage of feces or mucus from the anus on straining nor should there be any tissue protrusion.**

A Hemorrhoids: spherical, bluish lumps that appear suddenly at the anus and range in diameter from several millimeters to several centimeters. (Overlying anal skin may be tense, edematous, painful, and pruritic.)

P Dilatation of the superior and inferior hemorrhoidal veins

A Anal skin tags: excess anal or perianal tissue of varying sizes that is soft, pliable, and covered by normal skin

P Residual resolved thrombosed external hemorrhoids, pregnancy, anal operations

A Anal fissure: linear tear in the epidermis of the anal canal, beginning below the dentate line and extending distally to the anal orifice and possibly accompanied by pain; pruritus; bleeding; and a sentinel skin tag inferior to the fissure at anal margin

P Trauma such as that from anal intercourse (especially forced intercourse) or forced passage of a large, hard stool. (Use of local anesthetic may be necessary to thoroughly examine the area.)

A Anorectal abscesses: undrained collections of perianal pus from the tissue spaces in and adjacent to the anorectum

P Infection of the anal glands, usually posterior and between the internal and external sphincters

A Anorectal fistula: inflamed, red, raised area along with purulent or

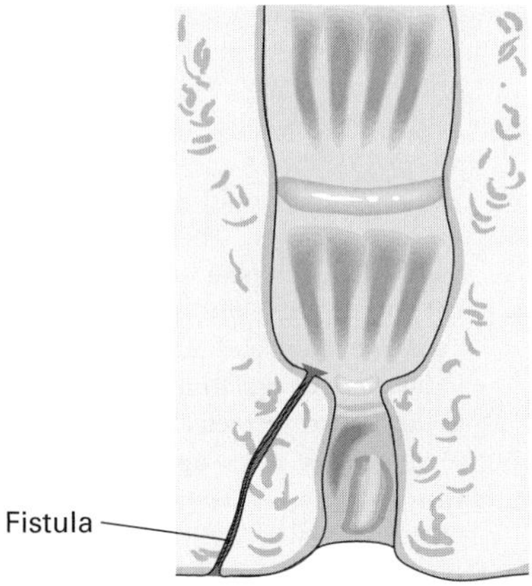

Figure 22-4 Anorectal Fistula

serosanguineous discharge on the perianal skin (Figure 22-4)

P Hollow fibrous tract lined by granulation tissue and having an opening inside the anal canal or rectum and one or more orifices in the perianal skin usually as a result of incomplete healing of a drained anorectal abscess

A Anal incontinence: gaping of the anus and soiling of the skin with stool

P Neurological disease, traumatic injury, surgical damage to the puborectalis or sphincter muscles

A Rectal prolapse: protrusion of the rectal mucosa (pinkish-red "doughnut" with radiating folds) through the anal orifice (Figure 22-5)

P Poor pelvic musculature tone, chronic straining to stool, fecal incontinence, neurological disease, traumatic damage to the pelvis

A Erythematous plaques that develop into vesicular lesions that may become pustules and ulcerate

P Herpes simplex virus (HSV)

A Condylomata acuminatum: warts or lesions that are beefy red, irregular, and pedunculated

P Human papillomavirus

A Mucoid or creamy exudate and possibly blood from the rectum

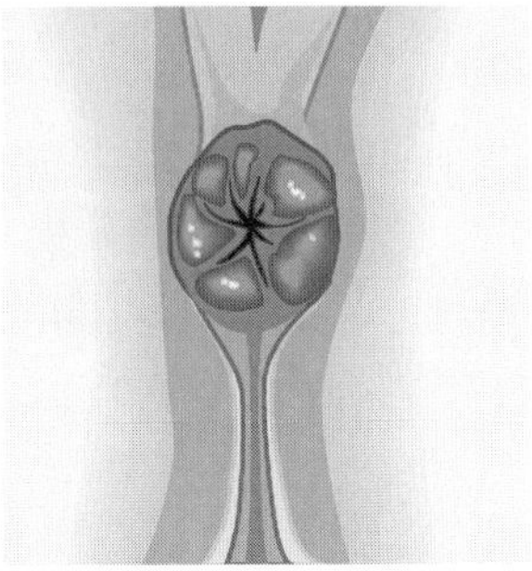

Figure 22-5 Rectal Prolapse

P Gonococcal proctitis

A Multiple perianal fissures and edematous skin tags

P Perianal disease

Palpation

Anus and Rectum

To perform anal and rectal wall palpation:

E **1.** Have the patient assume one of the positions described in Figure 22-3.

2. Reassure the patient that sensations of urination and defecation are common during the rectal assessment.

3. Lubricate a gloved index finger.

4. Place your gloved and lubricated finger near the anal orifice. Instruct the patient to bear down (Valsalva maneuver) as you gently insert the flexed tip of the finger into the anal sphincter, with the ball of the finger toward the anterior rectal wall (i.e., pointing toward the umbilicus, see Figure 22-6). The anus should never be approached from a right angle (i.e., with the index finger extended). If the patient tightens the sphincter, remove your finger, reassure the patient, and try again using a relaxation technique such as deep breathing.

5. Feel the sphincter relax. Insert the finger as far as it will go (Figure 22-7). Note anal sphincter tone.

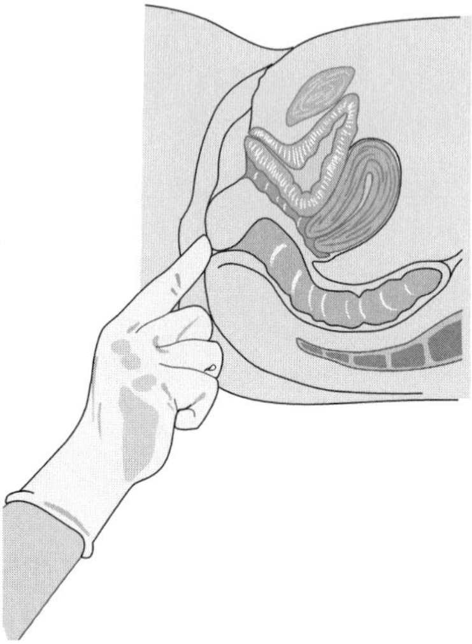

Figure 22-6 Position of the Index Finger for Anorectal Palpation

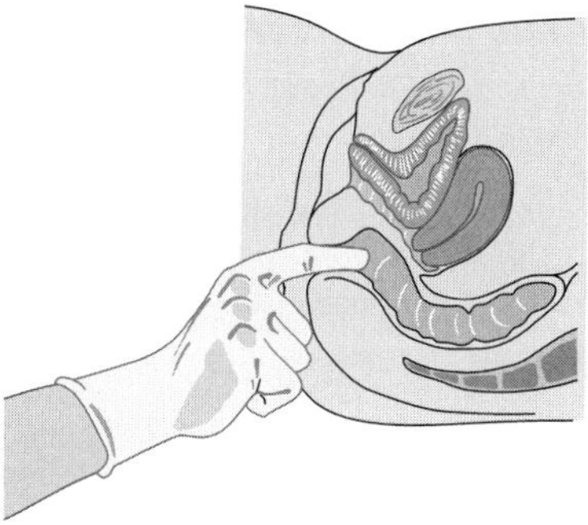

Figure 22-7 Position of the Index Finger in the Anorectum

6. Palpate the lateral, posterior, and anterior walls of the rectum in a sequential manner. The lateral walls are felt by rotating the finger along the sides of the rectum. Palpate for nodules, irregularity, masses, and tenderness.

7. Ask the patient to bear down again (to help palpate masses).

8. Slowly withdraw the finger. Inspect any fecal matter on your glove and test the fecal matter for occult blood. Table 22-1 lists common stool findings and etiologies. Table 22-2 lists the common causes of rectal bleeding.

9. Offer the patient tissues to wipe off the lubricant.

N **The rectum should accommodate the index finger. There should be good sphincter tone at rest and on bearing down. There should be no excessive pain and no tenderness, induration, irregularities, or nodules in the rectum or rectal wall.**

A Anal stenosis: a too-tight anal canal (Inserting the index finger causes pain and is very difficult or impossible.)

P Congenital; acquired: anorectal operation, diarrheal disease, inflammatory conditions, habitual use of laxatives, chlamydial infection, malignancy

A Internal masses of vascular tissue in the anal canal

P Internal hemorrhoids

A Rectal polyps: soft nodules in the rectum

P Rectal polyps: pedunculated (attached to a stalk) or sessile (adhering to the rectal mucosal wall)

A An indurated cord palpated in the anorectum

P Anorectal fistula tracts (may be palpated from the secondary orifice toward the anus)

A Rectal prolapse: small, symmetric projection 2 to 4 cm in length

P Lax anal sphincter (best assessed with the patient in a squatting position)

A Foreign bodies palpated in the rectum

P Thermometers, enema catheters, vibrators, bottles, phallic objects

A Hard mass in the anal canal

P Anal carcinoma

A Fecal impaction: firm, sometimes rocklike but often rubbery, puttylike mass

P Lack of colon response to the usual stimuli that promote evacuation; insufficient accessory stimuli (normally eating and physical activity) to promote evacuation

TABLE 22-1 Common Stool Findings and Etiologies

STOOL FINDING	ETIOLOGY
Black, tarry (melena)	Upper gastrointestinal bleeding
Bright red	Rectal bleeding
Black	Iron or bismuth ingestion
Gray, tan	Obstructive jaundice
Pale yellow, greasy, fatty (steatorrhea)	Malabsorption syndromes (e.g., celiac disease), cystic fibrosis
Mucus with blood and pus	Ulcerative colitis, acute diverticulitis
Maroon or bright red	Diverticulosis

TABLE 22-2

Common Causes of Rectal Bleeding

- Cancer of the colon
- Benign polyps of the colon
- Hemorrhoids
- Anal fissure
- Inflammatory bowel disease
- Forced or vigorous anal intercourse
- Traumatic sexual practices

Nursing Alert

Risk Factors for Colorectal Cancer

- Over 50 years of age
- Family history of colorectal cancer
- Personal history of adenomatous polyps
- Personal history of chronic inflammatory bowel disease (ulcerative colitis, Crohn's disease)
- Personal history of endometrial, ovarian, or breast cancer
- Lack of physical activity
- Low fruit and vegetable intake—high-fat diet
- Obesity
- Alchohol consumption
- Tobacco use

Prostate

To perform prostatic palpation:

E 1. Position the patient as tolerated (the standing position is preferred).

2. Reassure the patient that sensations of urination and defecation are common during the prostatic assessment.

3. Use a well-lubricated, gloved index finger.

4. Insert the finger and proceed as described in steps 4 and 5 on page 311.

5. Press your gloved thumb into the perianal tissue while pressing your index finger toward it (bidigital examination of the bulbourethral gland, see Figure 22-8). Assess for tenderness, masses, and swelling.

6. Release the pressure of your thumb and index finger. Remove the

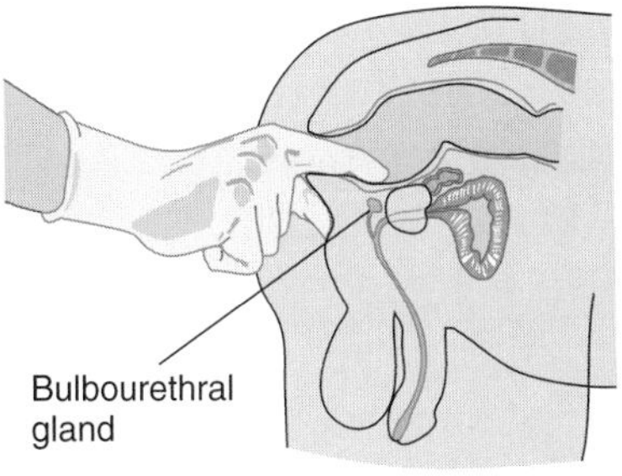

Figure 22-8 Bidigital Palpation of the Bulbourethral Gland

thumb from the perianal tissue and advance the index finger.

7. Palpate the posterior surface of the prostate gland (Figure 22-9). Note size, shape, consistency, sensitivity, and mobility of the prostate. Note whether the median sulcus is palpated.

8. Attempt to palpate the seminal vesicles by extending your index finger above the prostate gland. Assess for tenderness and masses.

9. Slowly withdraw your finger. Inspect any fecal matter on the glove and test the fecal matter for occult blood (if not previously done).

N **The prostate gland should be small, smooth, mobile, and nontender. The median sulcus should be palpable.**

A Benign prostatic hypertrophy (BPH): soft, nontender, enlarged prostate

P Aging and the presence of testosterone, which converts to dihydrotestosterone, leading to prostatic cell growth

A Prostatic abscess: firm, tender, or fluctuant mass on the prostate

P *Escherichia coli*

A Firm, hard, or indurated nodules on the prostate

P Prostate cancer

A Bacterial prostatitis: exquisitely tender and warm prostate

P *Escherichia coli*

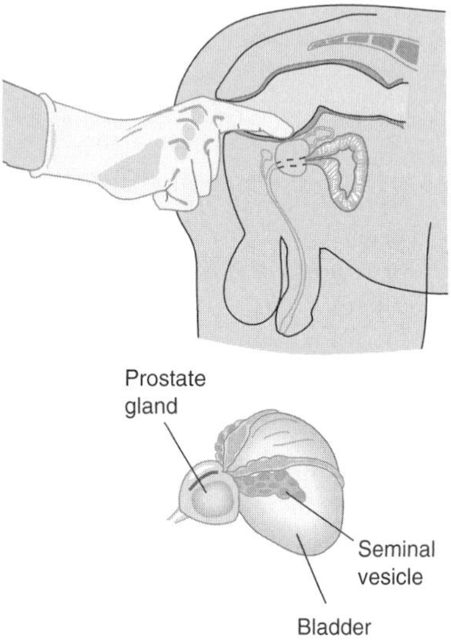

Figure 22-9 Prostatic Palpation

Nursing Alert

Risk Factors for Prostate Cancer

Males over the age of 50 are at the highest risk for developing prostate cancer. Other risk factors include: a first-degree relative with prostate cancer, African American race, high levels of serum testosterone, and high intake of dietary fat, oil, and sugar.

Unit 4 Special Populations

23

Pregnant Patient

Anatomy and Physiology

Pregnancy is subdivided into trimesters of a little more than 13 weeks each, and various symptoms and problems can be specific to certain trimesters. Common body system changes are listed here.

Skin and Hair

Increased subdermal fat deposit; thickening of the skin; possible development or improvement of acne; pigmentation increases in the nipples, areola, external genitalia, and anal region; possible development of melasma or chloasma on the face; possibly, linea nigra, or darkening of the linea alba on the abdomen; typically, development of striae gravidarum (stretch marks) on the abdomen, breasts, and upper thighs; skin tags; possibly, increased facial hair; possible shedding and thinning of the scalp hair; spider angiomas; hemangiomas, varicosities, and palmar erythema

Head and Neck

Possibly, enlarged thyroid gland after approximately 12 weeks' gestation

Eyes, Ears, Nose, Mouth, and Throat

Corneal thickening and edema; visual changes; nasal stuffiness; snoring; congestion; epistaxis; impaired hearing or fullness in the ears; decreased sense of smell; soft, edematous, bleeding gums; ptyalism (excessive salivation)

Breasts

Enlargement; tingling; tenderness; increase in number and size of alveoli; enlargement of Montgomery's tubercles, proliferation of lactiferous ducts; increased nodularity on palpation; possibly, darkened areolae; possibly, darkened and more erect nipples; secretion of colostrum (possibly as early as the second trimester)

Thorax and Lungs

Elevation of the diaphragm by approximately 4 cm; thoracic diameter expansion of 5 to 7 cm; majority of respiratory effort diaphragmatic; tidal volume increase of 30% to 40%; increased respiratory rate; hyperventilation or shortness of breath, especially on exertion

Heart and Peripheral Vasculature

Increased blood volume; more horizontal lie as well as upward and leftwise shift along with the apical impulse of maternal heart; heart rate increase of 10 to 15 beats per minute; possibly, a split first heart sound; physiological systolic murmurs of grade 2/6; varying blood pressure depending on position and trimester; commonly, supine hypotension; possibly, lowered diastolic pressure (by 5 mm Hg) in the second trimester with increase to first-trimester levels after midpregnancy; lower blood pressure in the second trimester; dependent edema in the feet, hands, and face

Abdomen

Decreased tone and motility; decreased bowel sounds; increased emptying time for the stomach and intestines; increased reflux, indigestion, flatulence, and constipation; hemorrhoids; nausea and vomiting; separation of the rectus muscle of the abdominal wall (diastasis recti)

Urinary System

Glomerular filtration rate (GFR) increases of approximately 50%; changes in reabsorption rates of various chemicals, especially sodium and water; increased urinary frequency; glycosuria (glucose in the urine); proteinuria; nocturia

Musculoskeletal System

Widening (and, occasionally, separation) of the symphysis pubis at approximately 28 to 32 weeks; increased pelvic mobility to accommodate vaginal delivery; unsteady gait known as the "waddle of pregnancy"; upper back, sternal, or rib pain; lordosis of the lumbar spine; sciatic nerve pain manifesting as lower back pain or a shooting pain down the leg or as leg weakness; increased fat deposits

Neurological System

Headaches; numbness and tingling; seizure activity with no prior history (suggestive of the development of eclampsia) or seizure activity associated with pregnancy-induced hypertension (PIH); dizziness and lightheadedness

Female Genitalia

Dilatation of uterine vessels; amenorrhea; transformation of pregnant uterus from a pelvic organ (palpably enlarged on bimanual examination at 6 to 7 weeks [Figure 23-1]) to an abdominal organ at approximately 12 weeks of gestation; at 16 weeks, uterine fundus midway between the symphysis pubis and the umbilicus; at 20 weeks, uterine fundus typically at the umbilicus; between 18 and 32 weeks, uterine fundal height above the symphysis pubis, measured in centimeters, and used to confirm gestational age in weeks; elongation of the round and broad ligaments to accommodate the growing fetus; lightening (also called dropping, a decrease in fundal height resulting from descent of the presenting fetal part into the pelvis and typically occurring approximately 3 weeks before the onset of labor in the nulliparous woman and possibly not until after active labor begins in the multiparous woman; Braxton Hicks contractions (irregular and usually painless) beginning as early as the first trimester; increased cervical vascularity and friability, or susceptibility to bleeding, especially after Pap smear or intercourse (Table 23-1 for additional cervical and uterine changes in pregnancy); an increase in the number and size of endocervical glands causes a softening of the cervix; mucus production resulting in formation of the endocervical protective plug; vaginal mucosa thickening secondary to hormonal changes; progressively increasing vaginal discharge that is typically of a white, milky consistency but that may become noticeably thicker from 36 weeks on and may contain clumps when the mucus plug is expelled; hormonally induced changes in the vaginal environment leading to increased risk of yeast infections

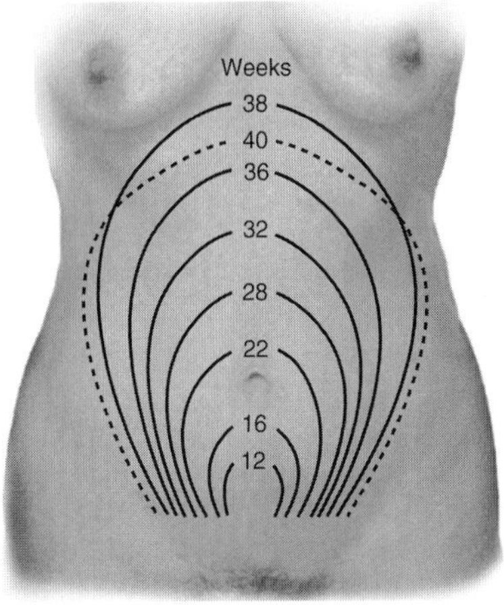

Figure 23-1 Uterine/Abdominal Enlargement of Pregnancy

Anus and Rectum

Decreased gastrointestinal tract tone and motility produce a sense of fullness, indi-

TABLE 23-1 Changes in Pelvic Organs in Pregnancy

NAME	GESTATIONAL AGE	DESCRIPTION
Ladin's sign	5–6 weeks	Softening of cervical-uterine junction
Goodell's sign	6 weeks	Cervical softening
McDonald's sign	7–8 weeks	Easy flexion of fundus on cervix
Chadwick's sign	8 weeks	Cervical bluish hue
Hegar's sign	8 weeks	Softening of uterine isthmus

gestion, constipation, bloating, and flatulence. Development of hemorrhoids is common and can become very problematic. As pregnancy progresses and the uterus enlarges, mechanical pressure may aggravate constipation and hemorrhoids. Vitamin and iron supplementation may increase the above symptoms and commonly darken the stool.

Hematological System

Increased white blood cell (WBC) count; increased total red blood cell (RBC) volume; increased plasma volume; decreased number and increased size of platelets; increased fibrinogen and factors VII through X; physiological anemia of pregnancy

Endocrine System

Increase in basal metabolic rate (BMR) of 15% to 25%; increased resistance to insulin; possibly, pregnancy-induced glucose intolerance (potential risk factor for future development of insulin-dependent diabetes mellitus); decreased resistance to infection

HEALTH HISTORY

See Tables 23-2 and 23-3.

Medical History

Asthma, diabetes mellitus, cardiac disease, renal disease, seizure disorder, autoimmune disorders

Surgical History

Uterine surgery, cone or excisional biopsy of the cervix, abdominal surgery leading to internal or external scarring or adhesions

Communicable Diseases

TORCH diseases (toxoplasmosis, rubella, cytomegalovirus, herpes), measles, varicella, mumps, human parvovirus, HIV, hepatitis. A rubella titer, RPR or VDRL, and hepatitis B surface antigen are routinely drawn on pregnant patients; HIV testing is recommended, if the patient allows it.

Family Health History

Preterm labor or delivery; hypertensive disorders of pregnancy; diethylstilbestrol (DES) exposure; multiple births (e.g., twins, triplets) in female relatives of patient's mother; chromosomal abnormalities such as Down syndrome; genetic disorders such as Tay-Sachs, Gaucher's, sickle cell diseases; inheritable diseases, congenital anomalies; blood disorders; neural tube defects; diabetes; cardiac deformities

continues

Social History

Alcohol use: can lead to fetal alcohol syndrome (FAS). The absolute safe level of alcohol consumption is unknown; problems have been documented with >2 oz of alcohol per day and with binge drinking.

Tobacco use: smoking can lead to a small-for-gestational age (SGA) infant, preterm labor, spontaneous abortions, and lower Apgar scores (system for evaluating newborn status, refer to Chapter 24). The effects are dose related, and tobacco use during pregnancy should be discontinued.

Drug use: effects on the fetus vary according to the drug(s) used and the gestational age at time of use. The most common complications are spontaneous abortion, preterm delivery, congenital anomalies, and stillbirth.

TABLE 23-2 Obstetric History

PRESENT OBSTETRIC HISTORY

Last menstrual period (LMP)

History since LMP (e.g., fever, rashes, disease exposures, abnormal bleeding, nausea and vomiting, medication use, toxic exposures)

Signs and symptoms of pregnancy

Use of fertility drugs

Estimated date of delivery (EDD) or estimated date of confinement (EDC)*

Genetic predispositions

PAST OBSTETRIC HISTORY

Gravidity/gravida (number of pregnancies)

Parity/para (number of births 20 weeks or greater; usually listed as term [37–42 weeks gestational age], preterm [20–37 weeks gestational age], or postterm [>42 weeks gestational age])

Spontaneous abortion

Therapeutic abortion

Ectopic pregnancy

Multiples or multiple births (more than one fetus or baby)

Number of living children

Pregnancy history (see Table 23-3 for high-risk factors):

- Complications during pregnancy
- Duration of gestation
- Date of delivery
- Type of delivery
  (vaginal versus cesarean)
  (if cesarean, reason)
  (forceps or vacuum extraction)
  (episiotomy or laceration, and degree)
- Length of labor
- Medications and anesthesia used
- Complications during labor and delivery
- Postpartum complications

Infant weight and sex, Apgar score

Type of feeding (breastfeeding versus bottle feeding)

Breastfeeding: difficulties

**Use Naegele's rule to determine EDD: subtract 3 months from the first day of the LMP, then add 7 days. This is based on a 28-day cycle and may have to be adjusted for shorter or longer cycles. For example, if the LMP is September 1, 9/1 – 3 months = 6/1*

6/1 + 7 days = 6/8

The EDD for this patient is June 8. A pregnancy wheel may also be used.

TABLE 23-3 Risk Factors for Pregnancy

There are many risk factor tools and scoring systems available with varying degrees of sensitivity and specificity. Some prenatal forms include a risk screen in the history.

MATERNAL

- Age less than 18 or older than 40
- Single
- Abusive relationship and other violence or family relationship stresses
- Low socioeconomic status, poverty, or low educational level
- Long work hours, long commute or long, tiring trip; excessive fatigue
- Stress or unusual anxiety, or both, per patient perception
- Unplanned pregnancy or conflict about pregnancy, or both
- Height of less than 5 ft.
- Weight of less than 100 lbs.
- Inadequate diet
- Habits: smoking, excessive caffeine (greater than six cups of coffee per day) or alcohol consumption, drug addiction

REPRODUCTIVE HISTORY

- More than one prior abortion (some risk tools differentiate first and second trimester)
- Uterine anomaly
- Molar pregnancy/hydatidiform mole
- Myomas (leiomyomas)
- Sexually transmitted infections or diseases
- Perinatal death
- Preterm delivery or premature labor, or both
- Delivery of infant less than 2500 g
- Delivery of infant greater than 4000 g
- Delivery of infant with congenital or perinatal disease
- Delivery of infant with isoimmunization or ABO incompatibility
- Gestational diabetes
- Operative delivery
- Cervical incompetence
- Prior cerclage

MEDICAL PROBLEMS

- Hypertension
- Renal disease, pyelonephritis, asymptomatic bacteriuria
- Diabetes mellitus
- Heart disease
- Sickle cell disease
- Anemia
- Pulmonary disease
- Endocrine disorder
- Neurological disorder
- Autoimmune disorder
- Hematological disorder

PRESENT PREGNANCY

- Late, inadequate, or no prenatal care
- Abdominal surgery
- Bleeding
- Placenta previa
- Premature rupture of membranes
- Anemia
- Hypertension
- Preeclampsia or eclampsia
- Hydramnios
- Multiple pregnancy
- Abnormal glucose screen
- Low or excessive weight gain
- Rh-negative sensitization
- Teratogenic exposure
- Viral infections (especially fever-rash within first trimester)
- Sexually transmitted infection(s) or disease(s)
- Bacterial infections (bacterial vaginosis and group B *streptococcus*, in particular)
- Protozoal infections
- Abnormal presentation (e.g., breech, transverse) at approximately 36 weeks
- Postdates

Nursing Tip

Obstetric Abbreviations

You can classify pregnant patients according to their prior obstetric outcomes by using the following abbreviations:

G: gravida
P: para
T: term
P: preterm
A: abortion (either therapeutic or spontaneous; may be listed separately)
E: ectopic pregnancy
LC: living children

Examples:

G:4, P:2, T:2, P:0, A:1, E:1, LC:2, = 4 pregnancies, 2 births, 2 term births, 0 preterm births, 1 abortion, 1 ectopic pregnancy, 2 living children

Equipment

- Stethoscope
- Doppler or fetoscope
- Centimeter tape measure
- Watch with a second hand
- Nonsterile gloves
- Speculum
- Genital culture supplies (see Chapter 20)
- Pap smear supplies (see Chapter 20)
- Sphygmomanometer
- Urine cup
- Urine dipsticks

Nursing Checklist

General Approach to Assessment of the Pregnant Patient

1. Greet the patient and explain how the assessment will proceed.
2. Ensure that the examination room is ready and supplies are at hand.
3. Use a quiet room that will be free of interruptions.
4. Ensure that there is adequate lighting, including a light that is appropriate for the pelvic assessment.
5. Before performing the physical assessment, complete the health history and the nutritional and psychosocial assessments. (These are usually done in an office before proceeding to the examination room.)
6. Ask the patient to void before the examination. The urine should be saved and checked for sugar and acetone.
7. For the physical assessment, instruct the patient to remove all street clothing, to don an examination gown, and to cover the lap with the sheet provided.
8. Perform the initial assessment in a head-to-toe manner. Be efficient to minimize the time the patient spends in the supine position. Use verbal guidance to assist the patient in assuming the lithotomy position; help her place her feet in the foot or leg stirrups. Always inform the patient before touching her of what you will be doing and what to expect ("this may pinch," "you may feel some pressure," and so on). The patient may be dizzy on sitting up or standing. It may be beneficial to assist her to a sitting position or to brace her arm. She should be cautioned not to stand or sit up abruptly.

Assessment of the Pregnant Patient

Assessment of the pregnant patient includes a complete initial assessment as well as subsequent specific follow-up prenatal visits. The American College of Obstetricians and Gynecologists (ACOG) recommends the following schedule for prenatal visits: every 4 weeks for weeks 6–28 of gestation, every 2 weeks for weeks 28–36 of gestation, and weekly from 36 weeks of gestation until delivery. Patients going beyond the 40th week of gestation (postdates) require additional evaluations.

General Assessment, Vital Signs, and Weight

E 1. Conduct a general assessment, including of vital signs, as described in Chapter 9.
2. Obtain the patient's weight as described in Chapter 7.

N **See Chapter 9 for normal general assessment findings and for vital sign changes that occur in pregnancy. See Chapter 7 for the recommended weight gain during pregnancy.**

A Hypertension at any time in pregnancy (systolic pressure greater than 140 mm Hg and a diastolic pressure greater than 90 mm Hg, or an increase in systolic pressure of 30 mm Hg or an increase in diastolic pressure of 15 mm Hg above prepregnancy levels)

P PIH secondary to vasospasms

A Weight gain more than the recommended amount

P Increased caloric intake, multiple pregnancies (e.g., twins), polyhydramnios, edema secondary to PIH

A Weight gain less than the recommended amount

P Hyperemesis gravidarum, decreased caloric intake, malabsorption syndromes

Skin and Hair

E/N See Chapter 10.

A Prurigo of pregnancy: highly pruritic, excoriated papules usually distributed on the hands and feet

P Idiopathic

A Papular dermatitis of pregnancy: erythematous, pruritic, widespread, soft papules

P Unknown but associated with increased risk of fetal loss

A Erythematous plaques that develop into vesicular lesions that may become pustular

P Primary herpes (if contracted in the first trimester, places the fetus at risk for abnormalities)

Head and Neck

E/N See Chapter 11.

A Hyperthyroidism; more rarely, hypothyroidism

P Neoplastic disorders such as choriocarcinoma, ovarian teratoma, and hydatidiform mole; single active thyroid nodule or multinodular goiter

Eyes, Ears, Nose, Mouth, and Throat

E/N See Chapters 12 and 13.

A Retinal arterial constriction

P PIH

A Any growth in the mouth

P Usually benign tumors secondary to hormonal changes

Breasts

E 1. Examine the breasts as described in Chapter 14.
2. Don gloves.
3. Assess the shape of each nipple by putting your thumb and forefinger on the areola and pressing inward to express any discharge. Observe whether the nipple protracts (becomes erect) or retracts (inverts).

N **See Chapter 14. Nipples normally protract when stimulated.**

A/P See Chapter 14 for additional information.

Thorax and Lungs

E/N/A/P See Chapter 15 for additional information.

Heart and Peripheral Vasculature

E/N See Chapter 16.

A Generalized edema (as opposed to dependent edema of pregnancy)

P PIH, kidney disease, cardiovascular disease

Abdomen

E/N See Chapter 17.

A Severe nausea and vomiting (hyperemesis gravidarum)

P Idiopathic

A Epigastric pain

P Liver inflammation or necrosis from PIH

Urinary System

E **1.** Obtain a complete urinalysis at the initial prenatal visit.
2. Obtain a urine culture if indicated by urinalysis or patient history.
3. It is common (but not proven to affect outcome) to assess urine for protein, glucose, leukocytes, and nitrates at each subsequent prenatal visit.

N **The urine may turn a brighter yellow as a result of prenatal vitamins. Trace amounts of protein may be noted. Glycosuria may be noted without pathology, but possibility of diabetes mellitus cannot be ignored. Leukocytes and nitrates are normally absent.**

A Nitrates or large amounts of leukocytes

P Urinary tract infection

A Dysuria (difficulty in initiating urinary flow, increased frequency, and feeling of being unable to empty the bladder)

P Bacterial infection, inflammation of the bladder (cystitis), urinary tract infection

A Pain in the flank area (CVA tenderness)

P Pyelonephritis

A Proteinuria greater than trace on a urine dipstick

P PIH, collagen disorder, kidney disease

Musculoskeletal System

E/N/A/P See Chapter 18 for additional information.

Neurological System

E/N See Chapter 19.

A Seizures

P Eclampsia (a subset of PIH), CVA, tumor, epilepsy

A Hyperreflexia and clonus

P PIH

Female Genitalia

E **1.** For the initial prenatal visit, perform the assessment as described in Chapter 20.
2. Perform cultures if indicated (see Chapter 20).
3. Postdate pregnancies and pregnancies complicated by preterm labor symptoms or preterm labor risk factors may require a cervical assessment with each visit.

N **See Chapter 20 for normal findings of the female genitalia assessment. In the multiparous woman, the vulva and vagina may appear more relaxed in tone, and the perineum may be shorter. There is often a visible, white, milky discharge, and the cervix may show more ectropion (eversion and friability). In ectropion, the columnar epithelium extends from the os past the normal squamocolumnar junction, often**

producing a red, possibly inflamed appearance. See Table 23-1 for additional changes in the pelvic organs.

Manual assessment should reveal uterine size appropriate for gestational age; assessment may be slightly more painful than that for the nonpregnant patient. A retroverted and retroflexed uterus may be more difficult to assess. Palpation of the adnexa may demonstrate a slight tenderness and enlargement of the ovulatory ovary secondary to the corpus luteum of pregnancy.

A Persistent abdominal pain or tenderness

P PIH, abruptio placenta

A Painful adnexal masses

P Ectopic pregnancy (pregnancy other than intrauterine, such as abdominal or in the fallopian tube), infection, cancerous growth

Uterine Size

Fundal Height by Centimeters

E 1. Place the patient in a supine position.
2. Place the zero centimeter mark at the symphysis pubis and in the midline of the abdomen.
3. Palpate the top of the fundus and pull the tape measure to the top.
4. Note the centimeter mark.

N **Uterine size is determined by internal pelvic exam on the initial prenatal visit, by palpation if less than 18 weeks, and by fundal height in centimeters for subsequent visits. If the initial visit is late in pregnancy, it will include the internal pelvic exam and fundal height. A 16-week uterus is between the symphysis and umbilicus; a 20-week uterus is at the umbilicus (20 cm); and between 18 and 32 weeks, the size is equal to the centimeter height of the uterine fundus. After 32 weeks, although still used, this measurement is less accurate.**

A Uterine size larger than expected given last menstrual period (LMP)

P Hydatidiform mole or molar pregnancy, especially in the absence of fetal heart tones (FHTs); multiple gestation; inaccurate dating; uterine pathology (fibroid); polyhydramnios; in later pregnancy, macrosomia (newborn weighing greater than 4000 g)

A Uterine size smaller than expected given LMP

P Nonviable pregnancy; inaccurate dating; intrauterine growth restriction (IUGR) or transverse lie of the fetus

Fetal Heart Rate (FHR)

E 1. Place the patient in a supine position.
2. Place the Doppler or fetoscope on the abdomen and move the instrument around until FHTs are heard.
3. Count the FHR for sufficient time to determine rate and absence of irregularity (optimally 1 minute).

N **During early gestation, the fetal heart is generally heard in the mother's midline area between the symphysis pubis and umbilicus. It can be heard via Doppler usually by approximately 12 weeks and sometimes as early as 9 weeks. Use a Doppler to auscultate FHTs before 20 weeks; a fetoscope can be used after 20 weeks. A Doppler is commonly used throughout pregnancy because it is convenient and allows the patient to hear as well. Normal FHR is 110 to 160 bpm. Near-term FHTs are generally heard at maximum intensity in the mother's left or right lower quadrant. If FHTs are best heard above the mother's umbilicus, suspect a breech presentation or placenta previa. The fetal heart is best heard through the fetal back, the location of which can be determined by performing Leopold's maneuver as described on page 325.**

Nursing Tip

Fetal Movement

At approximately 18 to 20 weeks, the first fetal movements (FMs) felt in utero, known as quickening, are noticed and interpreted by the pregnant woman as fluttering or kicking. They initially may be difficult to differentiate from other pregnancy symptoms such as gas and ligament stretching. Failure of the mother to notice fetal movement by approximately 20 weeks should alert you to the possibility of either inaccurate dating or, in the absence of FHTs, nonviable pregnancy. Beginning at approximately 28 weeks for an at-risk pregnancy (e.g., maternal diabetes, previous fetal or newborn demise, multiple fetuses, PIH) and approximately 32 weeks for a low-risk pregnancy, fetal kick or fetal movement self-monitoring should be introduced. The pregnant woman's sensation of fetal movement may change in the third trimester, going from "somersaults" to rolling from side to side to kicks or subtle shifts; however, the actual number of fetal movements felt should not decrease dramatically. Any decrease in fetal movement requires rapid evaluation.

A Bradycardia: FHR below 110 bpm
P Fetal distress, maternal drug use
A Absence of fetal heart activity
P Ectopic pregnancy, a blighted ovum, fetal demise, molar pregnancy
A Tachycardia: FHR above 160
P Cardiac dysrhythmia, maternal fever or drug use

Leopold's Maneuver

Beginning at 36 weeks, determine fetal presentation by performing Leopold's maneuver (Figure 23-2).

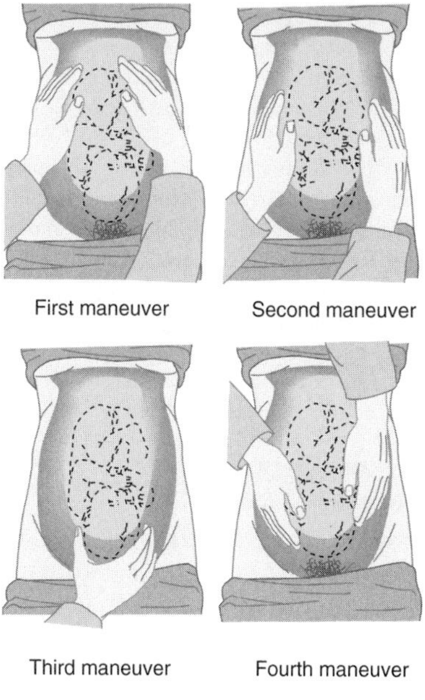

Figure 23-2 Leopold's Maneuver

First Maneuver

E 1. Place the patient in a supine position with the patient's knees bent.
2. Stand to the patient's right side and facing her head.
3. Keeping the fingers of your hand together, palpate the uterine fundus.
4. Determine which fetal part presents at the fundus.

Second Maneuver

E 1. Move both hands to the sides of the uterus.
2. Keep your left hand steady and use your right hand to palpate the patient's abdomen.
3. Determine the positions of the fetus's back and small parts.
4. Keep your right hand steady and use your left hand to palpate the patient's abdomen.

Third Maneuver

E 1. Place your right hand above the symphysis pubis, your thumb on one side of the fetus's presenting part and your fingers on the other side.
2. Gently palpate the fetus's presenting part.
3. Determine whether the buttocks or the head is the presenting part in the pelvis (should confirm the findings of the first maneuver).

Fourth Maneuver

E 1. Change your position so that you are facing the patient's feet.
2. Place your hands on each side of the uterus and above the symphysis pubis and attempt to palpate the cephalic prominence (forehead). This maneuver will assist you in determining the fetal lie (long axis of fetus in relation to long axis of mother) and attitude (head flexed or extended).

N **The fetus's head is usually the presenting part. It feels firm, round, and smooth. The head can move freely when palpated. In contrast, the buttocks (breech position) feel soft and irregular. On palpation, the fetus's whole body seems to move but not with as much facility as the head. The fetus's back is firm, smooth, and continuous. The limbs are bumpy and irregular. The long axis is vertical, and the fetal head is flexed. If the fetus is not in a vertex presentation, the type of delivery can be affected (e.g., the fetus in a persistent transverse or oblique lie will need to be delivered by cesarean section). A breech fetus may be delivered vaginally or by cesarean, depending on the health care provider's comfort and experience in facilitating a vaginal breech delivery. Breech presentation, if uncorrected (i.e., by external version [the manual turning of the fetus by the health care provider]), is associated with an increased rate of perinatal morbidity and mortality, prolapsed umbilical cord, placenta previa, fetal anomalies and abnormalities (which may not manifest immediately after birth), and uterine anomalies.**

A Inability to determine fetal outline

P Polyhydramnios and maternal obesity

Hematological System

See Table 23-4.

Endocrine System

See Table 23-4. See Table 23-5 for special antepartum tests and evaluations.

TABLE 23-4 Laboratory Tests and Values in Pregnancy

TEST	REFERENCE RANGE*	TIMING
Prenatal Panel		
Blood type	A, B, O, AB	Initial visit
Rh	Positive or negative	Initial visit
Antibody screen	Negative	Initial visit; as needed at 28 weeks
RPR (rapid plasma reagent) or VDRL (Venereal Disease Research Laboratories)	Nonreactive or negative. A positive result requires the more specific MHA-TP (microhemagglutination assay for *Treponema pallidum* antibodies) or FTA-ABS (fluorescent treponemal antibody absorbed)	Initial visit; may repeat at 36 weeks

continues

TABLE 23-4 Laboratory Tests and Values in Pregnancy

continued

TEST	REFERENCE RANGE*	TIMING
Cystic fibrosis screening	Noncarrier This disease is inherited in an autosomal recessive pattern and may not manifest with symptoms until later in childhood. Caucasian (non-Jewish) carry at a rate of 1 in 25, while Ashkenazi Jewish carry at a rate of 1 in 29; Hispanics are 1 in 46; African Americans are 1 in 65; and Asian Americans are 1 in 90.	Ideally, prior to pregnancy; if not, at initial prenatal visit
Rubella	Immune (nonimmune patients should be cautioned to avoid contact with any possible exposure during the first trimester and will require a postpartum immunization)	Initial visit
Hepatitis B surface antigen	Negative	Initial visit; may repeat at 36 weeks
HIV (many states are mandating this test or that it at least be offered)	Negative	Initial visit; repeat on basis of history or exposure
Varicella	Immune	Initial visit if uncertain history
Human parvovirus B19 (fifth disease)	Negative	May be done on initial visit or as indicated by exposure
Hepatitis C antibody	Negative	Initial visit if indicated by history
CBC to include:		Initial visit; repeat at 26–28 weeks and 36 weeks
HGB	10.0–14.0 g/dl	
HCT	32.0%–42.0%	
MCV	80.0–100.0 fL	
Platelets	50,000–400,000 mm^3	
Hemoglobin electrophoresis	Normal AA hemoglobin pattern	As indicated by race, ethnic background, or demonstrated anemia
Maternal serum alpha fetal protein (MSAFP) or triple marker screen	Both are maternal blood screening tests. MSAFP screens for neural tube defects and ventral wall defects, an elevation being a positive screen. As a screening test, there are false negatives (misses 20% of actual defects) and false positives, which may result from	15–20 weeks; 16–18 weeks is optimal

continues

TABLE 23-4 Laboratory Tests and Values in Pregnancy

continued

TEST	REFERENCE RANGE*	TIMING
	inaccurate dates, multiple fetus pregnancy, or bleeding with pregnancy. The MSAFP incidentally picks up 20% of Down-affected infants, as the alpha fetal protein will be diminished. Poorly understood is the association of an increased MSAFP with a normal fetus, but increased pregnancy complications such as preterm labor or delivery or PIH. The triple screen adds estradiol and HCG to the test and thus increases the detection of Down syndrome to approximately 60%.	
Genital Cultures or Probes		
Chlamydia by DNA probe or culture	Negative	Initial visit; may repeat at 36 weeks
Gonorrhea by DNA probe or culture	Negative	Initial visit; may repeat at 36 weeks
Genital bacterial/group beta *Streptococcus* (GBS)	Normal flora or negative for gonorrhea, bacterial vaginosis, GBS, and other pathogens	Initial visit; may repeat at 36 weeks
Urinalysis	Same as nonpregnant. Glycosuria is a normal variant.	Initial visit; as needed per symptoms and history
Urine culture	No notable pathogens	Initial visit; as needed per symptoms and history
Toxoplasma IgG	0–5 IU/ml	As indicated by any history of exposures and symptoms
Glucose screen: 1 hour post 50-g glucola glucose tolerance test	1 hour: 140 mg/dl or less (ACOG standard); may vary depending on regional variations; 130–135 mg/dl most common	26–30 weeks for all pregnant women and an early test, preferably with initial prenatal panel, for a woman with a family history of diabetes, a prior macrosomic baby, or who is 34 years or older or obese

**Reference range values may vary to some degree among laboratories.*

TABLE 23-5 Special Antepartum Tests and Evaluations

TEST	DESCRIPTION
Ultrasound	At any time for pregnancy dating, although more accurate for dates early in pregnancy. Confirm or rule out placenta previa, multiple pregnancy; confirm presenting fetal part. Evaluate amniotic fluid volume or fetal growth (especially to rule out intrauterine growth restriction or discordant growth with a multiple pregnancy). Evaluate for ectopic pregnancy or fetal demise.
Genetic testing: chorionic villi sampling (CVS), early amniocentesis, amniocentesis, chromosome studies	CVS for chromosome studies is best done at approximately 9-week gestational age; early amniocentesis is done at approximately 13–16 weeks, and traditional amniocentesis between 16 and 20 weeks, timing being the only difference between the two techniques. Early amniocentesis may carry a higher incidence of abortion. There may be an approximately 1% increased risk of limb deformities associated with CVS, as well as a 1% increased risk of spontaneous abortion. Blood or tissue chromosome studies can be done at any time and are best done with a known family history prior to conception.
Nonstress test (NST) or contraction stress test (CST) for fetal well-being; with decreased fetal movement, known decreased fluid volume, history of certain maternal diseases (insulin-dependent diabetes, collagen vascular disease), or obstetric complications, such as IUGR, postdates, preeclampsia, discordant twin or multiples	For a nonstress test, an electrical fetal monitor is applied to the woman's abdomen, with a tocodynamometer to monitor and record uterine activity and fetal movement and a Doppler to monitor and record FHR, looking at fetal heart response to fetal movement (and any spontaneous uterine contractions). Timing is typically 1 or 2 times per week and may start as early as 32 weeks depending on the risk factor. With a contraction stress test, uterine activity is induced by timed breast nipple stimulation (which induces uterine contractions), and, failing adequate uterine stimulation from nipple stimulation, pitocin intravenously via a pump is used to induce uterine activity. (Relative contraindications for contraction stress test include any risk for uterine rupture, such as previous vertical cesarean section; premature delivery risk; any bleeding risk such as known placenta previa; or any unexplained vaginal bleeding.) Timing is typically once per week after 36 weeks.
Amniotic fluid volume (AFV), which may be described as amniotic fluid index (AFI); most commonly ordered with postdates pregnancies	Ultrasound measurement of AFV using an index to determine normal, increased, or decreased fluid levels
Biophysical profile	A composite test including amniotic fluid volume, nonstress test, fetal breathing movements, fetal limb movements, and fetal tone; each rated on 0–2 score. This study is done most commonly for the same reasons as an NST or CST.

continues

TABLE 23-5 Special Antepartum Tests and Evaluations *continued*

TEST	DESCRIPTION
Fetal movement count	Can be done by all pregnant women; requires no equipment; and incurs no direct cost. There are many methods of doing fetal movement or kick counts (e.g., number of movements during the day or at certain times of the day, or noting the amount of time to discern 10 separate fetal movements after dinner).

Nursing Alert

Danger Signs of Pregnancy

- Vaginal bleeding*
- Leaking or gush of watery fluid*
- Abdominal or pelvic pain or cramping*
- Severe headaches or blurring of vision
- Persistent chills or fever greater than 102°F
- Persistent vomiting
- Decreased fetal movement or lack of fetal movement
- Change in vaginal discharge or pelvic pressure before 36–37 weeks*
- Frequent (more than four per hour) uterine contractions or painless tightenings between 20 and 37 weeks*

**Associated with preterm labor.*

24

Pediatric Patient

Physical Growth

One important set of parameters required for pediatric health assessment is physical growth parameters. The parameters of weight, length or height, and head circumference (dependent on age) are essential in serial physical growth measurement. (Chest circumference is of less importance.)

For infants (0–12 months), average birth weight is 7.5 pounds (3.5 kg), average birth length is 19 to 21 inches (48 to 53 cm), and average birth head circumference is 13 to 14 inches (33 to 35.5 cm). Infants should double birth weight at 6 months and triple birth weight by 1 year of age. An infant's height increases approximately 1 inch (2.5 cm) per month for the first 6 months; height increase then slows to ½ inch (1.3 cm) per month until 12 months of age. Growth in the toddler period (12–24 months) begins to slow. The birth weight usually quadruples by 2.5 years of age. The average weight gain during the toddler period is 4 to 6 pounds (1.8 to 2.7 kg) per year. The toddler usually grows 3 inches (7.6 cm).

Preschoolers (2–6 years) gain an average of 5 pounds (2.3 kg) per year. Height increases between 2.5 and 3 inches (6.4 to 7.6 cm) per year. The preschooler's birth length usually doubles by 4 years of age. In contrast, the school-age child (6–12 years) grows 1 to 2 inches (2.5 to 5 cm) per year and gains 3 to 6 pounds (1.3 to 2.7 kg) annually.

Infancy and adolescence (13–18 years) are two periods of rapid growth in the pediatric patient. Rapid growth in the adolescent is called the growth spurt. Females commonly experience this between ages 10 and 14, whereas males experience it somewhat later, between 12 and 16 years of age.

Anatomy and Physiology

Structural and Physiological Variations

Vital Signs

- Infants aged 6 months and younger are unable to shiver in lower ambient temperature. The absence of this important protective mechanism puts infants at risk for hypothermia, bradycardia, and acidosis.
- By age 4, temperature parameters are comparable to those seen in adults.
- Pulse rates and respiratory rates in children decline with age and reach adult levels by adolescence.

- In children 1 year of age and older, determine normal systolic blood pressure (BP) as follows:

  normal systolic BP (mm Hg) =
  80 + (2 × age in years)
- Normal diastolic BP is generally two-thirds the systolic BP.

Skin and Hair

- Lanugo, a fine, downy hair, can be present on a newborn's temples, upper arms, shoulders, back, and pinnae of the ears. The darker-skinned newborn has more lanugo.
- Vernix caseosa, a thick, cheesy, protective integumentary mechanism consisting of sebum and shed epithelial cells, is present on the newborn's skin.
- Relative to an adult, a child has a higher ratio of body surface area to body surface mass.

Head

- Suture ridges are palpable until approximately 6 months of age.
- The posterior fontanel, formed by the junction of the sagittal and lambdoidal sutures, usually closes by 3 months of age (Figure 24-1A).
- The junction of the sagittal, coronal, and frontal sutures forms the anterior fontanel, which closes by 19 months of age (see Figure 24-1B).

Eyes, Ears, Nose, Mouth, and Throat

- Newborns do not produce tears until their lacrimal ducts open, at around 2 to 3 months of age.
- For primary and secondary teeth eruption, see Figure 24-2.
- The external auditory canal is shorter and positioned more upward.
- The Eustachian tube is more horizontal, wider, and shorter than on the adult.
- The frontal sinuses develop at 7 years of age, the sphenoid sinuses at puberty.
- At birth, vision is 20/200.
- Salivation starts at 3 months.

Breasts

See Table 24-1 and Chapter 14.

Thorax and Lungs

- A newborn's chest is circular because the anteroposterior and lateral diameters are approximately equal. By 6 years of age, the ratio of anteroposterior to lateral diameter reaches adult values.
- Ribs are displaced horizontally in infants.
- Until 3 to 4 months of age, infants are totally dependent on breathing through their nose.
- During infancy and the toddler period, abdominal breathing is always prevalent over thoracic breathing.
- The trachea is short in the infant (2 inches), 18 months (3 inches), teen (4 to 5 inches).

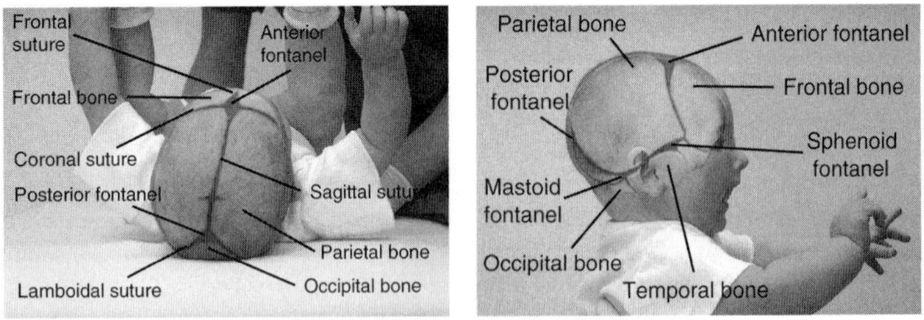

A. Superior View

B. Lateral View

Figure 24-1 Infant Head Structures

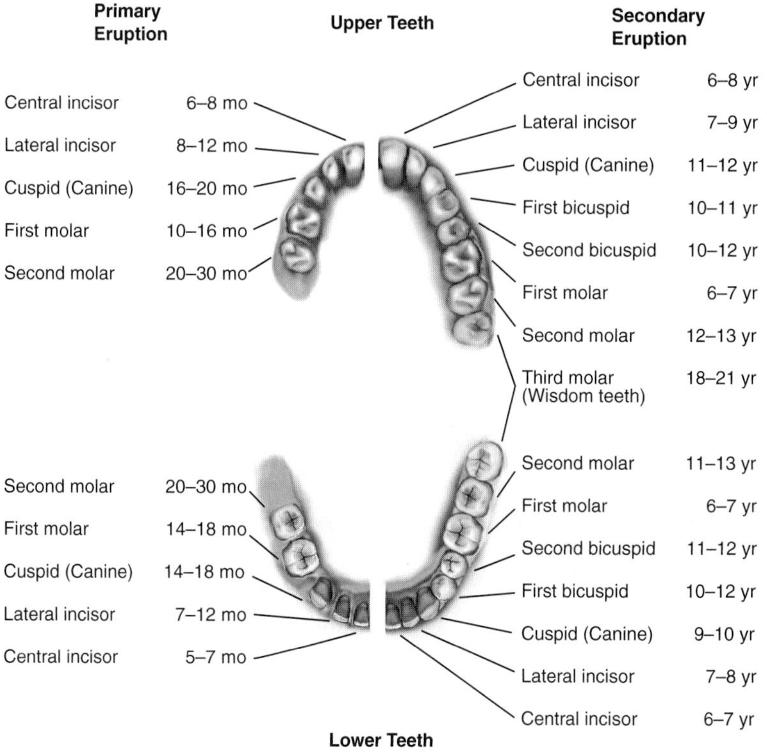

Figure 24-2 Deciduous and Permanent Teeth

Heart and Peripheral Vasculature

- The infant, toddler, and preschooler's heart lies more horizontally than an adult's heart; thus, the apex is higher, at about the left fourth intercostal space (ICS).
- The three fetal shunts (ductus venosus, foramen ovale, and ductus arteriosus) normally close at birth or shortly thereafter.

Abdomen

- At birth, the neonate's umbilical cord contains two arteries and one vein.
- The infant liver is proportionally longer than the adult's.

Musculoskeletal System

- Bone growth ends at age 20, when the epiphyses close.

Neurological System

- The neurological system of the infant is incompletely developed. The autonomic nervous system helps maintain homeostasis as the cerebral cortex develops.
- In the first year, the neurons become myelinated, and primitive motor reflexes are replaced by purposeful movement. The myelinization occurs in a cephalocaudal and proximodistal manner (head and neck, trunk, and extremities).

Urinary System

In infancy the urinary bladder is between the symphysis pubis and umbilicus.

Female Genitalia

See Table 24-2 and Chapter 20.

Male Genitalia

See Table 24-3 and Chapter 21.

TABLE 24-1 Sexual Maturity Rating for Female Breast Development

	DEVELOPMENTAL STAGE
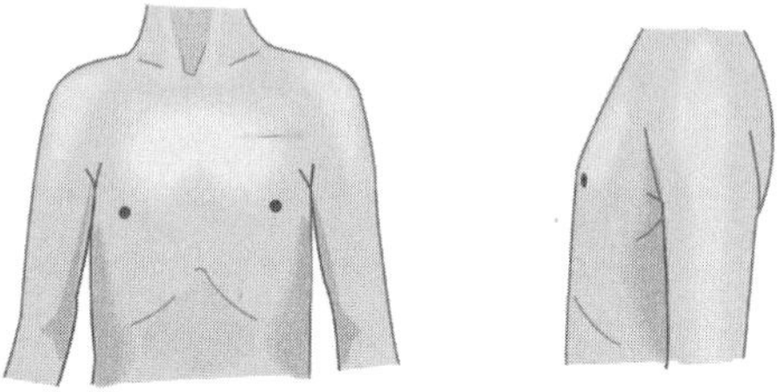	1. Preadolescent stage (before age 10). Nipple is small, slightly raised.
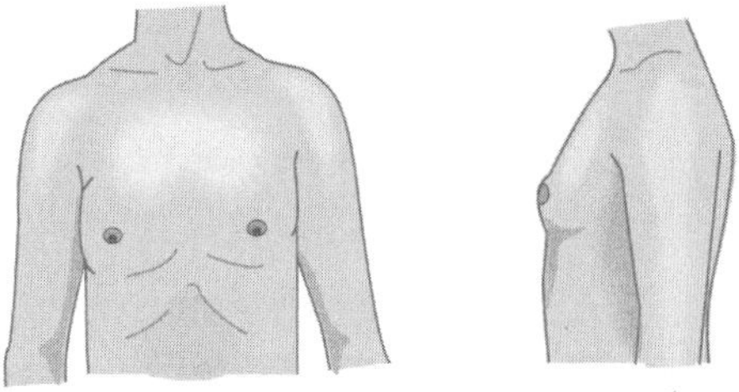	2. Breast bud stage (after age 10). Nipple and breast form a small mound. Areola enlarges. Height spurt begins.
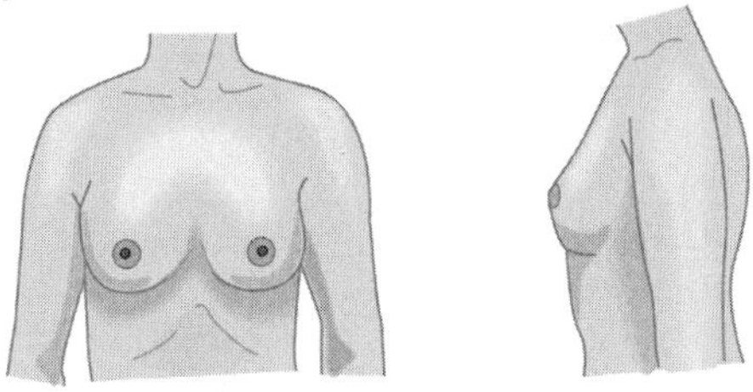	3. Adolescent stage (10–14 years). Nipple is flush with breast shape. Breast and areola enlarge. Menses begins. Height spurt peaks.
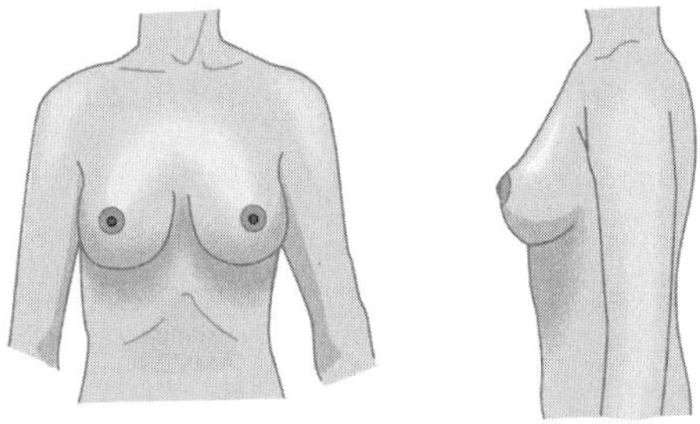	4. Late adolescent stage (14–17 years). Nipple and areola form a secondary mound over the breast. Height spurt ends.
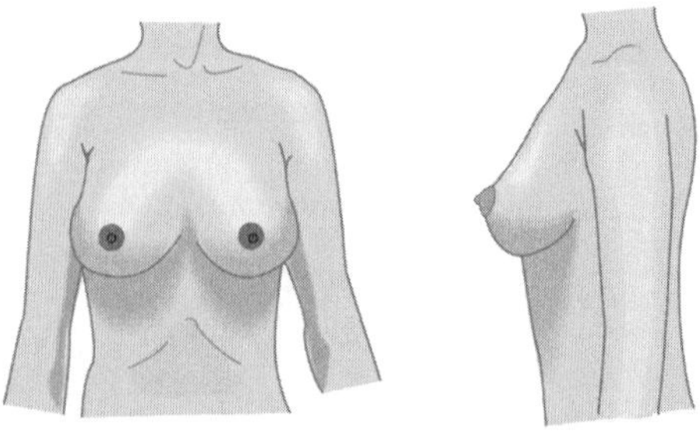	5. Adult stage. Nipple protrudes; areola is flush with the breast shape.

TABLE 24-2 Sexual Maturity Rating for Female Genitalia

DEVELOPMENTAL STAGE	DESCRIPTION
Stage 1 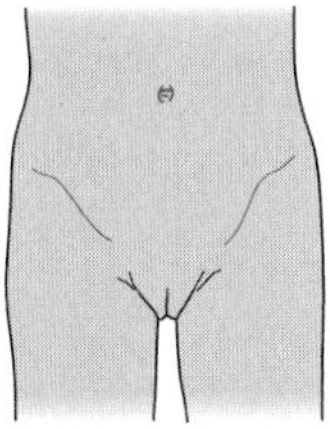	No pubic hair, only body hair (vellus hair)
Stage 2 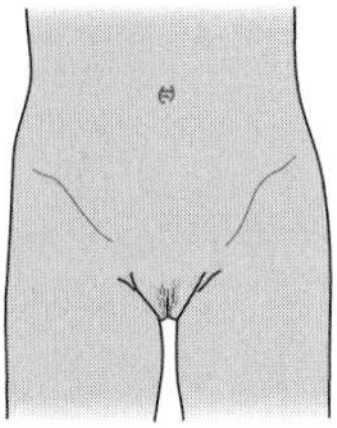	Sparse growth of long, slightly dark, fine pubic hair, slightly curly and located along the labia (ages 11 to 12)
Stage 3 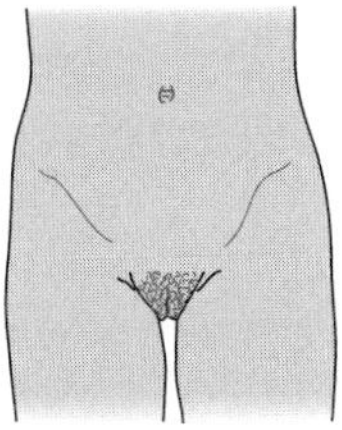	Pubic hair becomes darker, curlier, and spreads over the symphysis (ages 12 to 13)
Stage 4 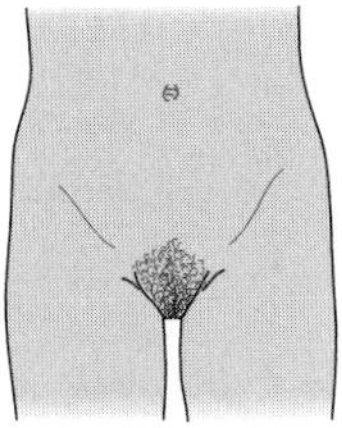	Texture and curl of pubic hair are similar to those of an adult but not spread to thighs (ages 13 to 15)
Stage 5 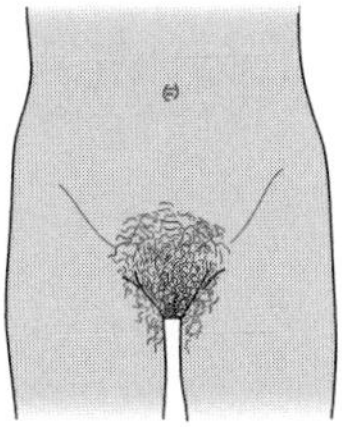	Adult appearance in quality and quantity of pubic hair; growth is spread to inner aspect of thighs and abdomen

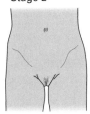

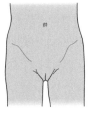

TABLE 24-3 Sexual Maturity Rating for Male Genitalia

DEVELOPMENTAL STAGE	PUBIC HAIR	PENIS	SCROTUM
1. 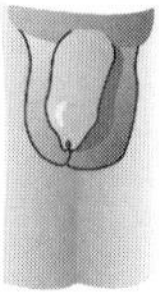	No pubic hair, only fine body hair (vellus hair)	Preadolescent; childhood size and proportion	Preadolescent; childhood size and proportion
2. 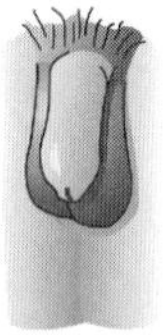	Sparse growth of long, slightly dark, straight hair	Slight or no growth	Growth in testes and scrotum; scrotum reddens and changes texture
3. 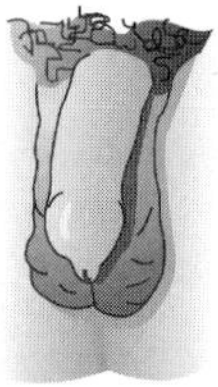	Becomes darker and coarser; slightly curled and spreads over symphysis	Growth, especially in length	Further growth
4. 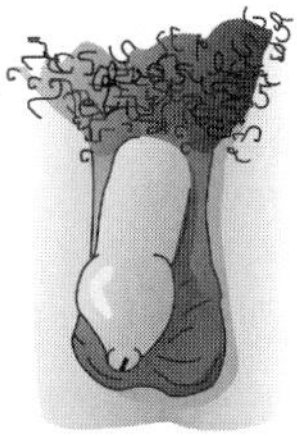	Texture and curl of pubic hair are similar to those of an adult but not spread to thighs	Further growth in length; diameter increases; development of glans	Further growth; scrotum darkens
5. 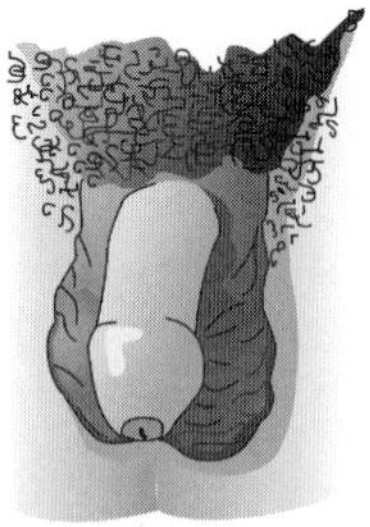	Adult appearance in quality and quantity of pubic hair; growth is spread to medial surface of thighs	Adult size and shape	Adult size and shape

HEALTH HISTORY

Pertinent information should be elicited regarding the birth history, including prenatal, labor and delivery, and postnatal history.

Prenatal

1. Did you plan your pregnancy for ___________ (insert current month)?
2. How many weeks after thinking that you were pregnant did you go to a health care provider for a check-up?
3. How many children have you carried to full term?
4. Were there any pregnancies that you were not able to carry to full term? What happened?
5. Did you take any prescribed or over-the-counter medications?
6. Did you drink alcohol, caffeine, or smoke cigarettes during pregnancy?
7. Did you take any drugs during pregnancy, such as marijuana, crack cocaine, amphetamines, hallucinogens such as LSD and mescaline? If so, what were the amounts and frequency of use?
8. Were there any problems or illnesses that either you or your health care provider were worried about during pregnancy (e.g., PIH, preterm labor, gestational diabetes, TORCH infection, group B streptococcus [GBS])?
9. Was the pregnancy conceived naturally?

Labor and Delivery

1. How many weeks did you carry the baby before delivering?
2. Was the labor spontaneous or induced?
3. How many hours was the labor?
4. Was the baby delivered vaginally or by cesarean section? If by cesarean section, why?
5. Was any analgesia or anesthetic used?
6. Did you hold your baby immediately after delivery? (The answer to this question provides information about the neonate's condition at delivery.)
7. Immediately after delivery, what was the baby's color?
8. What were the baby's Apgar scores at 1 and 5 minutes?
9. What were the birth weight and birth length of the baby?
10. Was the baby's father at the birth with you?
11. Where was the baby born (home, hospital, automobile, other location)?

Postnatal

1. Did you and your baby go home together? (If no, inquire about the reason for the separate discharges.)
2. If a hospital delivery, how long were you and the baby hospitalized?
3. Did the baby have any breathing or feeding problems during the first week?
4. To your knowledge, did your baby receive any medications during the first week?
5. How would you describe the baby's color at 1 week? (For light-skinned babies, ask whether the skin was pale, pale pink, blue, or yellow. For dark-skinned babies, inquire about the color of the sclera, oral mucosa, and nailbeds.)
6. Was the baby circumcised?
7. Did you start breast- or bottle-feeding your baby?
8. Were there any problems with your choice of feeding method?
9. Did you or the baby have a fever after delivery?
10. How did you feel 1 to 2 weeks after delivery?
11. Did you have anyone to help you care for the baby at home in the first few weeks after delivery?

continues

Medical History

Same as for an adult

Surgical History

Same as for an adult

Injuries and Accidents

Determine whether the child has a pattern of frequent injuries or accidents. Repeat trauma may indicate abuse.

Childhood Illnesses

Document past and current exposure to measles, mumps, rubella, pertussis, chickenpox, and respiratory syncytial virus (RSV).

Immunizations

Table 24-4 lists the schedule of immunizations recommended by the Advisory Committee on Immunization Practices (CDC, 2004).

Family Health History

Sudden infant death syndrome (SIDS), attention deficit hyperactivity disorder (ADHD), congenital disorders or defects, mental retardation

Growth and Development

Refer to Chapter 4

Equipment

- Equipment listed in Chapters 10–22
- Scale (infant or stand-up)
- Appropriately sized blood pressure cuff
- Snellen E and Tumbling E charts
- Allen cards
- Ophthalmoscope
- Otoscope speculums (2.5 to 4 mm), pneumatic attachment
- Pediatric stethoscope
- Growth chart
- Peanut butter, chocolate
- Small bell
- Brightly colored object
- Clean gloves
- Measuring tape

NURSING CHECKLIST

General Approach to Pediatric Physical Assessment

1. Assess the patient in a warm, quiet room. To prevent hypothermia, always keep infants under the age of 6 months warm during the examination.
2. Use natural lighting during the assessment, if available. Fluorescent lighting makes assessing varying degrees of cyanosis and jaundice difficult.
3. To help reduce anxiety and uncooperativeness (especially in young children), have a familiar caregiver present during the assessment.
4. Talk to the child in a soothing voice; even an infant who cannot understand your words will take comfort from a calm, supportive approach.
5. Explain all procedures and allow older infants, toddlers, preschoolers, and younger school-age patients to touch or manipulate medical equipment.
6. To promote the child's feeling of security, allow the infant who cannot sit up and the younger child to sit on the caregiver's lap for as much of the examination as possible.

continues

7. Until the infant or toddler is comfortable, maintain eye contact with the caregiver while the assessment is taking place. Making eye contact with the child who has stranger anxiety can be detrimental to completing the examination.
8. Interview the older school-age child or adolescent separately, without the caregiver. Talking to the individual without the caregiver present may yield important information not gained during a group interview (e.g., about drug use).
9. If the child is sleeping, take advantage of the situation by doing simple procedures (measuring length and head circumference) and performing system assessments that require a quiet room (such as the cardiac and respiratory assessments) first.
10. Do all invasive or uncomfortable procedures (ear inspection, hip palpation) last because they may cause discomfort, crying, fear, and increased heart rate.
11. To prevent falls, always keep one hand on any infant placed on the examination table.

Nursing Tip

Integrating Vital Signs into the Pediatric Examination

- Apical heart rate can be obtained during the cardiac assessment.
- Respiratory rate can be obtained when auscultating the lungs.
- Blood pressure and rectal temperature measurement are more threatening and thus should be performed toward the end of the assessment, preferably before using the otoscope.

Physical Assessment

Many assessment techniques for the child are similar to those for the adult. Refer to specific system chapters for detailed explanations of assessment techniques.

Vital Signs

See Chapter 9.

Temperature

Axillary

E 1. When taking an axillary temperature, have the child sit or lie on the caregiver's lap to free your hands to make other observations or to prepare for the next portion of the examination.

2. Explain to the patient that this type of temperature measurement does not hurt. To pass time, ask the caregiver to read the child a story.

N/A/P See Chapter 9.

Rectal

E 1. Children are not fond of rectal temperature measurement, so your explanation should be matter of fact: "I need to measure your temperature in your bottom. You need to hold very still while I do this. Your mommy (or other appropriate person) will be right here with you."

2. Place the patient in either a side-lying or prone position on the caregiver's lap, or place the patient on the back on the examination table; use your nondominant hand to firmly grasp the child's feet.

3. After lubricating the stub-tipped thermometer, insert it gently into the patient's rectum: ½ inch for a newborn, ¾ inch for infants, and 1 inch for preschoolers and older patients. Hold the thermometer firmly between your fingers to avoid accidentally inserting it too far.

N/A/P See Chapter 9.

TABLE 24-4 Recommended Childhood Immunization Schedule—United States, 2005

<table>
<tr><th>Age ▶
Vaccine ▼</th><th>Birth</th><th>1 month</th><th>2 months</th><th>4 months</th><th>6 months</th><th>12 months</th><th>15 months</th><th>18 months</th><th>24 months</th><th>4–6 years</th><th>11–12 years</th><th>13–18 years</th></tr>
<tr><td>Hepatitis B[1]</td><td>HepB #1</td><td colspan="3">HepB #2</td><td colspan="4">HepB #3</td><td colspan="4">HepB Series</td></tr>
<tr><td>Diphtheria, Tetanus, Pertussis[2]</td><td></td><td></td><td>DTaP</td><td>DTaP</td><td>DTaP</td><td></td><td colspan="2">DTaP</td><td></td><td>DTaP</td><td>Td</td><td>Td</td></tr>
<tr><td>Haemophilus influenzae type b[3]</td><td></td><td></td><td>Hib</td><td>Hib</td><td>Hib</td><td colspan="2">Hib</td><td></td><td></td><td></td><td></td><td></td></tr>
<tr><td>Inactivated Poliovirus</td><td></td><td></td><td>IPV</td><td>IPV</td><td colspan="4">IPV</td><td></td><td>IPV</td><td></td><td></td></tr>
<tr><td>Measles, Mumps, Rubella[4]</td><td></td><td></td><td></td><td></td><td></td><td colspan="2">MMR #1</td><td></td><td></td><td>MMR #2</td><td colspan="2">MMR #2</td></tr>
<tr><td>Varicella[5]</td><td></td><td></td><td></td><td></td><td></td><td colspan="3">Varicella</td><td colspan="4">Varicella</td></tr>
<tr><td>Pneumococcal Conjugate[6]</td><td></td><td></td><td>PCV</td><td>PCV</td><td>PCV</td><td colspan="2">PCV</td><td></td><td>PCV</td><td colspan="3">PPV</td></tr>
<tr><td>Influenza[7]</td><td></td><td></td><td></td><td></td><td colspan="4">Influenza (Yearly)</td><td colspan="4">Influenza (Yearly)</td></tr>
<tr><td colspan="13">Vaccines below this line are for selected populations</td></tr>
<tr><td>Hepatitis A[8]</td><td></td><td></td><td></td><td></td><td></td><td></td><td></td><td></td><td colspan="4">Hepatitis A Series</td></tr>
</table>

This schedule indicates the recommended ages for routine administration of currently licensed childhood vaccines, as of December 1, 2004, for children through age 18 years. Any dose not administered at the recommended age should be administered at any subsequent visit when indicated and feasible.

■ Indicates age groups that warrant special effort to administer those vaccines not previously administered. Additional vaccines may be licensed and recommended during the year. Licensed combination vaccines may be used whenever any components of the combination are indicated and other components of the vaccine are not contraindicated. Providers should consult the manufacturers' package inserts for detailed recommendations. Clinically significant adverse events that follow immunization should be reported to the Vaccine Adverse Event Reporting System (VAERS). Guidance about how to obtain and complete a VAERS form is available at **www.vaers.org** or by telephone, **800-822-7967**.

Range of recommended ages

Only if mother HBsAg(–)

Preadolescent assessment

Catch-up immunization

DEPARTMENT OF HEALTH AND HUMAN SERVICES
CENTERS FOR DISEASE CONTROL AND PREVENTION

The Childhood and Adolescent Immunization Schedule is approved by:
Advisory Committee on Immunization Practices www.cdc.gov/nip/acip
American Academy of Pediatrics www.aap.org
American Academy of Family Physicians www.aafp.org

FOOTNOTES

Recommended Childhood and Adolescent Immunization Schedule • United States • 2005

1. **Hepatitis B (HepB) vaccine.** All infants should receive the first dose of HepB vaccine soon after birth and before hospital discharge; the first dose may also be given by age 2 months if the infant's mother is hepatitis B surface antigen (HBsAg) negative. Only monovalent HepB can be used for the birth dose. Monovalent or combination vaccine containing HepB may be used to complete the series. Four doses of vaccine may be administered when a birth dose is given. The second dose should be given at least 4 weeks after the first dose, except for combination vaccines which cannot be administered before age 6 weeks. The third dose should be given at least 16 weeks after the first dose and at least 8 weeks after the second dose. The last dose in the vaccination series (third or fourth dose) should not be administered before age 24 weeks.

   Infants born to HBsAg-positive mothers should receive HepB and 0.5 mL of Hepatitis B Immune Globulin (HBIG) within 12 hours of birth at separate sites. The second dose is recommended at age 1–2 months. The last dose in the immunization series should not be administered before age 24 weeks. These infants should be tested for HBsAg and antibody to HBsAg (anti-HBs) at age 9–15 months.

   Infants born to mothers whose HBsAg status is unknown should receive the first dose of the HepB series within 12 hours of birth. Maternal blood should be drawn as soon as possible to determine the mother's HBsAg status; if the HBsAg test is positive, the infant should receive HBIG as soon as possible (no later than age 1 week). The second dose is recommended at age 1–2 months. The last dose in the immunization series should not be administered before age 24 weeks.

2. **Diphtheria and tetanus toxoids and acellular pertussis (DTaP) vaccine.** The fourth dose of DTaP may be administered as early as age 12 months, provided 6 months have elapsed since the third dose and the child is unlikely to return at age 15–18 months. The final dose in the series should be given at age ≥4 years. **Tetanus and diphtheria toxoids (Td)** is recommended at age 11–12 years if at least 5 years have elapsed since the last dose of tetanus and diphtheria toxoid-containing vaccine. Subsequent routine Td boosters are recommended every 10 years.

3. ***Haemophilus influenzae* type b (Hib) conjugate vaccine.** Three Hib conjugate vaccines are licensed for infant use. If PRP-OMP (PedvaxHIB or ComVax [Merck]) is administered at ages 2 and 4 months, a dose at age 6 months is not required. DTaP/Hib combination products should not be used for primary immunization in infants at ages 2, 4 or 6 months but can be used as boosters following any Hib vaccine. The final dose in the series should be given at age ≥12 months.

4. **Measles, mumps, and rubella vaccine (MMR).** The second dose of MMR is recommended routinely at age 4–6 years but may be administered during any visit, provided at least 4 weeks have elapsed since the first dose and both doses are administered beginning at or after age 12 months. Those who have not previously received the second dose should complete the schedule by the visit at age 11–12 years.

5. **Varicella vaccine.** Varicella vaccine is recommended at any visit at or after age 12 months for susceptible children (i.e., those who lack a reliable history of chickenpox). Susceptible persons aged ≥13 years should receive 2 doses, given at least 4 weeks apart.

6. **Pneumococcal vaccine.** The heptavalent **pneumococcal conjugate vaccine (PCV)** is recommended for all children aged 2–23 months. It is also recommended for certain children aged 24–59 months. The final dose in the series should be given at age ≥12 months. **Pneumococcal polysaccharide vaccine (PPV)** is recommended in addition to PCV for certain high-risk groups. See *MMWR* 2000;49(RR-9):1-35.

7. **Influenza vaccine.** Influenza vaccine is recommended annually for children aged ≥6 months with certain risk factors (including but not limited to asthma, cardiac disease, sickle cell disease, HIV, and diabetes), healthcare workers, and other persons (including household members) in close contact with persons in groups at high risk (see *MMWR* 2004;53[RR-6]:1-40) and can be administered to all others wishing to obtain immunity. In addition, healthy children aged 6–23 months and close contacts of healthy children aged 0–23 months are recommended to receive influenza vaccine, because children in this age group are at substantially increased risk for influenza-related hospitalizations. For healthy persons aged 5–49 years, the intranasally administered live, attenuated influenza vaccine (LAIV) is an acceptable alternative to the intramuscular trivalent inactivated influenza vaccine (TIV). See *MMWR* 2004;53(RR-6):1-40. Children receiving TIV should be administered a dosage appropriate for their age (0.25 mL if 6–35 months or 0.5 mL if ≥3 years). Children aged ≤8 years who are receiving influenza vaccine for the first time should receive 2 doses (separated by at least 4 weeks for TIV and at least 6 weeks for LAIV).

8. **Hepatitis A vaccine.** Hepatitis A vaccine is recommended for children and adolescents in selected states and regions and for certain high-risk groups; consult your local public health authority. Children and adolescents in these states, regions, and high-risk groups who have not been immunized against hepatitis A can begin the hepatitis A immunization series during any visit. The 2 doses in the series should be administered at least 6 months apart. See *MMWR* 1999;48(RR-12):1-37.

Courtesy of Centers for Disease Control and Prevention (CDC)

Physical Growth

Weight

To prevent variations in serial weight checks, use the same scale at each visit if possible.

E **1.** If using an infant scale, cover it with a paper cover protector.
2. Balance or zero the scale.
3. Place infants or young toddlers nude on the scale. Always keep one hand on the child to prevent falls; lift your hand slightly when obtaining the actual weight reading.
4. Preschoolers and young school-age children can wear street clothes to be weighed. Have the older child undress, don a paper or cloth gown, and step on the standard platform scale.
5. Note and record weight.

N **Neonates usually lose approximately 10% of birth weight by the third or fourth day after birth and regain it by 2 weeks of age. This expected change in weight is called physiological weight loss, and it is due to a loss of extracellular fluid and meconium, a dark-green, sticky, stool-like substance excreted from the rectum within the first 24 hours after birth.**

A Small for gestational age (SGA): newborn weight less than the 10th gestational age percentile

P Maternal alcohol, drug, or tobacco abuse, PIH, certain genetic syndromes

A Large for gestational age (LGA): newborn weight greater than the 90th gestational age percentile

P Diabetic mother, genetic predisposition

A Weight below 5th percentile

P Nonorganic failure to thrive (FTT), cyanotic heart disease (CHD), cystic fibrosis (CF), malabsorption syndrome, fetal alcohol syndrome

Length and Height

Recumbent length is measured for children under 2 years of age.

E **1.** Position the measuring board flat on the examination table.
2. Place the child's head at the top of the board and the heels at the foot of the board, making sure the legs are fully extended.
3. Measure and record the length.
4. If a measuring board is not available, place the child in a supine position, making sure the legs are fully extended, and mark lines on the paper at the tip of the head and at the heel.
5. Measure between the lines and record.

Height for all other age groups can be measured in the same fashion as for an adult.

N **Refer to standard growth charts.**

A A height below the 5th percentile or above the 95th percentile or a patient whose height falls 2 standard deviations below his or her own established curve

P Organic or nonorganic FTT, congenital heart disease, CHD, CF, malabsorption problems, fetal alcohol syndrome

Head Circumference

Head circumference is measured for all children less than 2 years of age or serially for patients with known or suspected hydrocephalus or suspected cessation of brain growth.

E **1.** Place the patient in a sitting or supine position.
2. Using a tape measure, measure anteriorly from above the eyebrows and around posteriorly to the occipital protuberance.

N **Normal average head growth is 1 to 1.5 cm per month during the first year. Premature infants often have a small head circumference.**

A Microcephaly, a small brain with a resultant small head

P Intrauterine infections, maternal drug or alcohol ingestion during pregnancy, fetal alcohol syndrome, genetic defects

A Hydrocephalus (enlarged head), head circumference above the 95th percentile

P Imbalance in CSF production and reabsorption

Chest Circumference

Chest circumference is measured until 1 year of age. It is a measurement that by itself provides little information but is compared with head circumference to evaluate the child's overall growth.

E 1. Stand in front of the supine patient.
2. Measure chest diameter by placing the tape measure around the chest at the nipple line.
3. Measure during exhalation.

N **From birth until approximately 1 year of age, head circumference is greater than chest circumference. After age 1, chest circumference is greater than head circumference.**

A Measured chest circumference below normal limits

P Prematurity

Apgar Scoring

The Apgar scoring system provides a quick method to assess the need for newborn resuscitation in the delivery room. An Apgar score is given to a newborn at 1 and 5 minutes after birth. Perform steps 1 through 5 at 1 minute after birth; add the score in each category for the total. Repeat at 5 minutes after birth.

E 1. Auscultate the heart rate for 1 full minute.
2. Measure the degree of respiratory effort.
3. Evaluate muscle tone by attempting to straighten each extremity individually.
4. Evaluate the newborn's reflex irritability. Use a flicking motion of two fingers against the newborn's sole to rate reflex irritability.
5. Inspect the newborn's color.

N **A score of 8 to 10 demonstrates that the newborn is in good condition. Table 24-5 outlines the scoring system for each of the five areas assessed.**

A A moderately depressed newborn earns a score of 4 to 7. A score of 0 to 3 indicates that the newborn is severely depressed and needs immediate resuscitation. Either finding is abnormal.

P A low score can be the result of one or numerous problems. Prematurity, central nervous system depression, blood or meconium in the trachea, maternal history of drug abuse, certain drugs that are given to the mother in preparation for delivery and that cross over and cause fetal depression, congenital complete heart block, and congenital heart disease are some of the potential etiologies for a low Apgar score.

TABLE 24-5 Apgar Scoring

HEART RATE	RESPIRATORY RATE	TONE	REFLEX IRRITABILITY	COLOR
Absent = 0 <100 = 1 >100 = 2	Apnea = 0 Slow, irregular rate = 1 Crying vigorously = 2	Flaccid = 0 Some degree of flexion = 1 Full flexion = 2	No response = 0 Grimace = 1 Crying = 2	Cyanosis = 0 Body pink, extremities acrocyanotic = 1 Completely pink = 2

Skin

Inspection

Color

E Observe the color of the body, especially noting the nose tip, external ear, lips, hands, and feet. These areas are prime locations for detecting cyanosis or jaundice.

N **The skin of the newborn is reddish for the first 24 hours then turns varying shades of pale-pink, pink, brown, or black, depending on the child's race. It is also normal for dark-skinned newborns to look ruddy and for light-skinned newborns to exhibit a bluish-purple color of the hands and feet, although the rest of the body is pink. This condition is called acrocyanosis and may disappear with warming. Mongolian spots, deep-blue pigmentations over the lumbar and sacral areas of the spine, the buttocks, and, sometimes, the upper back or shoulders in newborns of African, Latino, or Asian descent, are extremely common and not to be confused with ecchymosis.**

A Jaundice, yellowing of the skin or sclera

P Rh/ABO incompatibility, maternal infections (pathological jaundice), increased levels of serum bilirubin (physiological jaundice)

A Harlequin color change, dependent side turns ruddy

P Benign condition, poor vasomotor control

Lesions

E/N See Chapter 10.

A Eczema (atopic dermatitis)

P Inhaled allergens induce mast-cell responses

A Telangiectatic nevi (storkbites), flat, deep, irregular, pink, localized areas in light-skinned children and deeper red areas in dark-skinned children, found on the back of the neck, the lower occiput, the upper eyelids, and the upper lip

P Capillary dilatation

A Diaper dermatitis, diffuse redness to papules, vesicles, edema, scaling, and ulcerations on the area covered by a baby's diaper

P Bacteria and urea reaction on the skin

A Neural tube defects: a dark-black tuft of hair or a dimple over the lumbosacral area

P Failure of the neural tube to fuse at approximately the fourth week of gestation, resulting in vertebral defect (spina bifida occulta)

A Small maculopapular lesions on an erythematous base, wheals, and vesicles

P Erythema toxicum, a benign rash

Palpation

E See Chapter 10.

N **Skin of the pediatric patient normally is smooth and soft. Milia, plugged sebaceous glands, present as small, white papules; occur usually on the nose and cheeks.**

A/P See Chapter 10.

Hair

Inspection

Lesions

E/N See Chapter 10.

A Seborrheic dermatitis (cradle cap): yellow to gray, greasy-appearing scales on the scalp of a light-skinned infant

P Increased epidermal tissue growth

Head

Inspection

Shape, Symmetry, and Head Control

E With the patient sitting upright in the caregiver's arms or on the examination table, observe the symmetry of the frontal, parietal, and occipital prominences.

N **The patient's head is symmetric and without depressions or protrusions.**

The anterior fontanel may pulsate with every heartbeat. The Asian infant generally has a flattened occiput, more so than do infants of other races. At 3 months of age, the infant is able to hold the head steady without help.

A A flattened occipital bone with resultant hair loss over the area

P Prolonged supine position

A Lack of head control beyond 4 to 6 months

P Prematurity, hydrocephalus, developmental delay

Palpation

Fontanel

E **1.** Place the child in an upright position.
2. Using the second or third finger pad, palpate the anterior fontanel at the junction of the sagittal, coronal, and frontal sutures.
3. Palpate the posterior fontanel at the junction of the sagittal and lambdoidal sutures.
4. Assess for bulging, pulsations, and size. Accurate measurements can be obtained only if the patient is not crying. Crying produces a distorted, full, bulging appearance.

N **The anterior fontanel is soft and flat. Size ranges from 4 to 6 cm at birth. The fontanel gradually closes between 9 and 19 months of age. The posterior fontanel is also soft and flat. Size ranges from 0.5 to 1.5 cm at birth. The posterior fontanel gradually closes between 1 and 3 months of age. It is normal to feel pulsations related to the peripheral pulse.**

A Bulging, tense fontanel

P Increased intracranial pressure (meningitis and increased CSF)

A Sunken, depressed fontanel

P Dehydration

A Wide anterior fontanel in a child older than 2½ years

P Rickets, hypothyroidism, Down syndrome, hydrocephalus

Suture Lines

E **1.** With the finger pads, palpate the sagittal suture line, which runs from the anterior to the posterior portion of the skull in a midline position.
2. Palpate the coronal suture line, which runs along both sides of the head, starting at the anterior fontanel.
3. Palpate the lambdoidal suture, which runs along both sides of the head, starting at the posterior fontanel.
4. Ascertain if these suture lines are open, united, or overlapping.

N **Grooves or ridges between sections of the skull are normally palpated up to 6 months of age.**

A Suture lines that overlap or override one another

P Craniosynostosis (premature ossification of suture lines) due to metabolic disorders or secondary to microcephaly

Surface Characteristics

E **1.** Using the finger pads in the same manner as for palpating the fontanels and suture lines, palpate the skull.
2. Note cranial surface edema and contour.

N **The skin covering the cranium is flush against the skull and without edema.**

A Craniotabes, softening of the outer layer of the cranial bones behind and above the ears combined with a ping pong ball sensation as the area is pressed gently in with the fingers

P Rickets, syphilis, hydrocephaly, hypervitaminosis A

A Cephalhematoma, localized, subcutaneous swelling over one of the cranial bones of a newborn

P Forceps delivery

A Caput succedaneum, swelling over the occipitoparietal region of the skull

P Pressure over the occipitoparietal region during a prolonged delivery (self-resolving)

A Molding, parietal bone overriding the frontal bone

P Induced pressure during delivery (self-resolving)

Eyes

General Approach

1. From infancy through approximately 8 to 10 years of age, the eyes should be assessed toward the end of the assessment, with the exception of testing the vision, which should be done first. Children generally are not cooperative for eyes, ears, and throat assessments.
2. Place the young infant, preschooler, school-age, or adolescent patient on the examination table. The older infant and the toddler can be held by the caregiver.

Vision Screening

E See Chapter 12. For a child who cannot read the alphabet, use the Tumbling E chart.

N **Normal vision in the newborn is 20/200; from 2 to 6 years of age, normal vision is 20/40.**

A/P See Chapter 12.

Allen Test

E **1.** With the child's eyes both open, show each card to the child and elicit a name for each picture.

2. Place the 2- to 3-year-old child 4.5 m (15 feet) from where you will be standing. Place the 3- to 4-year-old child 6 m (20 feet) from you.

3. With one of the child's eyes covered, show the pictures one at a time, eliciting a response after each showing.

4. Show the same pictures in different sequence for the other eye.

5. To record findings, the denominator is always constant at 30, because a child with normal vision should see the picture on the card (target) at 9 m (30 feet). To document the numerator, determine the greatest distance at which three of the pictures are recognized by each eye, for example, right eye = 15/30, left eye = 20/30.

N **The child should correctly identify three of the cards in three trials. Two- to three-year-old children should have 15/30 vision. Three- to four-year-old children should be able to achieve a score of 15/30 to 20/30. Each eye should have the same score.**

A/P If scores for the right and left eyes differ by 1.5 m (5 feet) or more or either or both eyes score less than 15/30.

Strabismus Screening

The Hirschberg test and the cover-uncover test screen for strabismus. The latter is the more definitive test.

Hirschberg Test

E/N See Chapter 12.

A It is abnormal for the light reflection to be displaced to the outer margin of the cornea as the eye deviates inward.

P Esotropia is thought to be congenital. Some theories suggest that neurological factors contribute to its development.

A It is abnormal for the light reflection to be displaced to the inner margin of the cornea as the eye deviates outward.

P Exotropia can result from eye muscle fatigue or can be congenital.

Cover-Uncover Test

E See Chapter 12.

N **Neither eye moves when the occluder is being removed. Infants less than 6 months of age display strabismus due to poor neuromuscular control of eye muscles.**

A It is abnormal for one or both eyes to move to focus on the penlight during assessment. Assume strabismus is present.

P Strabismus after 6 months of age is abnormal and indicates eye muscle weakness.

Inspection

Eyelids

E Observe for symmetrical palpebral fissures and position of eyelids in relation to the iris.

N **Palpebral fissures of both eyes are positioned symmetrically. Upper eyelid normally covers a small portion of the iris, and lower lid meets the iris. Epicanthal folds are normally present in Asian children.**

A Portion of the sclera is visible above the iris

P Hydrocephalus

A A fold of skin covers the inner canthus and lacrimal caruncle

P Down syndrome; fetal alcohol syndrome

Lacrimal Apparatus

E/N See Chapter 12.

A Dacryocystitis: inability to produce tears by 3 months of age

P Failure of the distal end of the membranous lacrimal duct to open, blockage elsewhere

Anterior Segment Structures

Sclera

E See Chapter 12.

N **The newborn exhibits a blue-tinged sclera.**

A/P See Chapter 12.

Iris

E Conduct the examination in the same manner as for an adult.

N **Until approximately 6 months of age, the iris is blue or slate gray in light-skinned infants and brownish in dark-skinned infants. Between 6 and 12 months of age, complete transition of iris color occurs.**

A Brushfield's spots: small, white flecks around the perimeter of the iris

P Down syndrome

Pupils

E See Chapter 12.

N A newborn will normally blink and flex the head closer to the body in reaction to light (optical blink reflex).

A/P See Chapter 12.

Posterior Segment Structures

General Approach

1. If the patient is uncooperative for a full funduscopic exam, attempt to observe the red reflex, optic disc, and retina.
2. The assessment is easier to accomplish if the infant or toddler is lying supine on the examination table. The assistance of another individual, such as the caregiver, to hold the patient in position is essential. The older patient may be allowed to sit, if cooperative.

Inspection

Red Reflex

E/N See Chapter 12.

A Absent red reflex

P Chromosomal disorders, intrauterine infections, ocular trauma

A Yellowish or white reflex

P Retinoblastoma

Retina

E/N See Chapter 12.

A Red or dark-red color

P Hemorrhage due to trauma (shaken baby syndrome)

Optic Disc

E/N/A/P See Chapter 12.

Ears

Auditory Testing

General Approach

1. Perform auditory testing at approximately 3 to 4 years of age or when the child can follow directions. See Chapter 13.
2. Before 3 years of age, the following are a few parameters for evaluating hearing:
   a. Does the child react to a loud noise?

b. Does the child react to the caregiver's voice by cooing, smiling, or turning the eyes and head toward the voice?
c. Does the child try to imitate sounds?
d. Can the child imitate words and sounds?
e. Can the child follow directions?
f. Does the child respond to sounds not directed at him or her?

External Ear

Inspection of Pinna Position

E/N See Chapter 13.

A The top of the ear is below the imaginary line drawn from the outer canthus to the top of the ear.

P See Chapter 13.

Internal Ear

Inspection

E **1.** A cooperative patient may be allowed to sit for the assessment.
2. Restrain the uncooperative young patient by placing him or her supine on a firm surface. Instruct the caregiver or assistant to hold the patient's arms up by the head, embracing the elbow joints on both sides of each arm. Restrain the infant by having the caregiver hold the infant's hands down.
3. With your thumb and forefinger grasping the otoscope, use the lateral side of the same hand to prevent the child's head from jerking. Your other hand can also be used to stabilize the patient's head.
4. Until approximately 3 years of age, pull the lower auricle down and out to straighten the canal. Use the adult technique after age 3.
5. Insert the speculum approximately ¼ to ½ inch, depending on age.
6. Suspected otitis media must be evaluated (typically using a pneumatic bulb attached to the side of the otoscope's light source):
a. A larger speculum is selected to make a tight seal and prevent air from escaping from the canal.
b. If a light reflex is present, focus on the light reflection.
c. Gently squeeze the bulb attachment to introduce air into the canal. (Some nurses prefer to gently blow air through the tubing versus squeezing air into the canal.)
d. Observe the tympanic membrane for movement.

N/A/P See Chapter 13.

Mouth and Throat

Inspection

Lips and Buccal Mucosa

E **1.** Follow the technique described in Chapter 13.
2. Observe whether the lip edges meet.

N **See Chapter 13.**

A Cleft lip: lip edges do not meet

P Congenital malformation

A Curdlike coating

P Thrush

Teeth

E/N See Chapter 13.

A Lack of visible teeth by 16 months

P Genetic abnormalities

A Brownish or black tooth surface

P Caries, bottle mouth

Hard and Soft Palates

E Observe palate for continuity and shape.

N **The roof of the mouth is continuous and has a slight arch.**

A Cleft palate: roof of mouth not continuous

P Congenital malformation

A High hard and soft palates

P Trisomy 18 and trisomy 21, Noonan's syndrome

A Epstein's pearls, small white cysts on the hard palate and gums

P Epithelial tissue trapped during palate formation

Oropharynx

E See Chapter 13.

N **Up to age 12 years, a tonsil grade of 2+ is considered normal. Tonsils should not interfere with the act of breathing.**

A Excessive drooling, salivation, choking, and coughing during feeding

P Tracheoesophageal fistula (TEF)

A Exudative pharyngitis with fever, sore throat, petechiae on the palate

P Mononucleosis

Neck

Inspection

General Appearance

E 1. Observe the neck in a midline position when the patient is sitting upright.
2. Note shortening or thickness of the neck on both right and left sides.
3. Note any swelling.

N **There is a reasonable amount of skin tissue on the sides of the neck. There is no swelling.**

A Weblike tissue bilaterally from the ear to the shoulder

P Congenital syndromes (e.g., Turner syndrome)

A Unilateral or bilateral swelling of the neck below the angle of the jaw

P Enlargement of the parotid gland (parotitis, mumps)

Palpation

Lymph Nodes and Thyroid

E/N See Chapter 11.

A Enlargement of the anterior cervical chain

P Bacterial infections of the pharynx (strep throat)

A Enlargement of the occipital nodes or posterior cervical chain nodes

P Tinea capitis, acute otitis externa, mononucleosis

A/P See Chapter 11.

Breasts

See Chapter 14 and Table 24-1.

> **Nursing Alert**
>
> **Stridor**
>
> Stridor is indicative of upper airway obstruction, particularly edema in children. Inspiration accentuates stridorous sounds. Children who present with stridor should be promptly evaluated to rule out epiglottitis (a medical emergency).

Thorax and Lungs

Shape of Thorax

E/N See Chapter 15.

A Abnormal chest configuration

P Cystic fibrosis

Retractions

E Evaluate intercostal muscles for signs of increased work of breathing.

N **Retractions are not present.**

A Retractions in the suprasternal, supraclavicular, subcostal, and intercostal regions; respiratory distress; nasal flaring; stridor; expiratory grunting; and wheezing.

P Abnormal function or disruption of the respiratory pathway or within organs that control or influence respiration; respiratory syncytial virus (RSV).

Heart and Peripheral Vasculature

General Approach

1. It is best to perform the cardiac assessment near the beginning of the examination, when infants and young children tend to be relatively calm.
2. During the assessment, note physical signs of a syndrome, such as Down's facies of a child with trisomy 21 or Down syndrome. Many children with Down syndrome have associated atrioventricular (A-V) canal malformation.

This defect involves an atrial septal defect (ASD), ventricular septal defect (VSD), and a common A-V valve.

3. Cardiac landmarks change when a child has dextrocardia. In this condition, the apex of the heart points toward the right thoracic cavity; thus, heart sounds are auscultated primarily on the right side of the chest.

Inspection

Apical Impulse

E See Chapter 16.

N **In both infants and toddlers, the apical impulse is located at the fourth ICS and just left of the midclavicular line. The apical impulse of a child 7 years of age and older is at the fifth ICS and to the right of the midclavicular line.**

A/P See Chapter 16.

Precordium

E Observe the chest wall for any movements other than the apical impulse.

N **Movements other than the apical impulse are abnormal.**

A Heaves: lifting of the cardiac area

P Volume overload (congestive heart failure [CHF]): congenital heart disease, left-to-right shunts

Palpation

See Chapter 16.

Thrill

E 1. Palpate as for adult or use proximal one-third of each finger and the areas over the metacarpophalangeal joints.
2. Place hand vertically along heart's apex and move hand toward sternum.
3. Place hand horizontally along sternum, moving up the sternal border about ½ inch to 1 inch each time.
4. At the clavicular level, place hand vertically and assess for a thrill at heart's base.
5. Use finger pads to palpate a thrill at the suprasternal notch and along the carotid arteries.

N **No thrill is found.**

A/P See Chapter 16.

Peripheral Pulses

E 1. Use the finger pads to palpate each pair of peripheral pulses simultaneously, except for the carotid pulse.
2. Palpate the brachial and femoral pulses simultaneously.

N **Pulse qualities are the same in the adult and the child.**

A Brachial-femoral lag

P Coarctation, narrowing of the aorta

Auscultation

E 1. Have the child lie down. If this position is not possible, the child should be at a 45° angle in the caregiver's arms.
2. Use a Z pattern to auscultate the heart. Place the stethoscope in the apical area and gradually move it toward the right lower sternal border and up the sternal border in a right diagonal line. Move gradually from the patient's left to the right upper sternal borders.
3. With the child in a sitting position, perform a second evaluation.

N **Fifty percent of all children develop an innocent murmur at some time in their lives. Innocent murmurs are accentuated in high cardiac output states such as fever. When the patient is sitting they are heard early in systole and at the second or third ICS and along the left sternal border; they are soft and musical in quality, and they disappear when the child lies down. Be aware of sinus arrhythmias during auscultation of the heart's rhythm. On inspiration, the pulse rate speeds up; on expiration, it slows. To determine whether the rhythm is normal, ask the child to hold his or her breath while you aus-**

cultate the heart. If the pause stops, a sinus arrhythmia is present. S_1 is best heard at the apex of the heart, at the left lower sternal border. S_2 is best heard at the heart base.

A Split S_2 on inspiration

P ASD (negative pressure in the thoracic cavity)

A Holosystolic murmurs heard maximally at the left lower sternal border

P VSD

A Continuous murmurs

P Collateral blood flow murmurs (pulmonary atresia), palliative shunt murmurs

A S_3 "Kentucky"

P CHF, VSD

Abdomen

General Approach

1. If possible, ask the caregiver to refrain from feeding the infant before the assessment because palpation of a full stomach may induce vomiting.
2. Children who are physically able should be encouraged to empty the bladder before the assessment.
3. The young infant, school-age, or adolescent patient should lie on the examination table. The toddler or preschooler should lie supine in the caregiver's lap and let the lower extremities bend at the knees and dangle.
4. If the child is crying, encourage the caregiver to help calm the child before you proceed with the assessment.
5. Observe nonverbal communication in children who are not able to verbally express feelings. During palpation, listen for a high-pitched cry and look for a change in facial expression or for sudden, protective movements that may indicate a painful or tender area.

> **Nursing Tip**
>
> **Assessing for Umbilical Hernias in Children**
>
> If the child is upset and crying, assess the umbilicus for an outward projection, which is indicative of an umbilical hernia. If an umbilical hernia is present, palpate the area to determine whether the hernia reduces easily. Approximate the size of the inner ring (the diameter of the hernia).

Inspection

Contour

E See Chapter 17.

N **The young child may have a "potbelly."**

A/P See Chapter 17.

Peristaltic Wave

E/N See Chapter 17.

A Pyloric stenosis: visible, peristaltic waves moving across the epigastrium from left to right

P Obstruction at the pyloric sphincter

Auscultation

See Chapter 17.

Palpation

General Palpation

E/N See Chapter 17.

A An olive-shaped mass in the epigastric area and to the upper right of the umbilicus

P Pyloric stenosis

A Hirschsprung's disease, abdominal distension coupled with palpable stool over the abdomen and absence of stool in the rectum

P Aganglionic segment of the colon

A Intersusception, sausage-shaped mass that produces intermittent pain when palpated in the upper abdomen

P No clear etiology (ileocecal region of the intestine telescopes down into the ileum itself), rotavirus vaccine

A Diaphragmatic hernia, bowel sounds heard in the thoracic cavity, a scaphoid abdomen, an upwardly displaced apical impulse, and signs of respiratory distress

P Protrusion of the intestines into the thoracic cavity

Liver Palpation

E For infants and toddlers, use the outer edge of the right thumb to press down and scoop up at the right upper quadrant. For the remaining age groups, use the same technique as for an adult.

N **The liver is not normally palpable, although the liver edge can be found 1 cm below the right costal margin in healthy children. The liver edge is soft and regular.**

A Hepatomegaly: full liver edge with a firm, sharp border palpated greater than 2 cm below the right costal margin

P Viral or bacterial illness, tumor, CHF, fat and glycogen storage diseases

Musculoskeletal System

General Approach

See Chapter 18.

Inspection

Muscles

E **1.** For the lower spine and hips to be evaluated, have the child disrobe down to a diaper or to underwear.
2. To evaluate the small infant's shoulder muscles, place your hands under the axillae and pull the infant to a standing position. The infant should not slip through your hands. Be prepared to catch the infant if needed.
3. Evaluate the infant's leg strength with the infant in a semi-standing position; lower the infant to the examination table until the infant's legs touch the table.
4. Place the infant older than 4 months in a prone position. Observe the infant's ability to use the upper extremities to lift the upper body off the examination table.

N **Degree of joint flexibility and range of motion (ROM) are the same for the child as for the adult.**

A Cerebral palsy (CP): increased muscle tone (spasticity)

P Abnormality in the pyramidal motor tract, perinatal asphyxia

A Gower's sign: inability to rise from a sitting to a standing position

P Duchenne's muscular dystrophy (MD): genetic abnormality in the short arm of the X chromosome

Joints

E See Chapter 18.

N **The infant's spine is C shaped. Head control and standing create the normal S-shaped spine of the adult. Lordosis is normal as the child begins to walk. The toddler's protruding abdomen is counterbalanced by an inward deviation of the lumbar spine.**

A Supernumerary digits (polydactyly) or fusion between digits (syndactylism)

P Congenital syndromes (Carpenter, fetal hydantoin, orofaciodigital, Smith-Lemli-Opitz, trisomy 13, VATER)

Tibiofemoral Bones

E **1.** Have child stand on examination table with medial condyles together.
2. Measure the distance between the two medial malleoli, and the two medial condyles.

N **The distance between the medial malleoli is less than 2 inches (5 cm). The distance between the medial condyles is less than 1 inch (2.5 cm). Knock-knee, or genu valgum, is common between 2 and 4 years of age. Bowleg, or genu varum, is normally present in many infants up to 12 months of age.**

A Genu valgum

P Physiological

A Genu varum

P Rickets

Palpation

Joints

E/N See Chapter 18.

A Osgood-Schlatter disease: palpation of a slight elevation of the tibial tuberosity

P Deformed tubercle caused by repetitive stress on the area

A Swollen, inflamed joints

P Juvenile rheumatoid arthritis

Feet

E 1. Place the patient on the examination table or the caregiver's lap.
2. Stand in front of the child.
3. Use one hand to hold the child's right heel immobile while using the other hand to push the forefoot (medial base of great toe) toward a midline position.
4. Observe for toe and forefoot adduction and inversion.
5. Repeat on the left foot.

N **The toes and forefoot are not deviated.**

A Metatarsus varus (club foot): toes and forefoot medially adducted and inverted

P Abnormal intrauterine position of the fetal foot, heredity

Hip and Femur

Because it may induce crying, Ortolani's maneuver is always performed at the very end of the assessment. The test is performed on one hip at a time. Evaluate the hips until 18 months of age or until the child is an established walker.

E 1. Place the infant supine on the examination table with the infant's feet facing you.
2. Stand directly in front of the infant.
3. Use the thumb to hold the inner thigh of the femur and the index and middle fingers to hold the greater trochanter (Figure 24-3A). These two fingers should rest over the hip joint.
4. Slowly press outward and abduct until the lateral aspect of the knee nearly touches the table (Figure 24-3B). Use the tips of the fingers to palpate the femora's head as it rotates outward.
5. Listen for an audible click (positive Ortolani's sign).
6. With the fingers in the same locations, adduct the hip to elicit a palpable click (positive Ortolani's sign). As the hip is adducted, it lifts anteriorally into the acetabulum.

N **A click will not be audible or palpated.**

A Developmental dysplasia of the hip (DDH): positive Ortolani's sign; sudden, painful crying during the test; asymmetric thigh skin folds; uneven knee level; and limited hip abduction

P Familial factors; maternal hormones associated with pelvic laxity; firstborn children; breech presentations; oligohydramnios

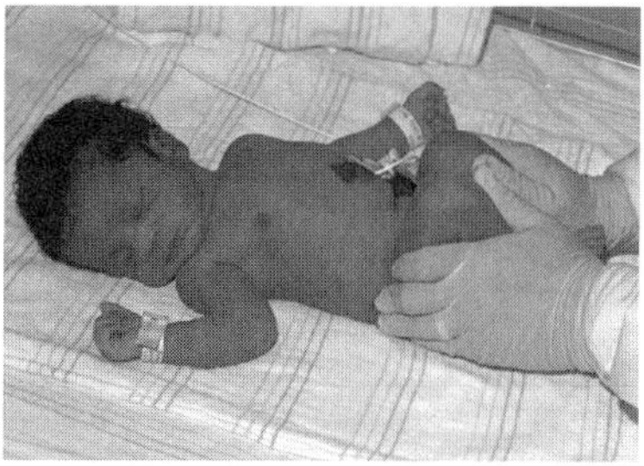

A. Hand Placement

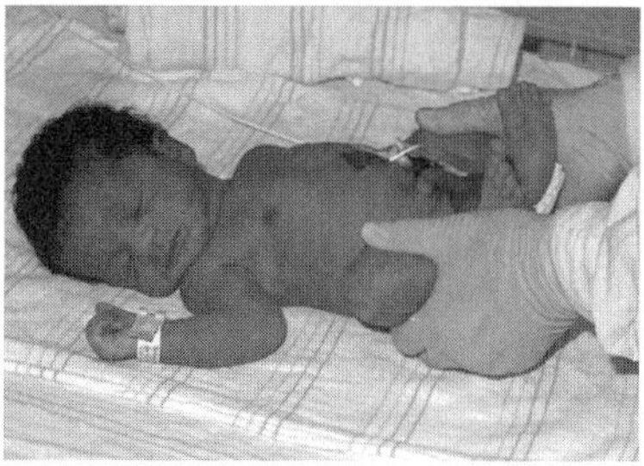

B. Hip Abduction

Figure 24-3 Ortolani Maneuver

Neurological System

General Approach

1. Some of the neurological assessment for the infant and the young child differs from that for the adult. An infant functions mainly at the subcortical level. Memory and motor coordination are approximately three-quarters developed by 2 years of age, when cortical functioning is acquiring dominance.
2. Incorporate findings of the fine and gross motor skills evaluation (previously performed during the musculoskeletal assessment). In addition, use the Denver II to assess personal-social and language skills. Refer to normal developmental milestones (see Chapter 4), and extrapolate warning signs of neurological developmental lag.
3. Because the infant cannot verbally express level of consciousness, assess instead the newborn's crying ability, activity level, positioning, and general appearance.
4. Only reflex mechanisms and cranial nerve (CN) testing are described in this section. Refer to the adult neurological assessment for all other testing.

Reflex Mechanisms of the Infant

Neonatal reflexes must be lost before motor development can proceed.

Rooting Reflex

E 1. Place the infant supine with the head in a midline position.
2. With your forefinger, stroke the infant's skin at one corner of the mouth.
3. Observe the movement of the infant's head.

N **Until 3 or 4 months of age, the infant will turn the head toward the side that was stroked. In the sleeping infant, the rooting reflex can be present normally until 6 months of age.**

A An absent rooting reflex from birth through 3 to 4 months of age

P Central nervous system disease such as frontal lobe lesions

Sucking Reflex

E 1. Place the infant supine.
2. Use your forefinger to touch the infant's lips to stimulate a response.
3. Observe for a sucking motion.

N **A sucking response occurs until approximately 10 months of age.**

A Absence of the sucking response

P Prematurity, breast-fed infant whose mother ingests barbiturates

Palmar Grasp Reflex

E 1. Place the infant supine with the head in a midline position.
2. Place the ulnar sides of your index fingers into the infant's hands while the infant's arms are in a semi-flexed position (Figure 24-4).
3. Press your fingers into the infant's palmar surfaces.

N **The infant grasps your fingers in flexion.**

A Palmar grasp reflex after 4 months of age

P Frontal lobe lesions

Tonic Neck Reflex

E 1. Place the infant in a supine position on the examination table.
2. Rotate the infant's head to one

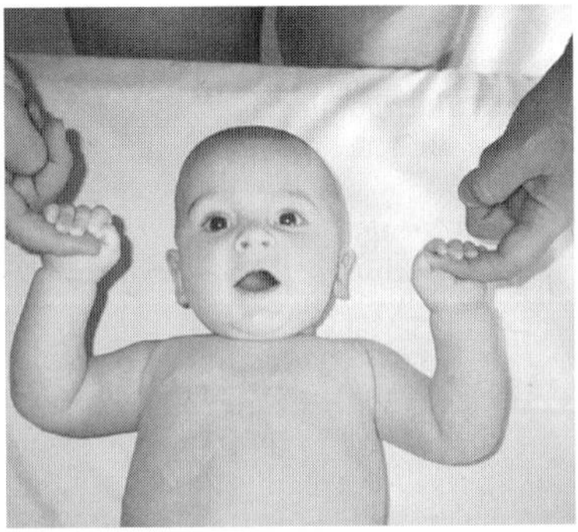

Figure 24-4 Palmar Reflex

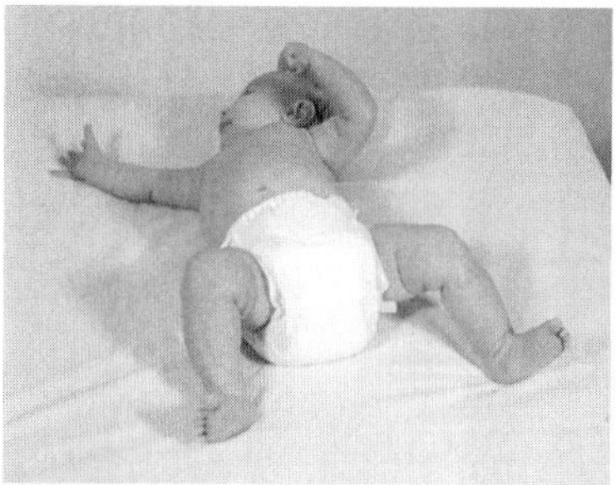

Figure 24-5 Tonic Neck Reflex

side and hold the jaw area parallel to the shoulder.

3. Observe for movement of the extremities.

N **The upper and lower extremities on the side to which the jaw is turned extend, and the opposite arm and leg flex (Figure 24-5). This reflex sometimes does not show up until 6 to 8 weeks of age.**

A Tonic neck reflex after 6 months of age

P Cerebral damage

Stepping Reflex

E **1.** Stand behind the infant and grasp the infant under the axillae to bring the infant to a standing position on a flat surface. Use the thumbs to support the back of the infant's head, if needed.

2. Push the infant's feet toward a flat surface and simultaneously lean the infant's body forward (Figure 24-6).

3. Observe the legs and feet for stepping movements.

N **Stepping movements are made by flexing one leg and moving the other leg forward. This reflex disappears at approximately 3 months of age.**

A Stepping response after 3 months of age

P CP

Plantar Grasp Reflex

E **1.** Position the infant supine on the examination table.

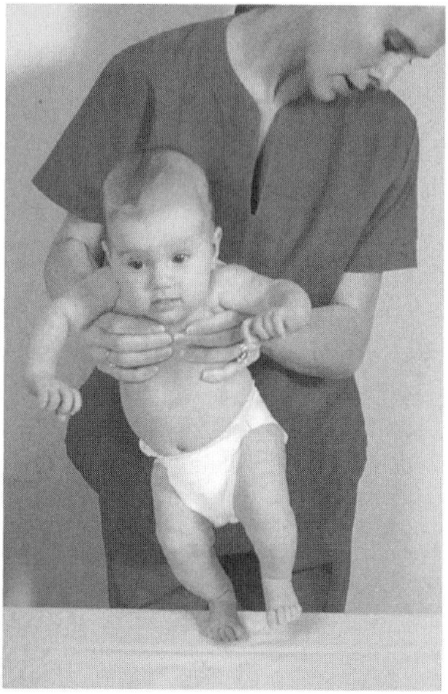

Figure 24-6 Stepping Reflex

2. Elevate the foot to be examined.

3. Touch the infant's foot on the plantar surface beneath the toes.

4. Repeat on the other side.

N **The toes curl down until 8 months of age.**

A Plantar grasp reflex absent on one or both feet

P Obstructive lesion (abscess, tumor), CP

Babinski's Reflex

E **1.** Position the infant supine on the examination table.

2. Elevate the foot to be examined.

3. With the tip of your thumbnail, stroke the plantar surface of the foot, from the lateral heel upward.

N **A child younger than 15 to 18 months normally fans the toes outward and dorsiflexes the great toe (Figure 24-7).**

A Babinski's reflex after learning to walk or after 18 months of age

P CP

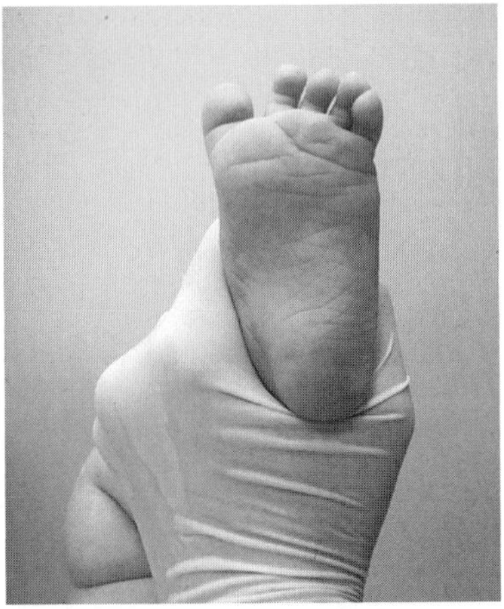

Figure 24-7 Babinski's Reflex

Moro (Startle) Reflex

E 1. Place the infant supine on the examination table.
2. Make a sudden, loud noise such as hitting your hand on the examination table.

N **The infant under 4 months of age quickly extends then flexes the arms and fingers in response to this maneuver. The thumb and index fingers form a C shape (Figure 24-8).**

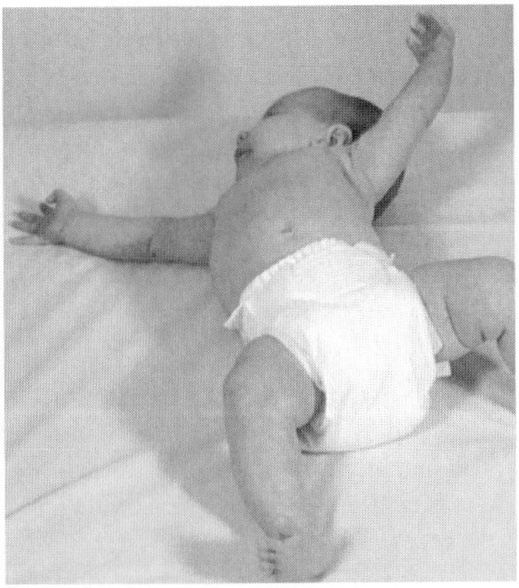

Figure 24-8 Moro Reflex

A Moro reflex after 4 to 6 months of age

P CP

Galant Reflex

E 1. Place the infant prone with the infant's hands under the abdomen.
2. Use your index finger to stroke the skin along the side of the spine.
3. Observe the stimulated side for any movement.

N **The infant under 1 to 2 months of age will turn the pelvis and shoulders toward the stimulated side.**

A No response in the patient under 2 months of age

P Spinal cord lesion

Placing Reflex

Do not test the placing and stepping reflexes at the same time because they are two different reflexes.

E 1. Grasp the infant under the axillae from behind and bring the body to a standing position. Use the thumbs to support the back of the head, if needed.
2. Touch the dorsum of one foot to the edge of the examination table.
3. Observe the tested leg for movement.

N **The infant's tested leg will flex and lift onto the examination table.**

A Lack of response is abnormal.

P It is difficult to elicit this reflex in breech-born babies and in those with paralysis or cerebral cortex abnormalities.

Landau Reflex

E 1. Carefully suspend the infant in a prone position, supporting the chest with your hand.
2. Observe for extension of the head, trunk, and hips.

N **The arms and legs extend during the reflex. The reflex appears at about 3 months of age.**

A Presence of the Landau reflex beyond 2 years of age is abnormal. Also, it is abnormal for the infant to assume a limp position.

P Mental retardation may account for an abnormality.

Cranial Nerve Function

A thorough assessment of CN function is difficult to perform on the infant under 1 year of age. Difficulty is also encountered with toddlers and preschoolers because they often either cannot follow directions or are unwilling to cooperate. Testing of the school-age child and the adolescent is carried out in the same manner as for an adult.

Infant (Birth to 12 Months)

E **1.** To test CN III, CN IV, and CN VI, move a brightly colored toy along the infant's line of vision. An infant older than 1 month responds by following the object with the eyes. Also evaluate pupillary response to a bright light in each eye.

2. CN V is tested by assessing the rooting reflex or sucking reflex.

3. Until 2 months of age, CN VII is tested by assessing the sucking reflex and observing symmetric sucking movements. After 2 months of age, an infant will smile, allowing assessment of facial symmetry.

4. In an infant less than 6 months of age, CN VIII is tested by assessing the Moro reflex.

5. CN IX and CN X are assessed by using a tongue blade to produce the gag reflex. Do not repeat testing if a positive response was already elicited when using a tongue blade to view the posterior pharynx.

6. To test CN XI, evaluate the infant's ability to lift the head up while in a prone position.

7. CN XII is assessed by allowing the infant to suck on a pacifier or a bottle, abruptly removing the pacifier or bottle from the infant's mouth, and observing for lingering sucking movements.

N/A/P See Chapter 19.

Toddler and Preschooler (1 to 5 Years)

E **1.** The older preschooler is able to identify familiar odors. Most children readily identify the smell of peanut butter and chocolate. Test CN I one side at a time by occluding the nostril on the opposite side and asking the child to close the eyes and identify the smell of peanut butter and chocolate. Use different substances to test each nostril.

2. Use Allen cards to test vision (CN II).

3. CN III, CN IV, and CN VI are tested in the same fashion as for the infant.

4. CN V is tested by giving the child something to eat and evaluating chewing movements. Sensory responses to light and sharp touch are not easily interpreted in these age groups.

5. Observe facial weakness or paralysis (CN VII) by making the child smile or laugh. An older preschooler may cooperate by raising the eyebrows, frowning, puffing the cheeks out, and tightly closing the eyes on command.

6. To evaluate CN VIII, observe the child's response to an unseen sound (e.g., ring a small bell out of the child's vision).

7. Test CN IX and CN X in the same manner as for an infant.

8. CN XII is difficult to assess in this age group.

N/A/P See Chapter 19.

Female Genitalia

E/N See Chapter 20 and Table 24-2.

A Pseudomenstruation: blood in the vaginal opening or on the diaper of an infant under 2 weeks of age

P Maternal hormones

Nursing Alert

Signs of Sexual Abuse in Children

The following are possible signs of sexual abuse in children:

- A strong fear of the examination
- Presence of STDs
- Abnormal discharge or odor
- Anorectal tears
- Absent or delayed anal reflex
- Anorectal ecchymosis, pruritus, HPV, scarring, or bleeding
- In the female, a broken hymen can be a sign of sexual abuse. Keep in mind, however, that a broken hymen can also result from foreign objects being placed into the vagina by the child, forceful use of diaper wipes during a diaper change, tampon use, and strenuous exercise such as gymnastics and horseback riding.
- Vaginal tears

Male Genitalia

E/N See Chapter 21.

A Cryptorchidism: undescended testis

P Result of embryonic development

A Hypospadias (ventral opening)

P Fetal development anomaly

A Epispadias (dorsal opening)

P Fetal development anomaly

Anus

See Chapter 22.

REFERENCE

Centers for Disease Control and Prevention. (2004). *Recommended childhood and adolescent immunization schedule, United States, 2005*. Retrieved May 11, 2005, from http://www.cispimmunize.org/IZschedule.pdf

Unit 5 Putting It All Together

25

The Complete Health History and Physical Examination

Performing a complete health history and physical examination is a skill that takes time and practice to develop. You must concentrate on perfecting interviewing techniques and assessment skills. Keep in mind that as assessment skills are perfected, the amount of time it takes to conduct them will decrease. Plan on spending between 30 and 90 minutes conducting the complete health history and physical examination.

Health History

Depending on the reason for the patient's visit, the health history can be complete, episodic, interval (follow-up), or emergency in nature.

Nursing Tip

General Documentation Guidelines

1. Ensure that you have the correct patient record or chart and that the patient's name and identifying information are on every page of the record.
2. Document as soon as the patient encounter is concluded to ensure accurate recall of data (follow institution's guidelines on frequency of charting).
3. Date and time each entry.
4. Sign each entry with your full legal name and with your professional credentials, or per your institution's policy.
5. Do not leave space between entries.
6. If an error is made while documenting, use a single line to cross out the error, then date, time, and sign the correction (check institutional policy); avoid erasing, crossing out, or using correction fluid.
7. Never correct another person's entry, even if it is incorrect.
8. Use quotes to indicate direct patient responses (e.g., "I feel lousy").
9. Document in chronological order; if chronological order is not used, state why.
10. Use legible writing.
11. Use a permanent ink pen. (Black is usually preferable because of its ability to photocopy well.)
12. Document in a complete but concise manner by using phrases and abbreviations as appropriate (see Abbreviations and Symbols in Appendix).
13. Document telephone calls that are related to the patient's case.
14. Remember, from a legal standpoint, if you didn't document it, it wasn't done.

> **Nursing Tip**
>
> **Tips for a Successful Assessment**
>
> 1. Ensure that the examination table is at a comfortable height for you and the patient and that there is easy access on all sides.
> 2. Respect the patient's modesty.
> 3. Have the patient make as few position changes as possible.
> 4. Ensure that all needed equipment is accessible and arranged in a logical manner.
> 5. Sit opposite the patient who is sitting or lying in bed.
> 6. Keep interruptions to a minimum.
> 7. Teach self-assessment techniques while the patient is gowned or during the corresponding system examinations.
> 8. Advise the patient about potential discomfort or sensations before performing procedures.
> 9. Ask the patient about pain or other sensations potentially associated with certain assessments.
> 10. Offer cleaning wipes or tissues to the patient after certain examinations (e.g., the pelvic and rectal examination).
> 11. Provide the patient with privacy for redressing.

Components of the developmental, cultural, and spiritual assessments are continually evaluated during the course of the patient interaction. Thorough assessments of any or all of these special areas can be completed if dictated by the patient's situation. The inspection component of the nutritional assessment is noted during the health history.

Sit opposite the patient who is sitting or lying in bed.

Physical Assessment

General Survey

The patient's general appearance is assessed during the health history. Incorporate the following into this assessment:

Physical Presence

Age: stated age versus apparent age
General appearance
Body fat
Stature: posture, proportion of body limbs to trunk
Motor activity: gait, speed and effort of movement, weight bearing, absence or presence of movement in different body areas
Body and breath odors

Psychological Presence

Dress, grooming, and personal hygiene
Mood and manner
Speech
Facial expressions

Distress

Physical
Psychological
Emotional

Neurological System

Assess mental status: facial expression, affect, level of consciousness, fund of information, attention span, memory, judgment, insight, spatial perception, calculations, abstract reasoning, and thought processes and content.

After the mental status assessment, ask the patient to undress and to don an examination gown (underwear may be worn). Ask the patient to empty the bladder and save urine for a specimen. Ask the patient to sit on the examination table and to hang the legs over the front of the table. A second drape may be provided to cover the patient's lap and legs. Stand in front of the patient.

Measurements

Record the patient's:

1. Height
2. Weight
3. Temperature
4. Pulse (radial preferred site in adult)
5. Respirations
6. Blood pressure (both arms)
7. Anthropometric measurements (if indicated)

Skin

Throughout the entire head-to-toe assessment, inspect the skin for the following characteristics:

1. Color
2. Bleeding
3. Ecchymosis
4. Vascularity
5. Lesions

Throughout the entire head-to-toe assessment, palpate the skin for:

1. Moisture
2. Temperature
3. Texture
4. Turgor
5. Edema

Head and Face

1. Inspect the shape of the head.
2. Inspect and palpate the head and scalp.
3. Inspect the color and distribution of the hair; note any infestations; palpate the hair.
4. Inspect the face for expression, shape, overall symmetry (cranial nerve [CN VII]), and symmetry of the eyes, eyebrows, ears, nose, and mouth.
5. Instruct the patient to raise the eyebrows, frown, smile, wrinkle the forehead, show the teeth, purse the lips, puff the cheeks, and whistle (CN VII).
6. Palpate the temporal pulses. Palpate the temporal muscles (CN V).
7. Palpate and auscultate the temporomandibular joints (CN V).
8. Palpate the masseter muscles (CN V).

Eyes

1. Test distance vision and near vision (CN II).
2. Test color vision.
3. Test visual fields via confrontation (CN II).
4. Assess extraocular mobility: cover-uncover test, corneal light reflex, and six cardinal fields of gaze (CN III, CN IV, and CN VI).
5. Assess direct and consensual light reflexes and accommodation (CN III).
6. Inspect the eyelids, eyebrows, palpebral fissures, and eye position.
7. Inspect and palpate the lacrimal apparatus of each eye.
8. Inspect the conjunctiva, sclera, cornea, iris, pupil, and lens of each eye.
9. Assess corneal reflex.
10. Conduct funduscopic assessment: retinal structures and macula

Ears

1. Test gross hearing: voice-whisper test or watch-tick test (CN VIII).
2. Inspect and palpate the external ear.
3. Assess ear alignment.
4. Conduct otoscopic assessment: EAC, and tympanic membrane.
5. Perform Weber and Rinne tests.

Nose and Sinuses

1. Inspect the external surface of the nose.
2. Assess nostril patency.
3. Test olfactory sense (CN I).
4. Use a nasal speculum to conduct internal assessment: mucosa, turbinates, and septum.
5. Inspect, percuss, and palpate the frontal and maxillary sinuses.

Mouth and Throat

1. Note breath odor.
2. Inspect the lips, buccal mucosa, gums, and hard and soft palates.
3. Inspect the teeth; count the teeth.
4. Inspect the tongue; ask patient to stick out the tongue (CN XII).
5. Inspect the uvula; note its movement when the patient says "ah" (CN IX and CN X).
6. Inspect the tonsils.
7. Inspect the oropharynx.
8. Test the gag reflex (CN IX and CN X).
9. Test taste (CN VII).
10. Palpate the lips and mouth, if indicated.

Neck

1. Inspect the musculature of the neck.
2. Inspect range of motion, shoulder shrug (CN XI), and strength of

sternocleidomastoid and trapezius muscles.
3. Palpate the musculature of the neck.
4. Inspect and palpate the trachea.
5. Palpate the carotid arteries (one at a time).
6. Inspect the jugular veins for distension; estimate jugular venous pressure (JVP), if indicated.
7. Inspect and palpate the thyroid gland (anterior approach).
8. Auscultate the thyroid gland and carotid arteries.
9. Inspect and palpate the cervical lymph nodes: preauricular, postauricular, occipital, submental, submandibular, tonsillar, anterior cervical chain, posterior cervical chain, supraclavicular, and infraclavicular.

Upper Extremities

1. Inspect nailbed color, shape, and configuration; palpate nailbed texture.
2. Assess capillary refill of the nailbeds.
3. Inspect muscle size and palpate muscle tone of the hands, arms, and shoulders.
4. Palpate the joints of the fingers, wrists, elbows, and shoulders.
5. Assess ROM and strength of the fingers, wrists, elbows, and shoulders.
6. Test position sense.
7. Palpate the radial and brachial pulses.
8. Palpate the epitrochlear node.

Move behind the patient. Untie the examination gown so that the patient's entire back is exposed. The gown should still cover the shoulders and the anterior chest.

Back, Posterior and Lateral Thoraxes

1. Palpate the thyroid gland (posterior approach).
2. Inspect and palpate the spinous processes; inspect cervical spine ROM.
3. Note thoracic configuration, symmetry of the shoulders, and position of the scapula.
4. Palpate the posterior thorax and the lateral thorax.
5. Assess posterior thoracic expansion.
6. Assess tactile fremitus of the posterior thorax and the lateral thorax.
7. Percuss the posterior thorax and the lateral thorax.
8. Assess diaphragmatic excursion.
9. Palpate the costovertebral angle (CVA); use your fist to percuss the CVA.
10. Auscultate the posterior thorax and the lateral thorax; assess voice sounds, if indicated.

Move in front of the patient. Drape the patient's gown at waist level (the female patient can cover her breasts).

Anterior Thorax

1. Inspect shape of the thorax, symmetry of the chest wall, presence of superficial veins, costal angle, angle of the ribs, intercostal spaces (ICSs), muscles of respiration, respirations, and sputum.
2. Palpate the anterior thorax.
3. Assess anterior thoracic expansion.
4. Assess tactile fremitus of the anterior thorax.
5. Percuss the anterior thorax.
6. Auscultate the anterior thorax; assess voice sounds, if indicated.

Heart

Auscultate the cardiac landmarks: aortic, pulmonic, mitral, and tricuspid areas and Erb's point.

Ask the female patient to uncover her breasts.

Female Breasts

1. Inspect the breasts for color, vascularity, thickness, edema, size, symmetry, contour, lesions, masses, and discharges with the patient in the following positions: arms at side, arms raised overhead, hands pressed into hips, and hands in front and patient leaning forward.
2. Palpate the breasts first with the patient's arms at her sides and then with her arms raised overhead.
3. Palpate the brachial, midaxillary, pectoral, and subscapular lymph nodes.
4. Teach breast self-examination.

Male Breasts

Repeat the sequence used for female breasts, but do not have the patient lean forward unless gynecomastia is present.

Assist the patient into a supine position with the patient's chest uncovered. Drape the patient's abdomen and legs. Stand at the right side of the patient.

Jugular Veins

As the patient changes from a sitting to a supine position for the breast assessment, observe the jugular veins when the patient is at a 45° angle. Assess again when the patient is supine.

Inspect the jugular veins for distension; estimate jugular venous pressure (JVP), if indicated.

Female and Male Breasts

1. Palpate each breast. The arm on the same side of the assessed breast should be raised over head.
2. Compress the nipple to express any discharge.

Heart

1. Inspect the cardiac landmarks for pulsations.
2. Palpate the cardiac landmarks for pulsations, thrills, and heaves.
3. Palpate the apical impulse.
4. Use the diaphragm of the stethoscope to auscultate the cardiac landmarks; count the apical pulse.
5. Use the bell of the stethoscope to auscultate the cardiac landmarks.
6. Have the patient turn onto the left side; repeat auscultation of the cardiac landmarks.

Return the patient to a supine position. Cover the patient's anterior thorax with the gown. Uncover the patient's abdomen, from the symphysis pubis to the costal margin.

Abdomen

1. Inspect contour, symmetry, pigmentation, and color.
2. Note scars, striae, visible peristalsis, masses, and pulsations.
3. Inspect the rectus abdominis muscles (with the patient supine and with the patient's head raised) and respiratory movement of abdomen.
4. Inspect the umbilicus.
5. Auscultate bowel sounds.
6. Auscultate for bruits, venous hum, and friction rub.
7. Percuss all four quadrants.
8. Percuss liver span and liver descent; use your fist to percuss the liver, if indicated.
9. Percuss the spleen, stomach, and bladder.
10. Lightly palpate all four quadrants.
11. Note any muscle guarding.
12. Deeply palpate all four quadrants.
13. Palpate the liver, spleen, kidney, aorta, and bladder.
14. Assess superficial abdominal reflexes.
15. Assess hepatojugular reflux, if indicated.

Inguinal Area

1. Inspect and palpate the inguinal lymph nodes.
2. Inspect for inguinal hernias.
3. Palpate the femoral pulses.
4. Auscultate the femoral pulses for bruits.

Use the gown to cover the exposed abdomen. Lift the drape from the bottom to expose the patient's lower extremities.

Lower Extremities

1. Inspect for color, capillary refill, edema, ulcerations, hair distribution, and varicose veins.
2. Palpate for temperature, edema, and texture.
3. Palpate the popliteal, dorsalis pedis, and posterior tibial pulses.
4. Inspect muscle size and palpate muscle tone of the legs and feet.
5. Palpate the joints of the hips, knees, ankles, and feet.
6. Assess ROM and strength of the hips, knees, ankles, and feet.

7. Test position sense.
8. Assess clonus.

Drape the lower extremities. Assist the patient to a sitting position and note the ease with which the patient sits up. Have the patient dangle the legs over the edge of the examination table.

Neurological System

1. Assess light touch: face, hands, lower arms, abdomen, feet, and legs (CN V).
2. Assess superficial pain (sharp and dull): face, hands, lower arms, abdomen, feet, legs (CN V).
3. Assess two-point discrimination: tongue, lips, fingers, dorsum of the hand, torso, and feet.
4. Assess vibration sense: fingers and toes.
5. Assess stereognosis, graphesthesia, and extinction.
6. Assess cerebellar function: finger to nose, rapid alternating hand movements, thumb to each finger, running heel down shin, foot tapping.
7. Assess deep tendon reflexes: biceps, triceps, brachioradialis, patellar, and Achilles.
8. Assess plantar reflex and Babinski reflex.

Ask the patient to stand barefoot on the floor. Remain physically close to the patient at all times.

Musculoskeletal System

1. Assess mobility: casual walk, heel walk, toe walk, tandem walk, backwards walk, stepping to the right and left, and deep knee bends (one knee at a time). Note any indications of discomfort.

Stand behind the patient.

2. Assess spinal ROM.

Open the patient's gown to expose the back. Ask the patient to bend forward at the waist.

3. Inspect the spine for scoliosis.

Close the patient's gown. Stand in front of the patient.

Neurological System

1. Perform the Romberg test; assess pronator drift.
2. Assess the patient's ability to hop on one foot, run heel down shin, and use the foot to draw a figure eight.

Assist the female patient back to the examination table. Ask her to assume the lithotomy position. Drape the patient. Sit on a stool in front of the patient's legs.

Female Genitalia, Anus, and Rectum

1. Inspect pubic hair distribution, presence of parasites, and skin color and condition: mons pubis, vulva, clitoris, urethral meatus, vaginal introitus, sacrococcygeal area, perineum, and anal mucosa.
2. Palpate the labia, urethral meatus, Skene's glands, vaginal introitus, and perineum.
3. Insert the vaginal speculum.
4. Inspect the cervix: color, position, size, surface characteristics, discharge, and shape of cervical os. Inspect the vagina.
5. Collect specimens for cytological smears and cultures.

Stand in front of the patient's legs.

6. Perform bimanual assessment of the vagina, cervix, fornices, uterus, and adnexa.
7. Perform rectovaginal assessment.
8. Palpate the anus and rectum.
9. If stool is on your glove, save the stool to test for occult blood.

Assist the patient to a sitting position. Offer her some tissues to wipe the perineal area. Ask her to redress.

Male Genitalia

Ask the male patient to stand. Sit on a stool in front of the patient. Have the patient lift the gown to expose the genitalia.

1. Inspect the hair distribution, penis, scrotum, and urethral meatus.
2. Palpate the penis, urethral meatus, and scrotum.
3. Palpate the inguinal area for nodes and hernias.

4. Auscultate the scrotum, if indicated.
5. Teach testicular self-examination.

Ask the patient to bend over the examination table. If the patient is bedridden, the knee-chest or left lateral decubitus position may be used. Expose the patient's buttocks. Stand behind the patient.

Male Anus, Rectum, and Prostate

1. Inspect the perineum, sacrococcygeal area, and anal mucosa.
2. Palpate the anus and rectum.
3. Palpate the prostate.
4. If stool is on your glove, save the stool to test for occult blood.

Cover the patient's buttocks. Assist the patient to stand up. Offer him some tissues to wipe the perianal area. Ask him to redress.

Give the patient a few minutes to redress in privacy before proceeding with the examination; the patient can also formulate questions during this time.

Completing the Assessment

When completing the assessment, ensure that you return the patient to the state you found him or her in at the beginning of the assessment. For example, for the bedridden patient, ensure that the side rails are up (if appropriate) and that the call bell is readily accessible. Ask the patient whether there is anything else that can be done to make him or her comfortable. Document all findings, and thank the patient for her or his time and cooperation.

Appendix

Abbreviations and Symbols

Abbreviations

A, A, & O ×3	awake, alert, & oriented times three (to person, place & time)
$\bar{a}$	before
AB	abortion
abd	abdomen; abdominal
ABG	arterial blood gas
Abx	antibiotic
$\overline{ac}$	before meals
AC>BC	air conduction is greater than bone conduction
AC<BC	air conduction is less than bone conduction
ACL	anterior cruciate ligament
AD*	right ear
ADL	activities of daily living
AEB	as evidenced by
AFI	amniotic fluid index
AGA	appropriate for gestational age
AIDS	acquired immunodeficiency syndrome
AKA	above the knee amputation
ALS	amyotrophic lateral sclerosis
ant	anterior
AOM	acute otitis media
AP	apical pulse; anteroposterior
A&P	anterior & posterior; auscultation & percussion
AROM	active range of motion; artificial rupture of membranes
AS	aortic stenosis
AS*	left ear
ASA	acetylsalicylic acid
ASD	atrial septal defect
Atb	antibiotic
AU*	both ears
AV	arteriovenous
A-V	atrioventricular
A&W	alive & well
AWMI	anterior wall myocardial infarction
ax	axillary
BF	black female
bid	twice a day
bil	bilateral
BKA	below the knee amputation
BM	black male; breast milk; bowel movement
BP	blood pressure
BPH	benign prostatic hypertrophy
BPM	beats per minute
BS	bowel sounds; breath sounds
b/t	between
BSE	breast self-examination
BUN	blood urea nitrogen
bx	biopsy
C	Celsius, centigrade
$\bar{c}$	with
CA	cancer
CABG	coronary artery bypass graft
CAD	coronary artery disease
CBS	capillary blood sugar
CC	chief complaint
cc*	cubic centimeter

**The Institute for Safe Medication Practices (ISMP) considers these abbreviations dangerous because of possible misinterpretation. For additional information, see ISMP List of Error-Prone Abbreviations, Symbols, and Dose Designations at http://www.ismp.org*

CCD	congenital cardiovascular defect
CHD	childhood diseases; congenital heart disease
CHF	congestive heart failure
CHI	closed head injury; creatinine height index
Cl	chloride
cm	centimeter
CMT	cervical motion tenderness
CMV	cytomegalovirus
CN I–XII	cranial nerves I–XII
CNS	central nervous system
c/o	complaining of; complaints of
CO_2	carbon dioxide
COA	coarctation of the aorta
COPD	chronic obstructive pulmonary disease
CP	chest pain; cerebral palsy
CPD	cephalopelvic disproportion
creat	creatinine
C/S	cesarean section delivery
CT	computerized tomography
CV	cardiovascular
CVA	costovertebral angle; cerebrovascular accident
CVP	central venous pressure
CVS	chorionic villi sampling
CXray	chest X ray
cx	cervix
d	day(s)
DBP	diastolic blood pressure
d/c*	discontinue; discharge
D&C	dilation & curettage
DDST II	Denver Developmental Screening Test II
DES	diethylstilbestrol
DM	diabetes mellitus
DOA	dead on arrival
DOB	date of birth
DOE	dyspnea on exertion
DTR	deep tendon reflex
DUB	dysfunctional uterine bleeding
DVT	deep vein thrombosis
DWM	divorced white male (DWF, DBM, DBF are variations of this)
dx	diagnosis
dz	disease
EAC	external auricular canal
EDC	expected date of confinement (delivery date)
EDD	estimated date of delivery
EEG	electroencephalogram
EENT	eyes, ears, nose, throat
EFM	electronic fetal monitoring
EKG	electrocardiogram
ENAP	examination, normal findings, abnormal findings, pathophysiology
EOM	extraocular muscle
ESR	erythrocyte sedimentation rate
ETOH	ethyl alcohol
F	Fahrenheit
FAS	fetal alcohol syndrome
Fe	iron
FHH	family health history
FHR	fetal heart rate
FHT	fetal heart tone
FLM	fetal lung maturity
FM	fetal movement
FOB	father of baby
FROM	full range of motion
FSH	follicle-stimulating hormone
FTT	failure to thrive
fx	fracture
Ⓖ	gallop
GC	gonorrhea and Chlamydia
GCS	Glasgow Coma Scale
GDM	gestational diabetes mellitus
GERD	gastroesophageal reflux disease
GI	gastrointestinal
GU	genitourinary
GYN	gynecologic
H/A	headache
HCG	human chorionic gonadotropin
HDL	high-density lipoprotein
HEENT	head, eyes, ears, nose, throat
HELLP	hemolysis, elevated liver enzymes, low platelets
H/H	hemoglobin & hematocrit
Hib	Haemophilus influenza b
HIV	human immunodeficiency virus
hl	health
HNP	herniated nucleus pulposus
h/o	history of
HOB	head of bed
HPI	history of present illness
HPV	human papillomavirus
HR	heart rate
hs*	at bedtime
HSV	herpes simplex virus
HT	height
HTN	hypertension
hx	history
IADL	instrumental activities of daily living
IBW	ideal body weight

ICP	intracranial pressure
ICS	intercostal space
IDDM	insulin-dependent diabetes mellitus
IDM	infant of diabetic mother
IICP	increased intracranial pressure
I&O	intake & output
IOP	intraocular pressure
IPPA	inspection, palpation, percussion, auscultation
IUD	intrauterine device
IUGR	intrauterine growth retardation
IUP	intrauterine pregnancy
IUPC	intrauterine pressure catheter
IV	intravenous
IWMI	inferior wall myocardial infarction
JVD	jugular venous distension
JVP	jugular venous pressure
K^+	potassium
kg	kilogram
KOH	potassium hydroxide
KUB	kidneys, ureters, bladder
L	liter
Ⓛ	left
LAD	left anterior descending (coronary artery)
lat	lateral
lbs	pounds
LBP	low back pain
LCM	left costal margin
LDL	low-density lipoprotein
LE	lower extremity
lg	large
LGA	large for gestational age
LH	leutinizing hormone
LLE	left lower extremity
LLL	left lower lobe (of lung)
LLQ	left lower quadrant (of abdomen)
LLSB	left lower sternal border
LMD	local medical doctor
LMP	last menstrual period
LOC	level of/loss of consciousness
LSB	left sternal border
LUE	left upper extremity
LUL	left upper lobe (of lung)
LUQ	left upper quadrant (of abdomen)
Ⓜ	murmur
MAC	mid-arm circumference
MAL	midaxillary line
MAMC	mid-arm muscle circumference
MCL	midclavicular line
MD	muscular dystrophy, doctor
Mec	meconium
MGR	murmur, gallop, rub
MI	myocardial infarction
MMR	measles, mumps, rubella
MMSE	Mini Mental State Exam
MN	midnight
MRI	magnetic resonance imaging
MS	multiple sclerosis
MSAFP	maternal serum alpha-fetal protein
MVA	motor vehicle accident
MVI	multivitamin
mets	metastasis of malignancy
ml	milliliter
mm Hg	millimeters of mercury
mo	month(s)
mod	moderate
mvt	movement
NA	not applicable
Na^+	sodium
NaCl	sodium chloride
NAD	no acute distress
NCP	nursing care plan
NGT	nasogastric tube
NIDDM	noninsulin dependent diabetes mellitus
NKA	no known allergies
NKDA	no known diagnosed or drug allergies
nl	normal
NPO	nothing by mouth
NS	normal saline
NSAID	nonsteroidal anti-inflammatory drug
NSR	normal sinus rhythm
NSVD	normal spontaneous vaginal delivery
N&V	nausea & vomiting
N, V, D	nausea, vomiting, diarrhea
O_2	oxygen
OB	obstetrics
OD*	right eye
OM	otitis media
OME	otitis media with effusion
OOB	out of bed
OPV	oral polio vaccine
OREF	open reduction with external fixation
ORIF	open reduction with internal fixation
OS*	left eye
OTC	over the counter (medications)
OU*	both eyes
Ø	no, none

oz	ounce
$\bar{p}$	after
Pap	Papanicolaou
$\overline{pc}$	after meals
PDA	patent ductus arteriosus
PE	physical examination, pulmonary embolus
PERRLA	pupils equally round, reactive to light and accommodation
PFT	pulmonary function test
PHH	past health history
PID	pelvic inflammatory disease
PIH	pregnancy-induced hypertension
PLT	platelets
PMH	past medical history
PMI	point of maximal intensity or impulse
PMS	premenstrual syndrome
PND	paroxysmal nocturnal dyspnea
po	by mouth
post	posterior
PP	patient profile
PPD	purified protein derivative; packs per day
PPH	postpartum hemorrhage
prn	as necessary
PROM	passive range of motion; premature rupture of membranes
PS	pulmonic stenosis
PT	physical therapy
pt	patient
PTA	prior to admission (arrival)
PTV	prior to visit
PUD	peptic ulcer disease
PVC	premature ventricular complex (or contraction)
PVD	peripheral vascular disease
q	every
qd*	every day
qh	every hour
qid	four times a day
qod*	every other day
Ⓡ	right; rectal
r	rectal
RCA	right coronary artery
RCM	right costal margin
RHD	rheumatic heart disease
RLE	right lower extremity
RLL	right lower lobe (of lung)
RLQ	right lower quadrant (of abdomen)
RML	right middle lobe (of lung)
ROM	range of motion
ROS	review of systems
RR	respiratory rate; red reflex
RSB	right sternal border
RT	related to, radiation therapy
RTC	return to clinic
RUE	right upper extremity
RUL	right upper lobe (of lung)
RUQ	right upper quadrant (of abdomen)
Rx	prescription drug
rx	reaction
$\bar{s}$	without
SAB	spontaneous abortion
SBE	subacute bacterial endocarditis
SBM	single black male (SBF, SWF, SWM are variations of this)
SBP	systolic blood pressure
SCA	sickle cell anemia
SDH	subdural hematoma
SEM	systolic ejection murmur
SEMI	subendocardial myocardial infarction
SGA	small for gestational age
SH	social history
SIDS	sudden infant death syndrome
sgy	surgery
sl	slight; slightly
SLE	systemic lupus erythematous
SOB	shortness of breath
s/p	status post
SQ*	subcutaneous
SROM	spontaneous rupture of membranes
SS#	social security number
s/s	signs & symptoms
SSCP	substernal chest pain
ST	sore throat
STD	sexually transmitted disease
sx	symptom
sz	seizure
T&A	tonsillectomy & adenoidectomy
TAB	therapeutic abortion
TAH	total abdominal hysterectomy
TB	tuberculosis
TENS	transcutaneous electrical nerve stimulation
THA	total hip arthoplasty
THR	total hip replacement
TIBC	total iron binding capacity
tid	three times a day
TKR	total knee replacement
TLC	total lymphocyte count

TM	tympanic membrane
TMJ	temporomandibular joint
TORCH	toxoplasmosis, other (syphilis, hepatitis B), rubella, cytomegalovirus, herpes simplex
TPR	temperature, pulse, respirations
tr	trace
TSE	testicular self-examination
TSF	triceps skin fold
TVH	total vaginal hysterectomy
tx	treatment
u/a	urinalysis
UC	uterine contraction
UCHD	usual childhood diseases
UE	upper extremity
URI	upper respiratory infection
U/S	ultrasound
UTI	urinary tract infection
UUN	urine urea nitrogen
VBAC	vaginal birth after cesarean
VE	vaginal examination
VS	vital signs
VSD	ventricular septal defect
VSS	vital signs stable
VTX	vertex
WBC	white blood cell
WD	well developed
WF	white female
wk	week
wkend	weekend
WM	white male
WN	well nourished
WNL	within normal limits
WT	weight
$\bar{x}$	except
X	times
yo	year old (age)
yr	year(s)

Symbols

~	similar
≅	approximately
@	at
✓	check
△	change
↑	increased
↓	decreased
=	equals
#	pounds
>	greater than
<	less than
%	percentage
+ or ⊕	positive
− or ⊖	negative
♀	female
♂	male
△1 △2 △3	trimester of pregnancy (one triangle for each trimester)
$\dot{\bar{\text{i}}}$	one
2°	secondary

Index

Note: Page numbers in **bold type** refer to boxed text, figures, and tables.

I

J

K

L

O

P

Q

R

U

V